Advances in Regional Anaesthesia and Acute Pain Management

Advances in Regional Anaesthesia and Acute Pain Management

Guest Editor

Eleni Moka

MDPI

Basel • Beijing • Wuhan • Barcelona • Belgrade • Novi Sad • Cluj • Manchester

Guest Editor
Eleni Moka
School of Health Sciences
Aristotle University
of Thessaloniki
Thessaloniki
Greece

Editorial Office
MDPI AG
Grosspeteranlage 5
4052 Basel, Switzerland

This is a reprint of the Special Issue, published open access by the journal *Journal of Clinical Medicine* (ISSN 2077-0383), freely accessible at: https://www.mdpi.com/journal/jcm/special_issues/252488N1H0.

For citation purposes, cite each article independently as indicated on the article page online and as indicated below:

Lastname, A.A.; Lastname, B.B. Article Title. *Journal Name* **Year**, *Volume Number*, Page Range.

ISBN 978-3-7258-6482-9 (Hbk)
ISBN 978-3-7258-6483-6 (PDF)
https://doi.org/10.3390/books978-3-7258-6483-6

Contents

About the Editor

Eleni Moka

Eleni Moka is an Ass. Professor of Anaesthesiology at the University of Thessaloniki in Greece. She is dedicated to regional anaesthesia and perioperative care, with a particular focus on UGRA, acute pain services, and transitional pain care. Her primary interests also encompass US application in daily clinical practice and enhancing recovery after surgery. She has been deeply involved in ESRA, serving as a Board member, Treasurer, and President of its Executive Board.

Preface

Regional anaesthesia (RA) and acute pain medicine have undergone exciting advances in the past few decades and have emerged as a transformative force to redefine the paradigms of patients' care. Ultrasound-guided RA techniques have become the gold standard, thanks to the associated improvements in efficacy, ease of performance and safety. As such, the accessibility, clinical use and popularity of RA have increased substantially. The seamless integration of RA with acute pain management protocols has far-reaching implications for patient outcomes. From minimizing opioid usage and associated side-effects to expediting recovery timelines, this holistic approach stands as a testament to the ever-evolving nature of medical science. As we navigate the complexities of this multidimensional landscape, it becomes increasingly apparent that RA and acute pain management are not merely adjuncts, but rather integral components in the continuum of patient-centered care. However, the fields have not yet reached their full potential. Emerging nerve blocks and updated acute pain management practices, though recent, have room for refinement, with certain techniques and protocols warranting meticulous scrutiny.

The goal of this Special Issue is to focus on contemporary evidence, underscore prevailing topics and highlight future directions in the aforementioned fields.

Eleni Moka
Guest Editor

Journal of
Clinical Medicine

MDPI

Editorial

Transforming Perioperative Care: Evolving Paradigms of the Expanding Role of Regional Anesthesia and Acute Pain Management

Eleni Moka

Faculty of Medicine, School of Health Sciences, Aristotle University of Thessaloniki, 54124 Thessaloniki, Greece; mokaeleni@hotmail.com

Over the past few decades, the field of regional anesthesia (RA) has witnessed a period of profound advances, extraordinary progress, and dynamic transformation. Once regarded as a niche domain within anesthesiology—primarily confined to selected surgical specialties—RA has evolved and has now emerged as a foundational pillar of modern anesthetic practice and a key enabler of individualized perioperative care. This evolution has been fueled by a confluence of scientific breakthroughs, clinical innovations, and technological advancements, all contributing to reshaping RA to be a refined, sophisticated, evidence–based, and widely implemented approach in contemporary medical practice. Its seamless integration into acute pain management protocols and perioperative clinical pathways has far-reaching implications on patient care, with recognized benefits that extend beyond superior analgesia to include enhanced recovery, greater patient satisfaction, reduced opioid dependence via opioid-sparing strategies, cost efficiency, and improved overall system performance. Ultrasound-guided RA (UGRA) techniques have revolutionized RA delivery, establishing a new "gold" standard of care thorough increased precision, safety, and ease of performance. Consequently, the accessibility, global clinical adoption, and popularity of RA have expanded dramatically. In the current era of patient-centered care, RA and acute pain management are no longer considered adjunctive tools but are viewed as integral components of a comprehensive, holistic, personalized perioperative strategy [1–3].

This progression has been propelled by the convergence of an expanding body of rigorous, high–quality clinical research, refined anatomical insights and complementary understanding, advanced pharmacologic options, and a shift towards value-based, outcome-driven healthcare. By minimizing opioid exposure and its associated risks while facilitating earlier mobilization and smoother recovery trajectories, the synergistic application of RA and acute pain management protocols exemplifies the principles of personalized and precision medicine. Yet, despite these strides, the field has not yet reached its full potential and continues to evolve. Emerging peripheral nerve blocks (PNBs), new-generation pharmacological adjuvants, and updated clinical protocols and practices still present opportunities for further refinement, validation, widespread dissemination, and broader implementation. The continued pursuit of innovation, safety, and patient-centered excellence will be essential to realizing the full potential of RA and acute pain management in the years ahead [2–4].

This Special Issue of the *Journal of Clinical Medicine* titled "Advances in Regional Anesthesia and Acute Pain Management" presents a timely, comprehensive, and multidimensional exploration and overview of this rapidly advancing discipline. Comprising eighteen rigorously peer-reviewed articles, authored by leading international experts, this collection offers an in-depth examination of the latest advances in RA and acute perioperative pain management. The contributions span a broad range of critical topics, including detailed anatomical considerations, technical innovations, pharmacologic developments, clinical applications and outcomes, safety protocols, and educational methodologies. Collectively, these studies not only synthesize current best practices but also illuminate ongoing challenges, emerging questions, and key opportunities that will shape the next phase of clinical evolution. At the core of this Special Issue lies the shared conviction that RA is uniquely positioned to advance the goals and support the evolving paradigm of modern perioperative medicine—delivering care that is not only effective and efficient but also individualized, humane, and grounded in the principles of precision and compassion. Unlike systemic analgesics, which affect the entire body and carry a higher burden of adverse effects, RA techniques enable site-specific interventions that can be adjusted to suit individual anatomy, the type of surgical procedure, patient comorbidities and individual characteristics, and recovery goals. These tailored strategies improve not only the physiological outcomes—such as pain control, reduction in postoperative nausea and vomiting, and early mobilization—but also psychological well-being and overall satisfaction. Importantly, in an era of escalating healthcare costs, RA contributes to value-based care through decreased hospital stays, reduced reliance on opioids, and improved long-term functional recovery.

The principle of a personalized approach to perioperative care is vividly exemplified in the population-based study by Cozowicz C. et al., which serves as a featured contribution within this Special Issue [5]. In this large-scale analysis encompassing data from over 1.3 million patients undergoing hysterectomy, the authors investigated outcomes associated with multimodal analgesia strategies, including RA implementation. Their findings revealed substantial improvements in postoperative outcomes, with multimodal analgesia being associated with a 35% reduction in overall complications, a 24% decrease in opioid consumption, and a 14% shorter hospital length-of-stay. A closer examination showed that respiratory complications were reduced by approximately 40%, cardiac complications decreased by 30%, and genitourinary complications declined by 40% when compared to patients who did not receive multimodal analgesia. Furthermore, the study demonstrated a stepwise reduction in opioid prescriptions, with the incremental application of additional analgesic modalities. The large-scale, high-volume, and real-world nature of this study offers compelling and generalizable evidence in support of multimodal pain management strategies. These findings make a persuasive case not only for the routine implementation of such protocols in gynecologic surgery but also for their broader adoption as a model of best practice across various surgical specialties. At a time when healthcare systems are striving to optimize outcomes within constrained resource environments, the implications of this research are both timely and highly consequential.

In orthopedic surgery—a field where postoperative pain is often profound and functional recovery depends on early mobilization—RA has consistently demonstrated substantial benefits. Multiple studies in this Special Issue reinforce the clinical value of PNBs in enhancing analgesia and reducing reliance on systemic opioids. Beric S. et al. provided clear evidence that supplementing spinal anesthesia with adductor canal and sciatic nerve blocks in patients undergoing anterior cruciate ligament reconstruction significantly improved immediate postoperative pain relief, preserved range of motion, and led to a marked reduction in opioid consumption [6]. As such, their study underscores the utility of targeted, site- and procedure-specific nerve blocks in optimizing recovery trajectories in procedures characterized by a high nociceptive burden. Complementing these findings, Viderman D. et al. conducted a comprehensive systematic review and meta-analysis, examining the use of gabapentinoids in joint arthroplasties [7]. While their analysis of over

1200 patients demonstrated a consistent, albeit modest, opioid-sparing effect, the overall benefit–risk profile of gabapentinoids remains a topic of ongoing debate and, according to the authors, pain reduction was not clinically relevant. Sedation was not evaluated in their study and, if taken into account, it might have influenced their conclusions. An important limitation of this study was that different gabapentinoids, their administration times, and dosages, as well as varying intraoperative management protocols, were pooled together. These agents have been incorporated into many multimodal analgesic regimens, based on early enthusiasm regarding their potential to reduce central sensitization and enhance postoperative pain control [8]. Nevertheless, more recent evaluations have highlighted concerns about their limited efficacy in reducing pain scores in the immediate and longer postoperative period and their association with side effects such as sedation, dizziness, and impaired balance—factors that could hinder early mobilization and increase the risk of falls in the orthopedic population [9,10]. As such, the role of gabapentinoids in orthopedic pain management is increasingly viewed as context-dependent, requiring careful patient selection, as well as dose titration and meticulous adjustment. Their inclusion in perioperative analgesia protocols should be informed by a nuanced understanding of both their pharmacodynamics and the evolving evidence base [10]. The juxtaposition of studies on RA techniques and gabapentinoids highlights the complexity of contemporary perioperative pain management, where no single approach or intervention suffices or can address the diverse needs of every patient. Instead, these findings reinforce the importance of individualized, evidence–based strategies that integrate pharmacologic, procedural, and functional considerations to achieve optimal outcomes while minimizing adverse effects.

Among the most clinically relevant and increasingly recognized challenges addressed in this Special Issue is the phenomenon of rebound pain (RP). Defined as a marked resurgence of intense pain following PNB resolution, RP has the potential to significantly disrupt the postoperative recovery process. It can impair patient satisfaction, delay functional rehabilitation, and in some cases, it may lead to increased reliance on rescue opioid analgesics [11]. Lee B. et al. provided valuable insights into this issue by directly comparing the efficacy of continuous versus single-shot superior trunk blocks in patients undergoing arthroscopic shoulder surgery [12]. Even when the analgesic efficacy of single-shot blocks was prolonged with intravenous dexmedetomidine as an adjuvant, their results demonstrated that continuous nerve blocks provided smoother, more stable, and more reliable postoperative analgesia while significantly reducing both the intensity and the frequency of RP following arthroscopic rotator cuff repair. These findings align with the growing clinical consensus that RP is a predictable phenomenon, and the expert opinion is that it must be anticipated and proactively managed, particularly in outpatient and ambulatory surgical settings, where patients are often discharged before PNBs wear off completely [13].

Indeed, the incidence of RP is notably higher in ambulatory patients and appears to be modulated and influenced by a combination of patient-specific, surgical, and anesthetic factors. Strategies to mitigate RP include thorough preoperative patient education, the implementation of multimodal analgesic protocols, the use of continuous PNB techniques, and the administration of systemic agents, such as intravenous dexamethasone. While RP may not universally lead to increased overall opioid consumption nor uniformly affect functional recovery or patient satisfaction scores, it is nonetheless a source of significant discomfort for surgical patients. Interestingly, despite experiencing RP, the majority of affected patients report that they would still opt for PNBs in future operative procedures, underscoring the perceived value and benefits of RA techniques. Moving forward, further research should aim to establish predictive models and tools to identify patients at higher risk for developing RP and to explore novel pharmacological or procedural modifications and strategies that may help reduce RP incidence and improve the continuity of postoperative analgesia [11,13,14].

The pharmacological enhancement of the RA technique efficacy represents another area of active investigation. Studies in this Special Issue explore the use of adjuvants to extend fascial plane block duration, improve postoperative analgesia quality, and mitigate side effects. Korkutata Z. et al. compared dexmedetomidine and tramadol as adjuvants to bupivacaine in transversus abdominis plane (TAP) blocks, finding dexmedetomidine to be superior in both analgesic duration and hemodynamic stability [15]. Urfalı S. et al. examined the impact of dexamethasone and dexmedetomidine on bupivacaine TAP blocks in cesarean section patients, observing longer-lasting analgesia and a reduced need for rescue medication [16]. Dexamethasone, due to its delayed onset but extended duration, was found to achieve lower pain scores and higher patient satisfaction scores. These findings are important not only for enhancing the RA efficacy but also for reducing the systemic opioid burden, a key public health priority in the context of the opioid epidemic.

In addition, fascial plane blocks—one of the fastest-growing areas in RA—are also well represented. M. et al. conducted a head-to-head comparison of the serratus anterior, erector spinae, and paravertebral blocks for breast cancer surgery [17]. Their results demonstrated comparable intraoperative analgesic efficacy across all three RA techniques, but with the serratus anterior block emerging as equally effective as the paravertebral block for reducing postoperative pain; it was determined to be the most practical option due to its ease of application and lower complication risks. Kim S. et al. extended the utility of the erector spinae plane block to cardiac surgery, showing its effectiveness, as a supplementary approach to cardiac anesthesia, in reducing opioid use and ICU length-of-stay in off-pump CABG patients [18]. These studies illustrate the versatility of fascial plane blocks and highlight their value in patients who are not suitable candidates for neuraxial techniques due to anticoagulation or hemodynamic instability.

Furthermore, the anatomical basis of PNBs is explored in detail in several contributions in this Special Issue. Bjorn S. et al. provided an important update on the medial femoral cutaneous nerve, demonstrating its anatomical consistency and clinical relevance in total knee arthroplasty (TKA) [19]. Inadequate coverage of this nerve may contribute to residual anteromedial knee pain postoperatively—a persistent issue in a subset of patients, although further trials are mandated to investigate whether its blockade translates into a clinical effect on postoperative pain after TKA or if it can be used for diagnosis and interventional pain management for chronic neuropathic pain due to its damage during surgery. Moreover, Staikou C. et al. examined the role of pericapsular nerve group (PENG) block in major hip surgery, concluding that it offers better postoperative analgesia with possibly less opioid consumption, prolonging the time to the first analgesic without the significant common side effects of anesthesia/analgesia or duration of hospital stay [20]. Similarly, Muse I. et al. reviewed the PENG block and its relevance to hip analgesia and highlighted a new block that anesthetizes nerves to the posterior capsule, superior gluteal nerve, and the nerve to the quadratus femoris muscle, called the posterior pericapsular deep-gluteal block, suggesting that complete analgesia for hip fracture surgery is possible, thus optimizing perioperative pain management [21]. These studies underscore the continued importance of anatomical precision in the development and refinement of RA techniques. As new blocks emerge and old ones are modified, anatomical validation remains essential to ensuring efficacy and avoiding inadvertent injury during PNB placement or surgery.

Notably, RA is no longer confined to adult surgical populations. Capuano P. et al. presented a compelling case study involving a pediatric renal transplant recipient, managed with a continuous erector spinae plane block [22]. The child experienced excellent pain relief, avoided systemic opioids, and had an uneventful recovery. This case, while limited in generalizability, offers a valuable template for expanding RA into pediatric and transplant populations—areas that have historically been underrepresented in RA clinical research. With proper training, institutional support, and vigilant monitoring, RA techniques can be safely employed in even the most vulnerable patient groups.

Education and training are also central to safe, consistent, and effective RA application. Seybold B. et al. explored the learnability of an ultrasound-guided cervical plexus blockade, used for carotid endarterectomy, and it demonstrated high success rates among anesthesia trainees, following brief yet structured instructional sessions [23]. Their findings highlight the rapid acquisition of this skill, a notably low failure rate, and a reduction in complications, particularly among anesthesiologists already familiar with other UGRA techniques. Their study affirms the critical role of simulation-based learning, hands-on mentorship, and stepwise skill-building in mastering anatomically complex and technically demanding PNBs [24,25]. As RA continues to expand in clinical scope and complexity, the standardization of educational frameworks will become increasingly important [26]. Incorporating simulation platforms [27], artificial intelligence (AI)-driven feedback systems [28], structured performance checklists, and objective competency assessments into training curricula will be essential for ensuring proficiency, quality, and patient safety. Furthermore, as RA becomes more advanced and widely accessible, remote learning solutions and virtual education models offer promising strategies to overcome geographical and institutional barriers to training [29]. These innovations may significantly expand global access to high-quality RA education, ultimately contributing to better outcomes and safer care across diverse practice settings.

Safety is a recurring theme in this Special Issue, particularly in relation to complex or controversial areas of practice. Hilber N. et al. addressed the concern that RA may mask symptoms of acute compartment syndrome in limb trauma surgery [30]. By reviewing 35 case reports and series, they concluded that RA techniques—especially when low-concentration local anesthetics are used—do not prevent timely diagnosis, especially when combined with vigilant clinical monitoring. Their analysis highlights the importance of interdisciplinary collaboration, patient education, and protocol-driven practice in high-risk settings. Safety is not a passive outcome but an active process requiring commitment, communication, and continual reassessment.

The international scope of this Special Issue deserves special mention. Authors from Europe, North America, Asia, and other regions bring diverse perspectives, practices, and innovations to the table. This geographic diversity underscores both the universal applicability of RA and the importance of context in its implementation. In low- and middle-income countries, for instance, barriers such as limited ultrasound machines access, staffing shortages, and insufficient training infrastructure must be addressed creatively. Solutions such as mobile simulation labs, remote mentoring platforms, and scalable educational programs may offer a roadmap for global equity in RA provision to our patients [31].

Technology is playing an increasingly important role in the evolution of RA. Emerging tools such as AI-assisted image interpretation, augmented reality-guided needle placement, and automated injection systems promise to enhance block accuracy, reduce operator variability, and improve patient safety. As these technologies mature, their integration into clinical practice must be guided by rigorous validation studies and cost-effectiveness analyses [32]. Moreover, the integration of RA data into electronic health records and clinical dashboards will enable real-time quality monitoring and performance improvement, ensuring that best practices are not only defined but also consistently implemented.

Looking forward, several strategic priorities emerge for this specialty. First, continued investment in high-quality research, including multicenter randomized trials and longitudinal outcome studies, is essential to answer remaining questions about block efficacy, safety, and comparative value [33,34]. Second, more attention must be paid to long-term outcomes, such as chronic postsurgical pain, return to function, and health-related quality of life [1,35]. Third, health economic studies should quantify the cost–benefit profile of RA techniques across different healthcare systems and patient populations. Fourth, efforts to standardize documentation, procedural nomenclature, and outcome reporting will enhance the comparability and generalizability of future research [1,35,36].

In conclusion, the articles presented in this Special Issue reflect the strength, depth, and maturity of RA as a discipline. They showcase a field that remains innovative, is evidence-based, and globally engaged; it is a field committed to improving patient care through precision, empathy, and scientific rigor. The knowledge shared herein not only advances the science of RA but also reaffirms its role as a cornerstone of modern perioperative medicine. The editorial team extends their sincere appreciation to all authors, peer reviewers, and collaborators who contributed to this issue. Their dedication, vision, and scholarly excellence have made this publication a valuable resource for clinicians, educators, and researchers alike. It is hoped that the insights gathered here will inspire continued inquiry, collaboration, and innovation in the service of better, safer, precise, and more personalized perioperative pain management worldwide.

Conflicts of Interest: The author declares no conflicts of interest.

References

1. Hutton, M.; Brull, R.; Macfarlane, A.J.R. Regional anaesthesia and outcomes. *BJA Educ.* **2018**, *18*, 52–56. [CrossRef]
2. Chitnis, S.S.; Tang, R.; Mariano, E.R. The role of regional analgesia in personalized postoperative pain management. *Korean J. Anesthesiol.* **2020**, *73*, 363–371. [CrossRef]
3. Mariano, E.R.; El-Boghdadly, K.; Ilfeld, B.M. Using postoperative pain trajectories to define the role of regional analgesia in personalized pain medicine. *Anaesthesia* **2021**, *76*, 165–169. [CrossRef]
4. Zeng, S.; Qing, Q.; Xu, W.; Yu, S.; Zheng, M.; Tan, H.; Peng, J.; Huang, J. Personalized anaesthesia and precision medicine: A comprehensive review of genetic factors, artificial intelligence, and patient—Specific factors. *Front. Med.* **2024**, *11*, 1365524. [CrossRef] [PubMed]
5. Cozowicz, C.; Gerner, H.D.; Zhong, H.; Illescas, A.; Reisinger, L.; Poeran, J.; Liu, J.; Memtsoudis, S.G. Multimodal Analgesia and Outcomes in Hysterectomy Surgery—A Population—Based Analysis. *J. Clin. Med.* **2024**, *13*, 5431. [CrossRef]
6. Berić, S.; Murselović, T.; Žižak, M.; Bulat, S.; Vrgoč, G. Comparative effects of spinal anasthesia and combined spinal with peripheral nerve blocks on postoperative outcomes in anterior cruciate ligament repair. *J. Clin. Med.* **2024**, *13*, 6845. [CrossRef] [PubMed]
7. Viderman, D.; Aubakirova, M.; Salamat, A.; Kaldybayev, D.; Sadir, N.; Tankacheyev, R.; Abdildin, Y.G. The impact of gabapentinoids on pain—Related outcomes after knee and hip surgery: A systematic review with meta—Analysis of randomized controlled trials. *J. Clin. Med.* **2024**, *13*, 4205. [CrossRef]
8. Tiippana, E.M.; Hamunen, K.; Kontinen, V.K.; Kalso, E. Do surgical patients benefit from perioperative gabapentin/pregabalin? A systematic review of efficacy and safety. *Anesth. Analg.* **2007**, *104*, 1545–1546. [CrossRef]
9. Verret, M.; Lauzier, F.; Zarychanski, R.; Perron, C.; Savard, X.; Pinard, A.-M.; Leblanc, G.; Cossi, M.-J.; Neveu, X.; Turgeon, A.F.; et al. Perioperative use of gabapentinoids for the management of postoperative acute pain: A systematic review and meta-Analysis. *Anesthesiology* **2020**, *133*, 265–279. [CrossRef] [PubMed]
10. Kharasch, E.D.; Clark, D.J.; Kheterpal, S. Perioperative gabapentinoids: Deflating the bubble. *Anesthesiology* **2020**, *133*, 251–254. [CrossRef]
11. Murphy, J.K.; O'Donnell, B. Rebound pain—Management strategies for transitional analgesia: A narrative review. *J. Clin. Med.* **2025**, *14*, 936. [CrossRef]
12. Lee, B.; Jang, J.; Lim, J.-R.; Kim, E.J.; Kim, D.; Chun, Y.-M.; Choi, Y.S. Continuous superior trunk block versus single—Shot superior trunk block with intravenous dexmedetomidine for postoperative analgesia in arthroscopic shoulder surgery: A prospective randomized controlled trial. *J. Clin. Med.* **2024**, *13*, 1845. [CrossRef]
13. Munoz-Leyva, F.; Cubillos, J.; Chin, K.J. Managing rebound pain after regional anaesthesia. *Korean J. Anesthesiol.* **2020**, *73*, 372–383. [CrossRef] [PubMed]

14. Dada, O.; Zacarias, A.G.; Ongaigui, C.; Echeverria-Villalobos, M.; Kushelev, M.; Bergese, S.D.; Moran, K. Does rebound pain after peripheral nerve block for orthopaedic surgery impact postoperative analgesia and opioid consumption? A narrative review. *Int. J. Environ. Res. Public Health* **2019**, *16*, 3257. [CrossRef] [PubMed]
15. Korkutata, Z.; Esen Tekeli, A.; Kurt, N. Intraoperative and postoperative effects of dexmedetomidine and tramadol added as an adjuvant to bupivacaine in transversus abdominis plane block. *J. Clin. Med.* **2023**, *12*, 7001. [CrossRef] [PubMed]
16. Urfalı, S.; Hakimoglu, S.; Turhanoglu, S.; Koyuncu, O. Transversus abdominis plane block following caesarean section: A prospective randomized controlled study comparing the effects on pain levels of bupivacaine, bupivacaine + dexmedetomidine, and bupivacaine + dexamethasone. *J. Clin. Med.* **2024**, *13*, 4270. [CrossRef]
17. But, M.; Wernicki, K.; Zielinski, J.; Szczecinska, W. A comparison of the effectiveness of the serratus anterior plane block and erector spinae plane block to that of the paravertebral block in the surgical treatment of breast cancer—A randomized, prospective, single-blinded study. *J. Clin. Med.* **2024**, *13*, 4836. [CrossRef]
18. Kim, S.; Woo Song, S.; Jeon, Y.G.; Song, S.A.; Hong, S.; Park, J.H. Evaluating the efficacy of the erector spinae plane block as a supplementary approach to cardiac anaesthesia during off–pump coronary bypass graft surgery via median sternotomy: A randomized clinical trial. *J. Clin. Med.* **2024**, *13*, 2208. [CrossRef]
19. Bjørn, S.; Nielsen, T.D.; Jensen, A.E.; Jessen, C.; Kolsen-Petersen, J.A.; Moriggl, B.; Hoermann, R.; Bendtsen, T.F. The anterior branch of the medial femoral cutaneous nerve innervates cutaneous and deep surgical incisions in total knee arthroplasty. *J. Clin. Med.* **2024**, *13*, 3270. [CrossRef]
20. Staikou, C.; Rekatsina, M.; Leoni, M.L.G.; Chamos, C.; Kapsokalyvas, I.; Varrassi, G.; Karmaniolou, I. Efficacy and safety of pericapsular nerve group block (PENG) in hip surgery under general anaesthesia: A systematic literature review and meta-analysis. *J. Clin. Med.* **2025**, *14*, 468. [CrossRef]
21. Muse, I.O.; Deiling, B.; Grinman, L.; Hadeed, M.M.; Elkassabany, N. Peripheral nerve blocks for hip fractures. *J. Clin. Med.* **2024**, *13*, 3457. [CrossRef]
22. Capuano, P.; Burgio, G.; Abbate, S.; Ranucci, G.; Bici, K.; Cintorino, D.; Arcadipane, A.; Martucci, G. Continuous erector spinae plane block for pain management in a paediatric kidney transplant recipient: A case report and review of the current literature. *J. Clin. Med.* **2024**, *13*, 1128. [CrossRef] [PubMed]
23. Seybold, B.; Gaier, N.; Ofenloch, A.; Boeckler, D.; Kalenka, A.; Fiedler-Kalenka, M. Learnability of Ultrasound—Guided locoregional anaesthesia for carotid endarterectomy. *J. Clin. Med.* **2024**, *13*, 7557. [CrossRef] [PubMed]
24. Ashokka, B.; Law, L.S.-C.; Areti, A.; Laurent, D.B.-S.; Zuercher, R.O.; Chin, K.-J.; Ramlogan, R. Educational outcomes of simulation-based training in regional anaesthesia: A scoping review. *Br. J. Anaesth.* **2025**, *134*, 523–534. [CrossRef] [PubMed]
25. Ramlogan, R.R.; Chuan, A.; Mariano, E.R. Contemporary training methods in regional anaesthesia: Fundamentals and innovations. *Anaesthesia* **2021**, *76* (Suppl. S1), 53–64. [CrossRef]
26. Johnston, D.F.; Turbitt, L.R. Defining success in regional anaesthesia. *Anaesthesia* **2021**, *76* (Suppl. S1), 40–52. [CrossRef]
27. Satapathy, A.R.; Khalid, I.B.; Fathil, S.M. Simulation in Regional Anaesthesia: A Narrative Review of Its History, Evolution and Future Prospects. *J. Clin. Med.* **2024**, *14*, 67. [CrossRef]
28. McKendrick, M.; Yang, S.; McLeod, G.A. The use of artificial intelligence and robotics in regional anaesthesia. *Anaesthesia* **2021**, *76* (Suppl. S1), 171–181. [CrossRef]
29. Chequer, S. Innovative technologies in regional anaesthesia education: A scoping review. *BJA Open* **2025**, *15*, 100473. [CrossRef]
30. Hilber, N.; Dodi, A.; Blumenthal, S.; Bruppacher, S.; Borgeat, A.; Aguirre, J. The impact of regional anaesthesia in masking acute compartment syndrome after limb trauma. *J. Clin. Med.* **2024**, *13*, 1787. [CrossRef]
31. Cozowicz, C.; Poeran, J.; Memtsoudis, S.G. Epidemiology, trends, and disparities in regional anaesthesia for orthopaedic surgery. *Br. J. Anaesth.* **2015**, *115* (Suppl. S2), ii57–ii67. [CrossRef]
32. Swain, B.P.; Nag, D.S.; Anand, R.; Kumar, H.; Ganguly, P.K.; Singh, N. Current evidence on artificial intelligence in regional anaesthesia. *World J. Clin. Cases* **2024**, *12*, 6613–6619. [CrossRef] [PubMed]
33. Ferry, J.; Lewis, O.; Lloyd, J.; El-Boghdadly, K.; Kearns, R.; Albrecht, E.; Altermatt, F.; Ashokka, B.; Ayad, A.E.; Aziz, E.S.; et al. Research priorities in regional anaesthesia: An international Delphi study. *Br. J. Anaesth.* **2024**, *132*, 1041–1048. [CrossRef] [PubMed]
34. Grant, S.A.; Kopp, S.; Albrecht, E. Research priorities in regional anaesthesia: Where should we focus? *Br. J. Anaesth.* **2024**, *133*, 1–2. [CrossRef] [PubMed]
35. Hopkins, P.M. Does regional anaesthesia improve outcome? *Br. J. Anaesth.* **2015**, *115* (Suppl. S2), ii26–ii33. [CrossRef]
36. Admiral, M.; Marhofer, P.; Hopkins, P.M.; Hollmann, M.W. Peripheral regional anaesthesia and outcomes: A narrative review of the literature from 2013 to 2023. *Br. J. Anaesth.* **2024**, *132*, 1082–1096. [CrossRef]

Journal of
Clinical Medicine

MDPI

Article

Intraoperative and Postoperative Effects of Dexmedetomidine and Tramadol Added as an Adjuvant to Bupivacaine in Transversus Abdominis Plane Block

Zeki Korkutata [1], Arzu Esen Tekeli [2,*] and Nurettin Kurt [2]

[1] Department of Anesthesiology and Reanimation, Bingol State Hospital, Bingol 12000, Turkey; zeki.korkutata@hotmail.com

[2] Department of Anesthesiology and Reanimation, Faculty of Medicine, Van Yuzuncu Yil University, Van 65080, Turkey; dr.nurettinkurt@gmail.com

* Correspondence: esentekeli190807@hotmail.com

Abstract: Background: We aimed to evaluate the intraoperative hemodynamics, opioid consumption, muscle relaxant use, postoperative analgesic effects, and possible adverse effects (such as nausea and vomiting) of dexmedetomidine and tramadol added as adjuvants to bupivacaine in the transversus abdominis plane block (TAP block) to provide postoperative analgesia. **Materials and Methods:** This was a prospective, randomized, controlled trial on patients who underwent laparoscopic cholecystectomy. After obtaining ethical approval at the Van Yuzuncu Yil University and written informed consent, this investigation was registered with ClinicalTrials.gov (NCT05905757). The study was conducted with 67 patients with ASA I–II physical status, aged 20–60 years, of either sex who were scheduled for an elective laparoscopic cholecystectomy under general anesthesia. Exclusion criteria were the patient's refusal, ASA III and above, a history of allergy to the study drugs, patients with severe systemic diseases, pregnancy, psychiatric illness, seizure disorder, and those who had taken any form of analgesics in the last 24 h. The patients were equally randomized into one of two groups: Group T (TAP Block group) and Group D (Dexmedetomidin group). Standard general anesthesia was administered. After intubation, Group T (Bupivacaine + adjuvant tramadol) = solutions containing 0.250% bupivacaine 15 mL + adjuvant 1.5 mg/kg (100 mg maximum) tramadol 25 mL and Group D (Bupivacaine + adjuvant dexmedetomidine) = solutions containing 0.250% bupivacaine 15 mL + 0.5 mcg/kg and (50 mcg maximum) dexmedetomidine 25 mL; in total, 40 mL and 20 mL was applied to groups T and D, respectively. A bilateral subcostal TAP block was performed by the same anesthesiologist. Intraoperative vital signs, an additional dose of opioid and muscle relaxant requirements, complications, postoperative side effects (nausea, vomiting), postoperative analgesic requirement, mobilization times, and the zero-hour mark (patients with modified Aldrete scores of 9 and above were recorded as 0 h), the third-hour, and sixth-hour visual analog scale (VAS) scores were recorded. The main outcome measurements were the effect on pain scores and analgesic consumption within the first 6 h postoperatively, postoperative nausea and vomiting (PONV), and time to ambulation. The secondary aim was to evaluate intraoperative effects (on hemodynamics and opioid and muscle relaxant consumption). **Results:** It was observed that dexmedetomidine and tramadol did not have superiority over each other in terms of postoperative analgesia time, analgesic consumption, side effect profile, and mobilization times ($p > 0.05$). However, more stable hemodynamics were observed with dexmedetomidine as an adjuvant. **Conclusions:** We think that the use of adjuvant dexmedetomidine in the preoperative TAP block procedure will provide more stable intraoperative hemodynamic results compared with the use of tramadol. We believe that our study will be a guide for new studies conducted with different doses and larger numbers of participants.

Keywords: bupivacaine; transversus abdominis plane block; dexmedetomidine; tramadol; cholecystectomy

1. Introduction

Today, cholecystectomy can be performed with open and laparoscopic techniques [1]. After laparoscopic surgery, most patients have severe abdominal pain and feel the need for effective analgesia [2]. Pain is a factor that causes a delay in postoperative discharge [3]. One of the most important goals of anesthesia applications is perioperative pain control. The development of different methods for pain control reduces the incidence of side effects due to high-dose analgesics. The use of locoregional anesthesia has spread during the last few years as it can be useful to reduce the time of hospitalization, the incidence of adverse events related to general anesthesia, and pain; moreover, it can be useful to achieve, almost, opioid-free anesthesia. It can be used as a substitute for general anesthesia or as an adjuvant to general anesthesia to achieve better pain control and lessen the use of intra- and postoperative analgesics (most all opioids), thus resulting in less nausea and vomiting risk, faster mobilization and recovery, and more rapid hospital discharge [4,5]. The use of ultrasonography (USG) increases the success of nerve blocks and plane blocks and reduces the amount of drugs used, as well as the possibility of side effects and complications [6,7]. The transversus abdominis plane block is one of the most frequently used regional approaches to provide analgesia in the anterior abdominal wall after laparoscopic abdominal surgery. Local anesthetic is injected into the planar space between the internal oblique and transversus abdominus muscles, and the afferent nerves are blocked [8]. By providing effective analgesia, this method significantly reduces the postoperative stress response and facilitates postoperative recovery [9].

Dexmedetomidine, a highly selective α2-adrenergic agonist that has sedative, analgesic, sympatholytic, and anesthetic effects, is an interesting agent that prolongs the block time with its adjuvant use with local anesthetics. Its central mediated analgesia, the mechanism by which dexmedetomidine enhances the quality of regional anesthesia when used as an adjuvant to local anesthetic, can be explained by two peripheral mechanisms. First is the vasoconstrictor effect around the site of injection, which leads to a delay in the absorption of the local anesthetic and prolongs the duration of the local anesthetic effect. The second mechanism is the direct action of dexmedetomidine on the activity of peripheral nerves [10]. Parenterally or orally administered tramadol is effective in the treatment of acute postoperative pain in adults, and it can also block potassium channels. Also, the serotonin (5-hydroxytryptamine, 5-HT) subtype 3 (5-HT3) receptors situated on peripheral nerve endings and in the dorsal laminae of the spinal cord are possibly peripheral sites of analgesic action for tramadol [11]. There are many studies evaluating the effects of tramadol as an adjuvant to local anesthetics [12–14]. We acted with the idea that comparing the effectiveness of such interesting and effective drugs as adjuvants in regional anesthesia would be valuable and contribute to the literature.

In ultrasound-guided TAP block applications, adjuvants can be added to the local anesthetic agent in order to increase the analgesic efficiency and reduce the potential side effects and toxic effects of the drug used. This prospective, randomized study aimed to evaluate the efficacy of perineural tramadol and dexmedetomidine added to the local anesthetic solution in prolonging postoperative analgesia, maintaining stable hemodynamic parameters, and reducing intraoperative opioid and muscle relaxant consumption, postoperative side effects, and postoperative mobilization time in patients undergoing laparoscopic cholecystectomy cases.

2. Methods

2.1. Study Design

The study was initiated after Van Yuzuncu Yil University Faculty of Medicine Ethics Committee's approval (15.12.2020/06), registered with ClinicalTrials.gov (NCT05905757). Sixty-seven patients who applied to the anesthesiology and reanimation clinic for elective laparoscopic cholecystectomy were included. The patients were informed in detail about the study and possible complications before the operation, and their verbal and written consents were obtained. All study patients were described on a 10 cm visual analog scale

(VAS) preoperatively with VAS 0–2: no pain, 3–4: mild pain, 5–6: moderate pain, 7–8: severe pain, and 9–10: unbearable pain. The inclusion criteria included patients aged 20–60 years, undergoing elective laparoscopic cholecystectomy surgery, having ASA I–II physical status, and giving consent. Patients outside the 20–60 age range; with ASA III and above physical status; with severe heart, lung, or liver disease; with kidney failure; with bleeding diathesis; who developed complications during the procedure; with fever and active infection; allergic to the drugs to be used in the study; who refused to participate; who had hypothermia or acid-base disorder; and who were taking antibiotics, anticonvulsants, antiarrhythmics, or cholinesterase inhibitors; as well as pregnant women; bleeding cases; emergency cases; and those with a BMI of 30 and above were excluded from the study (Figure 1).

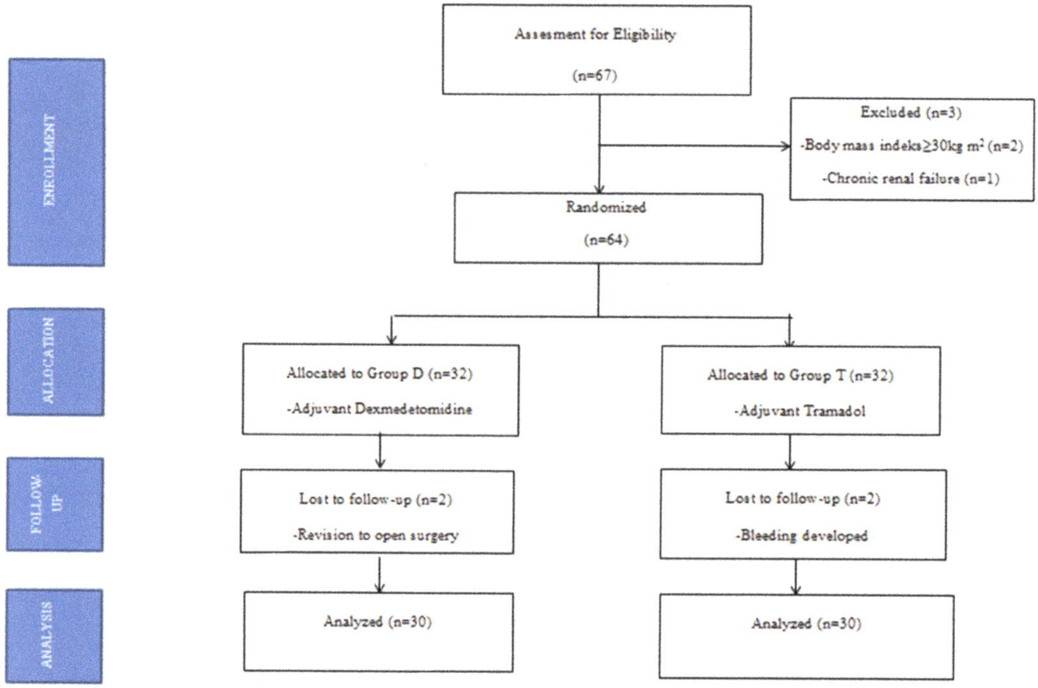

Figure 1. Flowchart of the study.

2.2. Sample Size Calculation

The purpose of adding dexmedetomidine (Sedadomid®, Kocak Farma, Istanbul, Turkey) or tramadol (Ramadex®, Haver, Tekirdag, Turkey) as an adjuvant to the local anesthetic is to observe the effect on the analgesic duration. According to the results of previous similar studies on this subject [15,16], at least 30 patients were required to detect a significant difference between the groups in terms of 180 min analgesia duration with a power of 80% and an α error of 0.05. Considering the patients who might be excluded from the study, the study started with 67 patients.

2.3. Anesthesia Application

A 22-gauge intravenous line was placed, and 10 mL kg^{-1} isotonic saline infusion was started. All patients were premedicated with 0.3 mg/kg midazolam. Standard monitoring with electrocardiography, non-invasive blood pressure, peripheral oxygen saturation, and bi-spectral index monitoring (Datex-Ohmeda S/5 monitor MBIS module, Helsinki, Finland) was applied to all patients in the operating room. Anesthesia induction was performed with intravenous propofol 2–3 mg kg^{-1}, fentanyl 2 μg kg^{-1}, and rocuronium bromide 0.6 mg kg^{-1} by the same anesthesiologist. Endotracheal intubation was performed when the BIS score was 40–60. Maintenance of anesthesia was provided with 4–6% end-tidal desflurane in 3 L of 40% O_2 and 60% air mixture. The minimum alveolar concentration of desflurane was targeted to reach a BIS value between 40 and 60. All patients were administered 20 mg/kg paracetamol IV as a standard analgesic before extubation.

2.4. Patient Randomization

The patients were randomly allocated into two groups using the single-blind closed-envelope method by a researcher who was not involved in the study.

2.5. Block Application

Following intubation, patients received a TAP block with an oblique subcostal approach in the supine position. The same anesthesiologist placed the ultrasound (Esaote® MyLab 5, Florence, Italy) probe (12MHz, linear probe; LA4 35) obliquely on the upper abdominal wall along the subcostal margin in the midline of the abdomen. The landmarks were the rectus abdominis muscle and transversus abdominis muscle. The probe was moved until the aponeurosis of the external, internal oblique, and transversus abdominis were seen. Then, the transversus abdominis muscle was identified by moving the probe laterally. The anesthesiologist directed the peripheral block needle (100 mm 22 G Echoplex, Vygon, Ecouen, France) toward the transversus abdominis fascia and injected 20 mL solution between the rectus abdominis and transversus abdominis muscles along the subcostal line. The same procedure was repeated on the contralateral side.

Group T (Bupivacaine (Buvicaine® 0.5%, Polifarma, Tekirdag, Turkey) + Adjuvant tramadol): 0.250% bupivacaine 15 mL + adjuvant 1.5 mg/kg (100 mg maximum) tramadol 25 mL, 40 mL in total, 20 mL was applied to each side.

Group D (Bupivacaine + adjuvant dexmedetomidine): 0.250% bupivacaine 15 mL + 0.5 mcg/kg and (50 mcg maximum) dexmedetomidine 25 mL, 40 mL in total, 20 mL was applied to each side.

Demographic data (age, weight, height, body mass index (BMI)), systolic arterial pressure (SAP), diastolic arterial pressure (DAP), mean arterial pressure (MAP), HR values, and operation times of the patients were recorded. Heart rate, non-invasive blood pressure, and SpO_2 measurements were taken immediately before induction, at 15 min intervals after intubation, and 5 min after extubation. Postoperative nausea and vomiting were noted as 'present or absent' only once, at the sixth postoperative hour. The patients were evaluated with a 0–10 verbal rating scale visual analog scale (VAS) at 0 h (modified Aldrete score > 9 in the recovery unit), 3 h, and 6 h after the operation, and the data were recorded. In the postoperative period, VAS value > 4 was evaluated in favor of analgesic need in all groups, and 50 mg Dexketoprofen IV bolus was administered in accordance with conventional treatment. There was no need for additional analgesia postoperatively at 6 h.

3. Statistical Data Analysis

In the descriptive statistics of the data, mean, standard deviation, median minimum and maximum, frequency, and ratio values were used. The distribution of variables was measured with the Kolmogorov–Smirnov test. Independent sample *t*-test and Mann–Whitney U test were used in the analysis of quantitative independent data. The Chi-square test was used in the analysis of qualitative independent data. The SPSS 28.0 software (SPSS Inc., Chicago, IL, USA) program was used in the analysis.

4. Results

T and D groups did not differ significantly in terms of demographic data and ASA scores ($p > 0.05$) (Table 1).

Table 1. Demographic data.

		Group T		Group D		p
		Mean ± sd/n%		**Mean ± sd/n%**		
Age		45.9 ± 10.1		42.7 ± 10.9		0.428 ^{t}
Gender	*Female*	21	70.0%	25	83.3%	0.222 $^{X^2}$
	Male	9	30.0%	5	16.7%	
Height (cm)		162.7 ± 9.9		162.5 ± 7.8		0.562 ^{m}
Weight (kg)		77.3 ± 15.1		74.0 ± 13.1		0.375 ^{t}
BMI		29.2 ± 5.7		28.0 ± 4.8		0.371 ^{m}
ASA	*I*	16	53.3%	13	43.3%	0.438 $^{X^2}$
	II	14	46.7%	17	56.7%	

^{t} Independent sample *t*-test/^{m} Mann–Whitney U test/$^{X^2}$ Chi-square test.

When the groups were compared in terms of intraoperative heart rate, it was found that there was no statistically significant ($p > 0.05$) difference between the groups until the 30th minute, and the intraoperative 30th-minute values were higher in favor of the T group ($p < 0.05$) (Figure 2).

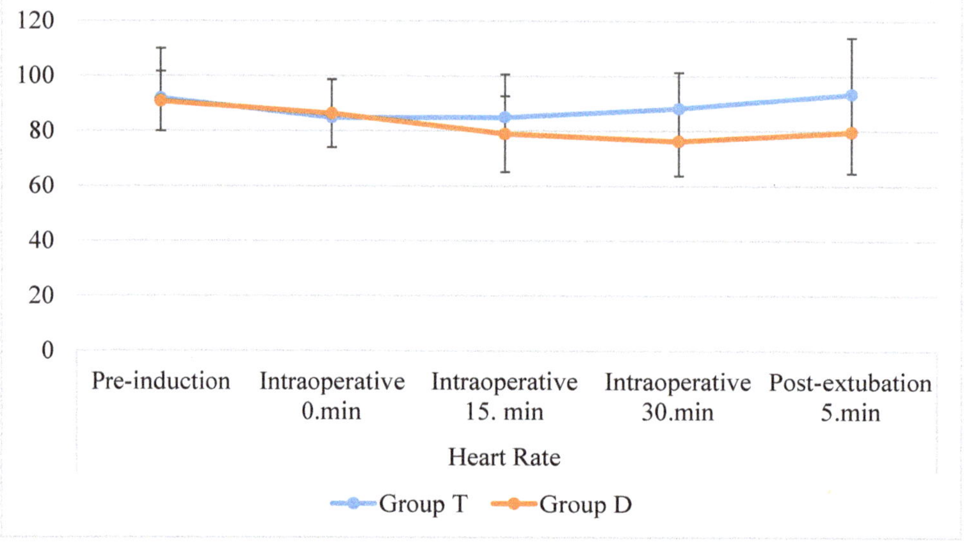

Figure 2. Heart rate changes.

Systolic and diastolic blood pressures did not differ significantly ($p > 0.05$) between the groups for the pre-induction, intraoperative, and post-extubation periods. While the mean arterial pressures at the pre-induction and intraoperative 15th minutes did not differ between the groups ($p > 0.05$), the intraoperative 0 min and 30 min values were found to be significantly lower, in favor of the T group ($p < 0.05$). The mean arterial pressure at the fifth minute after extubation was found to be significantly higher in group T ($p < 0.05$) (Table 2).

Table 2. Evaluation of blood pressures.

	Group T	Group D	p
	Mean ± sd	Mean ± sd	
Systolic Blood Pressure (SBP)			
Pre induction	143.5 ± 19.6	143.5 ± 17.9	0.935 [m]
Intraoperative 0 min	116.0 ± 21.2	128.1 ± 19.5	***0.011*** [m]
Intraoperative 15 min	122.9 ± 30.3	119.3 ± 21.4	0.605 [m]
Intraoperative 30 min	126.2 ± 21.8	112.7 ± 19.7	0.053 [m]
Post extubation 5 min	136.1 ± 18.6	128.3 ± 17.6	0.156 [m]
Diastolic Blood Pressure (DBP)			
Pre induction	78.9 ± 11.6	82.0 ± 13.0	0.339 [t]
Intraoperative 0 min	70.7 ± 14.6	77.5 ± 12.8	0.058 [t]
Intraoperative 15 min	78.9 ± 24.0	76.9 ± 17.2	0.703 [t]
Intraoperative 30 min	78.6 ± 13.5	71.0 ± 14.5	***0.042*** [t]
Post extubation 5 min	83.2 ± 12.6	78.5 ± 13.8	0.173 [t]
Mean Arterial Pressure (MAP)			
Pre induction	104.8 ± 13.0	104.7 ± 14.1	0.988 [m]
Intraoperative 0 min	89.1 ± 15.1	96.6 ± 14.2	***0.017*** [m]
Intraoperative 15 min	96.7 ± 23.7	93.4 ± 17.4	0.451 [m]
Intraoperative 30 min	96.4 ± 14.1	87.5 ± 15.6	***0.043*** [m]
Post extubation 5 min	103.9 ± 14.5	96.3 ± 15.1	***0.037*** [m]

[t] Independent samples *t* test/[m] Mann–Whitney U test. (Bold numbers are significant values).

VAS scores did not differ between the groups in all evaluated time periods (0 h, 3 h, and 6 h postoperatively) ($p > 0.05$) (Figure 3).

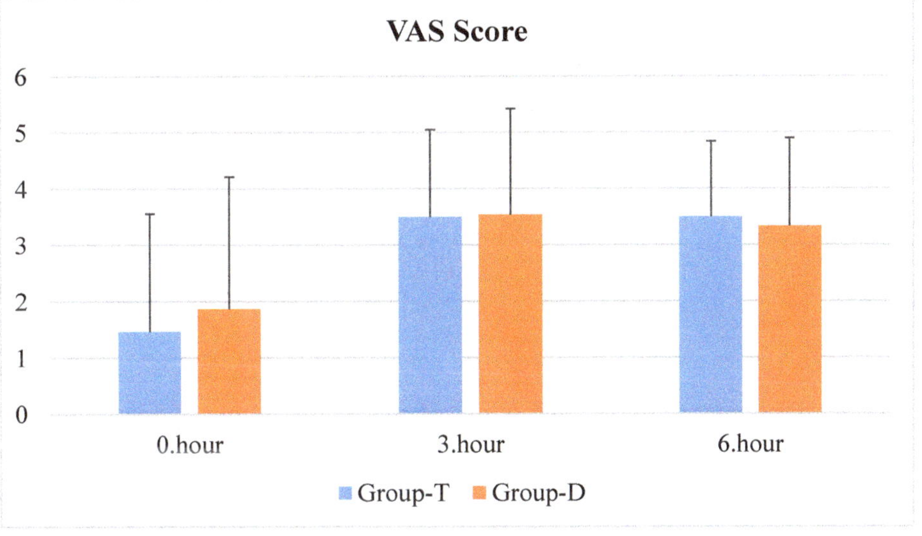

Figure 3. VAS scores for all groups.

The groups were also compared in terms of additional opioid and muscle relaxant needs (fentanyl, rocuronium), postoperative non-opioid analgesic consumption, mobilization times, and side effects (nausea, vomiting, etc.), and no statistically significant difference was observed ($p > 0.05$) (Table 3).

Table 3. Additional dose requirement, analgesic consumption, mobilization times, and side effects.

		Group T		Group D		p
		Mean ± sd/n-%		Mean ± sd/n-%		
Additional dose requirement	(-)	22	73.3%	27	90.0%	0.095^{X^2}
	(+)	8	26.7%	3	10.0%	
Rocuronium (mg)		10.0 ± 0.0		10.0 ± 0.0		1.000^{m}
Fentanyl (μcg)		56.3 ± 17.7		50.0 ± 0.0		0.540^{m}
Postoperative consumption of nonopioid analgesics						
1 h	(-)	24	80.0%	26	86.7%	0.488^{X^2}
	(+)	6	20.0%	4	13.3%	
2 h	(-)	30	100.0%	30	100.0%	1.000^{X^2}
	(+)	0	0.0%	0	0.0%	
3 h	(-)	20	66.7%	20	66.7%	1.000^{X^2}
	(+)	10	33.3%	10	33.3%	
4 h	(-)	30	100.0%	30	100.0%	1.000^{X^2}
	(+)	0	0.0%	0	0.0%	
5 h	(-)	30	100.0%	30	100.0%	1.000^{X^2}
	(+)	0	0.0%	0	0.0%	
6 h	(-)	18	60.0%	20	66.7%	0.592^{X^2}
	(+)	12	40.0%	10	33.3%	
Postoperative mobilization time		4.0 ± 1.8		4.0 ± 1.4		0.862^{m}
Nausea Vomiting	(-)	23	76.7%	19	63.3%	0.260^{X^2}
	(+)	7	23.3%	11	36.7%	

^{m} Mann–Whitney U test/$^{X^2}$ Chi-square test.

5. Discussion

Transversus abdominis plane block can be applied as part of a good perioperative hemodynamic and analgesic regimen in appropriate abdominal surgeries. This situation has brought with it efforts to increase the effectiveness and duration of the action of peripheral nerve blocks made for analgesic purposes. This study aimed to evaluate the efficacy of adjuvant tramadol and dexmedetomidine in addition to bupivacaine in the TAP block procedure, which was performed to increase postoperative analgesic efficacy, reduce the incidence of side effects, reduce the need for additional intraoperative doses (neuromuscular blocker, opioid), and shorten mobilization time. The doses to be used were determined based on different studies in the literature, and the minimum dose and maximum effect were targeted. This study, which is among the few studies evaluating the adjuvant efficacy of dexmedetomidine and tramadol, showed that dexmedetomidine provided stable intraoperative hemodynamics and showed similar efficacy to tramadol in terms of analgesic efficacy.

Postoperative analgesia management is a topic that remains popular today. Inadequate use of analgesics in the treatment of pain causes unmanageable pain, and unnecessary use of analgesics causes side effects [17]. Neethirajan et al. [18] used 1 μg/kg dexmedetomidine as an adjuvant to bupivacaine in TAP block in their randomized controlled study conducted in 2020. Heart rate and blood pressure values in the dexmedetomidine group were significantly lower than in the control group. In their study, the median value for the 30th-min heart rate was 56/min, and the mean arterial pressure was 72 mmHg. Similarly, in our study, heart rate and mean arterial pressure values at the 30th minute intraoperatively and after extubation were found to be lower in D-group patients than in T-group patients. The heart rate and blood pressure values were closer to the physiological limits in the D group because of the adjuvant dexmedetomidine for the dose we used. This suggests that it provides a more stable perioperative process in terms of hemodynamics.

In a large-scale meta-analysis by Abdallah et al. [19], in which a minimum of 0.75 μg/kg dexmedetomidine was added to local anesthetic as an adjuvant in peripheral block applications, it was reported that dexmedetomidine caused transient bradycardia despite its analgesic efficacy and time advantages. It was stated that cases with bradycardia were transient and reversible with atropine. On the contrary, in our study, there were no cases of bradycardia and hypotension as complications at a dose of 0.5 μg/kg dexmedetomidine, results that were more stable in terms of hemodynamics and closer to the physiological limits that were obtained in the dexmedetomidine group.

Basavarajaiah et al. [20] applied TAP block by adding tramadol and dexmedetomidine as adjuvants to levobupivacaine in pediatric laparoscopic orchiopexy surgeries in 2022. In their study evaluating the analgesic efficacy, they added 1 μg/kg dexmedetomidine and 1 mg/kg tramadol to levobupivacaine. They used the Face, Legs, Activity, Cry, and Consolability (FLACC) pain scale in the postoperative period and showed that the postoperative analgesia time was significantly longer in the dexmedetomidine-added group. This differs from our study in that the local anesthetic doses applied, the doses of tramadol and dexmedetomidine added as adjuvants, and the pain scale used for follow-up were different. In our study, postoperative 0 h, 3 h, and 6 h VAS scores did not differ significantly ($p > 0.05$) in T- and D-group patients. It was observed that they provided more effective analgesia with the high-dose dexmedetomidine they used in their studies. In this respect, the current study is important in terms of shedding light on new studies that will provide more effective analgesia and stable hemodynamics at different doses than those used in our study. In our study, no difference was observed between the tramadol and dexmedetomidine groups in terms of side-effect profiles, in line with the study of Basavarajaiah et al.

Elyazed et al. [21] investigated the effects of tramadol and dexmedetomidine added to ropivacaine as an adjuvant in supraclavicular brachial plexus block in a study they conducted on 105 patients in 2015. Compared with the control group, the analgesia duration of the groups with tramadol and dexmedetomidine was found to be significantly longer. While their study is a peripheral nerve block study, our study is a facial plane block study. Therefore, it would not be correct to compare the peripheral nerve block with the facial plane block. Additionally, the difference in local anesthetics used is also an important issue. The purpose of sharing this study here is to draw attention to the fact that both dexmedetomidine and tramadol are used as adjuvants in the supraclavicular block, which is a peripheral nerve block.

There are some limitations to this study. The main limitation of this study is the lack of a no-intervention control group. Secondly, postoperative pain perception is a subjective phenomenon that is burdensome to quantify. Thirdly, since there are not many studies with similar features in the literature, the doses we determined are minimal doses that provide effectiveness. Working with different doses and more participants may change the results. Finally, clinical signs or symptoms of neurotoxicity were not assessed.

As a result, we found that tramadol and dexmedetomidine did not have significant differences in postoperative analgesia, postoperative analgesic consumption, side effect profile, and postoperative mobilization time when added as an adjuvant to local anesthetic drugs in TAP block applications. However, we observed that the dexmedetomidine group provided more physiological hemodynamics in terms of heart rate and mean arterial pressure. We think that adjuvant dexmedetomidine would be appropriate when applying a TAP block for more stable hemodynamic results. In addition, we believe that new studies with the use of dexmedetomidine over 50 μg as an adjuvant to increase the duration of sensory and motor blockade in adults may yield more meaningful results on the duration of postoperative analgesia.

Author Contributions: Conceptualization, A.E.T. and Z.K.; methodology, A.E.T.; software, N.K. and Z.K., validation, A.E.T., Z.K. and N.K..; formal analysis, A.E.T. and N.K.; resources, A.E.T., Z.K. and N.K., writing—original draft preparation, A.E.T. writing—review and editing, A.E.T., Z.K. and N.K.; visualization, A.E.T. and Z.K., supervision, A.E.T. and N.K.; All authors have read and agreed to the published version of the manuscript.

Funding: This research received no external funding.

Institutional Review Board Statement: The study was approved by ethics committee of the Van Yüzüncü Yıl University Faculty of Medicine 15.12.2020/06, registered with ClinicalTrials.gov (NCT05905757).

Informed Consent Statement: Informed consent was obtained from all subjects involved in the study.

Data Availability Statement: If required, our data can be submitted.

Conflicts of Interest: The authors declare no conflict of interest.

References

1. Naja, M.Z.; Ziade, M.F.; Lönnqvist, P.A. General anaesthesia combined with bilateral paravertebral blockade (T5-6) vs. general anaesthesia for laparoscopic cholecystectomy: A prospective, randomized clinical trial. *Eur. J. Anaesthesiol.* **2004**, *21*, 489–495. [PubMed]
2. Sharami, S.H.; Sharami, M.B.; Abdollahzadeh, M.; Keyvan, A. Randomised clinical trial of the influence of pulmonary recruitment manoeuvre on reducing shoulder pain after laparoscopy. *J. Obstet. Gynaecol.* **2010**, *30*, 505–510. [CrossRef] [PubMed]
3. Gurusamy, K.S.; Vaughan, J.; Toon, C.D.; Davidson, B.R. Pharmacological interventions for prevention or treatment of post-operative pain in people undergoing laparoscopic cholecystectomy. *Cochrane Database Syst. Rev.* **2014**, CD008261. [CrossRef] [PubMed]
4. Mulier, J.P. Perioperative opioids aggravate obstructive breathing in sleep apnea syndrome: Mechanisms and alternative anesthesia strategies. *Curr. Opin. Anaesthesiol.* **2016**, *29*, 129–133. [CrossRef] [PubMed]
5. Ibrahim, M.; Elnabtity, A.M.; Hegab, A.; Alnujaidi, O.A.; El Sanea, O. Combined opioid free and loco-regional anaesthesia enhances the quality of recovery in sleeve gastrectomy done under ERAS protocol: A randomized controlled trial. *BMC Anesthesiol.* **2022**, *22*, 29. [CrossRef] [PubMed]
6. Zhang, J.W.; Feng, X.Y.; Yang, J.; Wang, Z.H.; Wang, Z.; Bai, L.P. Ultrasound-guided single thoracic paravertebral nerve block and erector spinae plane block for perioperative analgesia in thoracoscopic pulmonary lobectomy: A randomized controlled trial. *Insights Imaging* **2022**, *13*, 16. [CrossRef] [PubMed]
7. Sessler, D.I.; Pei, L.; Huang, Y.; Fleischmann, E.; Marhofer, P.; Kurz, A.; Mayers, D.B.; A Meyer-Treschan, T.; Grady, M.; Tan, E.Y.; et al. Recurrence of breast cancer after regional or general anaesthesia: A randomised controlled trial. *Lancet* **2019**, *394*, 1807–1815. [CrossRef] [PubMed]
8. Mavarez, A.C.; Ahmed, A.A. Transabdominal Plane Block. In *Stat Pearls*; Stat Pearls Publishing: Treasure Island, FL, USA, 2023.
9. Rafi, A.N. Abdominalfieldblock: A new approach via the lumbar triangle. *Anaesthesia* **2001**, *56*, 1003–1029. [CrossRef]
10. Sun, Q.; Liu, S.; Wu, H.; Ma, H.; Liu, W.; Fang, M.; Liu, K.; Pan, Z. Dexmedetomidine as an Adjuvant to Local Anesthetics in Transversus Abdominis Plane Block:A Systematic Review and Meta-analysis. *Clin. J. Pain* **2019**, *35*, 375–384. [CrossRef] [PubMed]
11. Mert, T.; Gunes, Y.; Guven, M.; Gunay, I.; Gocmen, C. Differential effects of lidocaine and tramadol on modified nerve impulse by 4-aminopyridine in rats. *Pharmacology* **2003**, *69*, 68–73. [CrossRef] [PubMed]
12. Nagpal, V.; Rana, S.; Singh, J.; Chaudhary, S. Comparative study of systemically and perineurally administered tramadol as an adjunct for supraclavicular brachial plexus block. *J. Anaesthesiol. Clin. Pharmacol.* **2015**, *31*, 191–195. [PubMed]
13. Khosa, A.H.; Asad, N.; Durrani, H. Does the addition of Tramadol to local anaesthetic mixture improve the quality of axillary brachial plexus block: A comparative study at the teaching hospital, Dera Ghazi Khan. *Pak. J. Med. Health Sci.* **2015**, *9*, 1120–1123.
14. Shin, H.W.; Ju, B.J.; Jang, Y.K.; You, H.S.; Kang, H.; Park, J.Y. Effect of tramadol as an adjuvant to local anesthetics for brachial plexus block: A systematic review and meta-analysis. *PLoS ONE* **2017**, *12*, e0184649. [CrossRef] [PubMed]
15. Swami, S.S.; Keniya, V.M.; Ladi, S.D.; Rao, R. Comparison of dexmedetomidine and clonidine (α2 agonist drugs) as an adjuvant to local anaesthesia in supraclavicular brachial plexus block: A randomised double-blind prospective study. *Indian J. Anaesth.* **2012**, *56*, 243–249. [CrossRef] [PubMed]
16. Alemanno, F.; Ghisi, D.; Fanelli, A.; Faliva, A.; Pergolotti, B.; Bizzarri, F.; Fanelli, G. Tramadol and 0.5% levobupivacaine for single-shot interscalene block: Effects on postoperative analgesia in patients undergoing shoulder arthroplasty. *Minerva Anestesiol.* **2012**, *78*, 291–296.
17. Diaz, G.; Flood, P. Strategies for effective postoperative pain management. *Minerva Anestesiol.* **2006**, 145–150.
18. Neethirajan, S.G.R.; Kurada, S.; Parameswari, A. Efficacy of Dexmedetomidine as an Adjuvant to Bupivacaine in Ultrasound-Guided Transverse Abdominis plane Block for Laparoscopic appendicectomy: A Randomised Controlled Study. *Turk. J. Anaesthesiol. Reanim.* **2020**, *48*, 364–370. [CrossRef] [PubMed]
19. Abdallah, F.W.; Brull, R. Facilitatory effects of perineural dexmedetomidine on neuraxial and peripheral nerve block: A systematic review and meta-analysis. *Br. J. Anaesth.* **2013**, *110*, 915–925. [CrossRef] [PubMed]

20. Basavarajaiah, S.; Patel, P.; Sharma, K. A Comparative Study of Dexmedetomidine and Tramadol as an Adjuvant to Levobupivacaine in Ultrasound Guided Transverse Abdominus Plane Block in Pediatric Patients Undergoing Laproscopic Orchidopexy. *Arch. Anesth. Crit. Care* **2022**, *8*, 270–273. [CrossRef]
21. Elyazed, M.M.A.; Shaimaa, F.M. Dexmedetomidine Versus Tramadol as Adjuvants to Ultrasound Guided Supraclavicular Brachial Plexus Block in Patients Undergoing Hand and Forearm Surgery. *Al-Azhar Assiut Med. J.* **2015**, *13*, 80–91.

Journal of
Clinical Medicine

MDPI

Case Report

Continuous Erector Spinae Plane Block for Pain Management in a Pediatric Kidney Transplant Recipient: A Case Report and Review of the Current Literature

Paolo Capuano [1], Gaetano Burgio [1], Serena Abbate [2], Giusy Ranucci [2], Kejd Bici [3], Davide Cintorino [3], Antonio Arcadipane [1] and Gennaro Martucci [1,*]

1 Department of Anesthesia and Intensive Care, Istituto Mediterraneo per i Trapianti e Terapie ad alta Specializzazione (IRCCS-ISMETT), UPMCI (University of Pittsburgh Medical Center Italy), 90127 Palermo, Italy; pcapuano@ismett.edu (P.C.); gburgio@ismett.edu (G.B.); aarcadipane@ismett.edu (A.A.)

2 Pediatric Unit, Pediatric Center, Istituto Mediterraneo per i Trapianti e Terapie ad alta Specializzazione (IRCCS-ISMETT), UPMCI (University of Pittsburgh Medical Center Italy), 90127 Palermo, Italy; sabbate@ismett.edu (S.A.); granucci@ismett.edu (G.R.)

3 Surgical Unit, Pediatric Center, Istituto Mediterraneo per i Trapianti e Terapie ad alta Specializzazione (IRCCS-ISMETT), UPMCI (University of Pittsburgh Medical Center Italy), 90127 Palermo, Italy; kbici@ismett.edu (K.B.); dcintorino@ismett.edu (D.C.)

* Correspondence: gmartucci@ismett.edu

Abstract: Pain management in patients undergoing kidney transplantation requires careful consideration due to their altered physiology, and potential risks associated with certain analgesic options. In recent years, personalized and multimodal approaches have proven to be pivotal in perioperative pain management, as well as in children. Implementing regional analgesia methods offers a valuable solution in many pediatric surgical settings and the erector spinae plane block (ESPB) could represent a possible analgesic strategy in pediatric patients undergoing renal transplantation. Here, we report the case of a 13-year-old child who underwent living-donor kidney transplantation (LDKx) and received continuous erector spinae plane block (ESPB) for perioperative pain management. This multimodal approach with continuous ESPB resulted in optimal pain control without the need for opioids, allowing for early mobilization and for an optimal postoperative course.

Keywords: fascial plane blocks; erector spinae plane block; kidney transplantation

1. Introduction

Kidney transplantation is the most effective treatment for children affected with end-stage renal disease [1]. When available, living-donor kidney transplantation (LDKx) carries several advantages, principally when performed as a pre-emptive strategy. These recipients often experience improved quality of life, better growth and development, and a reduced risk of complications associated with dialysis. Furthermore, having a kidney from a living donor tends to offer a longer lifespan for the transplanted organ due to less ischemic injury to the organ and lower rates of rejection [2].

Designated transplant centers for LDKx should construct multidisciplinary approaches to optimize outcomes and mitigate potential risks associated with the surgery and the hospital stay [3]. Pain is one of the main complications during the hospital stay for children because of its impact on general recovery and inflammation, and to the stress it causes for the family and caregivers. In cases of kidney disease, there are further challenges in pain management since impaired kidney function significantly limits the array of available analgesic options due to potential toxicity and altered drug metabolism related to alterations in drug distribution volume, modifications in protein binding, and delayed clearance [4]. In recent years, personalized and multimodal approaches have proven to be pivotal in perioperative pain management, as well as in children [5]. Implementing regional analgesia methods offers a valuable solution in many pediatric surgical settings; however, the use of a central regional anesthesia technique such as epidural blockade has been traditionally limited by concerns about bleeding—either primary or secondary to combining regional analgesia and anticoagulants after transplantation.

Today, a new generation of regional anesthesia techniques, called "fascial plane blocks", are emerging as an effective alternative to conventional techniques such as paravertebral, epidural, or spinal blocks [6]. The primary target of fascial plane blocks is the deep fascia, a dense membrane of connective tissue that extends throughout the body. It surrounds and encases muscles, nerves, and other structures, including mechanoreceptors and nervous fibers [7].

These blocks, by avoiding direct injection into the nerve or toward the neural axis, can minimize the risk of serious complications such as neural injury and neuraxial hematoma and can potentially represent a valid alternative option in high-risk patients.

However, despite the use of fascial plane blocks becoming increasingly widespread even in the context of high-risk surgeries such as cardiothoracic surgery, there are still no specific guidelines on their use and management in patients at risk of bleeding [8].

Here, we report the case of a 13-year-old child who underwent LDKx and received continuous erector spinae plane block (ESPB) for perioperative pain management.

The parents of the child gave their consent for anonymous publication of the case report.

2. Case Presentation

A 13-year-old boy, with a weight of 38 kg and height of 152 cm, suffering from renal failure due to a dysplastic single kidney was referred to our institute for work up for a kidney transplant. The mother was identified as a possible compatible donor.

Blood creatinine was 6.8 mg/dL, BUN was 158 mg/dL, while daily urine output was still 2500 mL. Platelet count was 325 ($\times 10^3$/uL), and coagulation values were in the normal range.

In November 2023, the patient was scheduled for a pre-emptive kidney transplant from a living donor. General anesthesia was achieved according to standard practice (fentanyl 100 mcg, propofol 120 mg, cisatracurium 8 mg), including the monitoring of neuromuscular blockade and the depth of anesthesia with Bispectral Index (BIS), blood pressure monitoring via radial artery, and placement of a central venous catheter.

After induction of anesthesia, the patient was placed in the left lateral position, and ultrasound-guided ESPB was performed for perioperative analgesia. A linear ultrasound transducer was placed on the parasagittal plane about 2 cm lateral to the T9-T10 transverse process and rhomboid major, and erector spinae muscles were identified superior to the hyperechoic transverse process (Figure 1).

Using an in-plane approach, an 18-gauge, 100 mm Contiplex Ultra 360® needle (B.Braun, Melsungen, Germany) was inserted in the caudal–cephalad direction, with the tip of the T10 transverse process below the erector spinae muscle as the endpoint for the needle tip. After hydrodissection with 2 mL of normal saline, 20 mL of 0.375% ropivacaine was injected into the area. Then, a peripheral nerve catheter was inserted into the fascial plane, and placement was checked with ultrasound (Figure 2).

The operation lasted 3 h, and a hockey-stick incision into the right iliac fossa was performed for retroperitoneal access to the iliac vessels. Apart from the fentanyl administered at induction, no additional analgesics drugs were used. The patient was extubated in the operating room and then transferred to the intensive care unit for postoperative monitoring. He was moved to the surgery ward on postoperative day one.

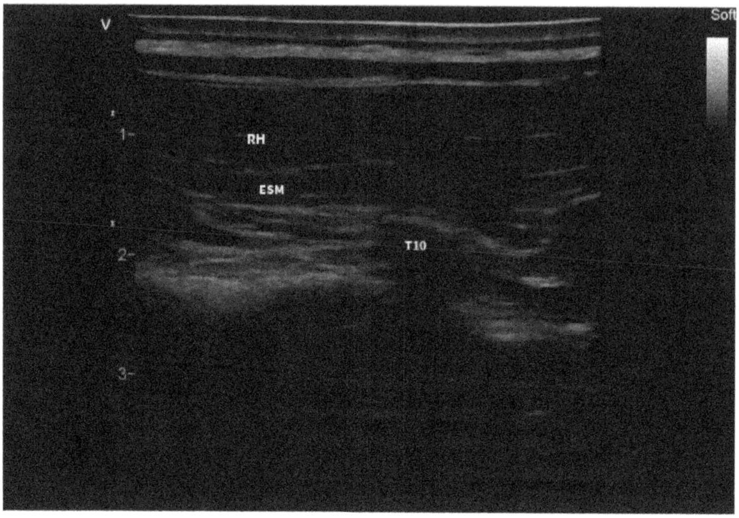

Figure 1. Sono-anatomy of the erector spinae plane block; RH: rhomboid muscle; ESM: erector spinae muscle; T10: transverse process.

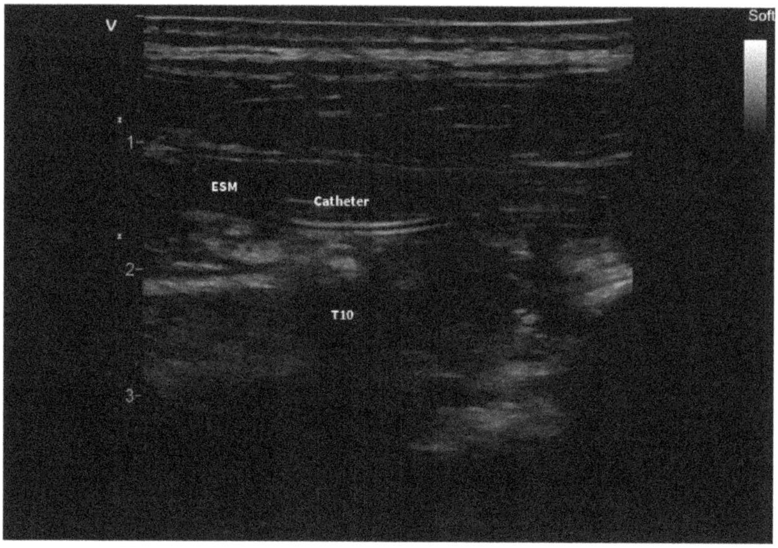

Figure 2. Ultrasound visualization of the ESPB catheter; ESM: erector spinae muscle; T10: transverse process.

Postoperative analgesia was achieved with paracetamol 500 mg every 6 h, together with ropivacaine 0.2% 20 mL every 8 h. With this multimodal approach, consistent good-quality analgesia (NRS < 3) was achieved, without side-effects such as constipation and postoperative nausea and vomiting. Postoperative physiotherapy was started immediately, and the patient was positioned out of bed on the second day and began walking early (Table 1).

Table 1. Ropivacaine administration, lab values, and progress indicators in the postoperative period.

	Operative Day	POD 1	POD 2	POD 3	POD 4
	Catheter placement				
Ropivacaine dose	0.375% 20 mL pre-operative	0.2% 20 mL × 3	0.2% 20 mL × 3	0.2% 20 mL × 3	Catheter removed
NRS at rest		0	0	0	0
NRS at movement		3	2	0	0
Gas canalization		x	x	x	x
Stool canalization			x	x	x
Creatinine mg/dL	6.8	2.52	1.2	1.21	0.69
Platelet ($\times 10^3$/uL)	325	271	285	299	301
INR	1.03	1.01	1	0.98	0.95
Diet		Sips of water	Soft diet	Regular diet	Regular diet
Movement		In the bed	Out of bed	Ambulating	Regular activity

In the first postoperative day, preventive anticoagulant treatment was initiated as per protocol (unfractionated heparin in continuous infusion in the range of 2–5 units/kg/h) until the fourth postoperative day, with no adverse effects observed.

Overall, the postoperative course was uneventful, complicated only by a urinary tract infection on day 8, promptly treated with piperacillin/tazobactam, and the patient was discharged on postoperative day 14.

3. Discussion

Pain management in patients with chronic kidney disease, particularly those who have undergone kidney transplantation, requires careful consideration due to their altered physiology, and potential risks associated with certain analgesic options. Drug metabolism and elimination can be significantly affected, leading to potential toxicity concerns with many pain medications.

Generally, morphine is still the most used drug for postoperative pain control, though its use, like other derivative opioids, is not without risk, because of the accumulation of toxic metabolites [9]. On the other hand, the use of other drugs such as gabapentinoids and NSAIDs, commonly administered in multimodal approaches, is also inadvisable in patients with chronic renal failure.

Consequently, the use of fascial plane blocks can be considered as a potential alternative in nephropathic patients, providing a valuable option for a multimodal approach to pain management.

The ESPB is a relatively new technique in the field of regional anesthesia and pain management. It was first described by Forero in 2016 and has gained attention in several surgical settings. In fact, the erector spinae is made up of three muscles (Spinalis, Longissimus, and Iliocostalis) that run from the sacrum to the skull, extending throughout the lumbar, thoracic, and cervical regions [10].

ESPB has gained attention and sparked debates over its mechanism of action since its first description. According to cadaveric studies and magnetic resonance imaging, it has been observed to provide analgesia for both somatic and visceral pain [11,12].

By injecting the local anesthetic into the interfascial plane between the erector spinae muscle and the transverse process, it can spread through channels in the intertransverse connective tissues. This spreading allows the local anesthetic to reach the ventral and dorsal rami of the thoracic spinal nerves, as well as the sympathetic ramus communicans at the intervertebral foramen level.

Furthermore, the involvement of lateral cutaneous branches of intercostal nerves is mentioned, suggesting that these nerve branches also contribute to the analgesic effect of the block [13].

ESPB has recently been described as a possible analgesic strategy in adult patients undergoing renal transplantation. When performed at the T9-10 level, ESPB provides analgesia without motor blocks in the abdominal–pelvic region: in the present case, a decreased sensation to pinprick and analgesia from T7 to T12 was recorded. In fact, ESPB provides both somatic and visceral analgesia by blocking both dorsal and ventral rami of the spinal nerves, and because of the transforaminal spread of local anesthetic into the paravertebral space and a variable amount of epidural spread [10].

In the 2019, Temirov et al. [14] first reported the successful use of a multimodal approach with a single ESPB shot in a 36-year-old man who underwent kidney transplantation. Continuous ESPB has also been described in the adult population for postoperative management in kidney transplantation. In a case series of 28 patients, Sharipova et al. [15] reported less pain and less opioid consumption, together with a lower incidence of nausea and vomiting, in 14 patients treated with continuous ESPB.

Similar results were reported by Vishwanath et al. [16]: in their quality improvement project, they switched from epidural catheters to erector spinae plane catheters in managing postoperative pain in 13 kidney transplantations. They reported a better safety profile, minimal use of opioids, and lesser adverse effects.

Though the use of the ESPB in children has been described for various types of surgery [17–20], to the best of our knowledge, this is the first report describing the use of continuous ESPB for pediatric kidney transplantation.

The importance of minimizing opioid use during the perioperative period for kidney transplant recipients has recently been addressed in the literature. As known, Enhanced Recovery After Surgery (ERAS) protocols focus on multimodal analgesia strategies aimed at reducing opioid consumption in various surgical settings, including kidney transplantation [21]. Therefore, adopting alternative or complementary analgesic strategies becomes crucial in mitigating opioid-related risks, and improving postoperative outcomes.

In the present case, a multimodal approach with continuous ESPB resulted in optimal pain control without the need for opioids, thus allowing for early mobilization. By eliminating the need for opioids, we observed a rapid recovery of intestinal function, without side-effects such as constipation and vomiting. Though desirable in all patients, a rapid and regular course is particularly desirable in pediatric cases, in which it is necessary to try to eliminate as much trauma as possible. Moreover, ESPB demonstrated a good safety profile, despite the need to initiate anticoagulant therapy with heparin, and no complications were observed. This is consonant with what is reported in the literature regarding the efficacy and the safety of fascial plane blocks in patients at high risk of bleeding in the cardiothoracic setting [8,22]. Specifically, Toscano et al. investigated the safety of fascial plane blocks, specifically continuous ESPB and SAPB in patients receiving anticoagulation and coagulopathy. They analyzed 70 patients undergoing minimally invasive mitral valve surgery through a right mini-thoracotomy. These patients received either continuous ESPB or SAPB for perioperative pain control. No adverse outcomes attributable to SAPB or ESPB in terms of vascular puncture, active bleeding, or hematoma formation were reported.

In fact, one of the advantages often highlighted with the Erector Spinae Plane Block is its anatomical location, which is deep in the erector spinae muscle plane and superficial to the transverse processes. This positioning is thought to contribute to a reduction in certain risks when compared to other regional anesthesia techniques [22].

Due to the distance of the ESP from major vessels and the spinal cord (medulla), there is a decreased risk of complications such as hypotension and hematoma when compared to techniques like Thoracic Epidural Analgesia (TEA) and Paravertebral Block (PVB) [8].

Furthermore, thanks to the interforaminal spread of the injectate in the ESPB, the risk of pneumothorax is reduced compared with PVB, where the needle is advanced closer to the pleura [22].

These anatomical considerations are also in line with a recent review that analyzed the safety and risk profiles of thoracic PVB and ESPB in patients receiving anticoagulant or antiplatelet therapy for cardiothoracic surgery or thoracic procedures [23]. The authors analyzed 15 articles and evidenced a low risk of bleeding associated with PVB and minimal or absent risk for ESPB, suggesting their favorable safety profiles for patients receiving anticoagulant or antiplatelet therapy, particularly in the context of cardiothoracic surgery or thoracic procedures.

Similar considerations were made by a panel of Canadian experts on regional anesthesia: they reviewed the evidence and classified the risk of bleeding complications following regional nerve blocks [24]. The ESPB was considered low-risk.

In the present case, the ESPB catheter was removed without stopping UFH infusion and no complications were observed.

There are currently no specific guidelines available on the management of the ESPB catheter during anticoagulation therapy. However, Adhikary et al. [25] reported the use of continuous ESPB for pain management in five patients undergoing left thoracotomy for left ventricular assist device placement. Despite the need for prolonged postoperative heparinization, they reported no complications in the management of catheters.

Similarly, in the study by Toscano et al. [8], regional catheters were removed at 48 hours irrespective of the international normalized ratio (INR) value and no complications were reported.

Finally, in the context of a multimodal approach in renal surgery, a possible alternative is represented by the quadratus lumborum block (QLB), which targets the somatic and visceral fibers on the anterolateral abdominal wall, achieving sensory block [26].

Onay et al. recently compared QLB and ESPB in terms of their effects on postoperative pain in open nephrectomy: they found that both approaches achieve similar results for at-rest and at-movement pain scores and opioid consumption during the postoperative period [27].

In our opinion, QLB is a valid option for pain management in kidney surgery but has some limitations in the field of renal transplantation. First, the QLB is considered a deeper block at high risk of bleeding, with a needle trajectory into a noncompressible space. Consequently, the risk of bleeding and complications is similar to that of the lumbar plexus block. Moreover, the postoperative catheter placement is probably more comfortable with the ESPB, with less impediment regarding early mobilization.

4. Conclusions

Continuous ESPB appears to be a valid and safe option in the multimodal analgesia of patients undergoing renal transplantation, even in the pediatric population, allowing good analgesia with a sparing of opioids. Future randomized trials will be needed to confirm our preliminary report.

Author Contributions: Conceptualization, G.B., P.C. and G.M.; methodology, P.C.; formal analysis, S.A. and G.R.; resources, G.M.; data curation, P.C., K.B. and D.C.; writing—original draft preparation, P.C. and G.M.; writing—review and editing, P.C., G.M., G.B. and A.A.; visualization, S.A., G.R., K.B. and D.C.; supervision, G.B. and A.A.; project administration, G.M.; funding acquisition, G.M. All authors have read and agreed to the published version of the manuscript.

Funding: This research was funded by Italian Ministry of Health, Ricerca Corrente—Linea di Ricerca ISMETT n 1.

Institutional Review Board Statement: Not applicable.

Informed Consent Statement: The parents of the child gave their consent for anonymous publication of the case report.

Data Availability Statement: Data are contained within the article.

Conflicts of Interest: The authors declare no conflicts of interest.

References

1. Chua, A.; Cramer, C.; Moudgil, A.; Martz, K.; Smith, J.; Blydt-Hansen, T.; Neu, A.; Dharnidharka, V.R.; the NAPRTCS investigators. Kidney transplant practice patterns and outcome benchmarks over 30 years: The 2018 report of the NAPRTCS. *Pediatr. Transplant.* **2019**, *23*, e13597. [CrossRef]
2. Chandar, J.; Chen, L.; Defreitas, M.; Ciancio, G.; Burke, G. Donor considerations in pediatric kidney transplantation. *Pediatr. Nephrol.* **2020**, *36*, 245–257. [CrossRef] [PubMed]
3. Abu-Sultaneh, S.; Hobson, M.; Wilson, A.; Goggins, W.; Nitu, M.; Lutfi, R. Practice Variation in the Immediate Postoperative Care of Pediatric Kidney Transplantation: A National Survey. *Transplant. Proc.* **2017**, *49*, 2060–2064. [CrossRef]
4. Lambourg, E.; Colvin, L.; Guthrie, G.; Walker, H.; Bell, S. Analgesic use and associated adverse events in patients with chronic kidney disease: A systematic review and meta-analysis. *Br. J. Anaesth.* **2022**, *128*, 546–561. [CrossRef]
5. Gai, N.; Naser, B.; Hanley, J.; Peliowski, A.; Hayes, J.; Aoyama, K. A practical guide to acute pain management in children. *J. Anesthesia* **2020**, *34*, 421–433. [CrossRef]
6. Elsharkawy, H.; Pawa, A.; Mariano, E.R. Interfascial Plane Blocks. *Reg. Anesthesia Pain Med.* **2018**, *43*, 341–346. [CrossRef] [PubMed]
7. Findley, T.; Chaudhry, H.; Stecco, A.; Roman, M. Fascia research—A narrative review. *J. Bodyw. Mov. Ther.* **2012**, *16*, 67–75, Erratum in Mov. Ther. 2012, 16, 270. [CrossRef]
8. Toscano, A.; Capuano, P.; Galatà, M.; Tazzi, I.; Rinaldi, M.; Brazzi, L. Safety of Ultrasound-Guided Serratus Anterior and Erector Spinae Fascial Plane Blocks: A Retrospective Analysis in Patients Undergoing Cardiac Surgery While Receiving Anticoagulant and Antiplatelet Drugs. *J. Cardiothorac. Vasc. Anesthesia* **2022**, *36*, 483–488. [CrossRef]
9. Dean, M. Opioids in renal failure and dialysis patients. *J. Pain Symptom Manage* **2004**, *28*, 497–504. [CrossRef]
10. Pawa, A.; King, C.; Thang, C.; White, L. Erector spinae plane block: The ultimate 'plan A' block? *Br. J. Anaesth.* **2023**, *130*, 497–502. [CrossRef]
11. Chin, K.J.; El-Boghdadly, K. Mechanisms of action of the erector spinae plane (ESP) block: A narrative review. *Can. J. Anaesth.* **2021**, *68*, 387–408. [CrossRef] [PubMed]
12. Schwartzmann, A.; Peng, P.; Maciel, M.A.; Alcarraz, P.; Gonzalez, X.; Forero, M. A magnetic resonance imaging study of local anesthetic spread in patients receiving an erector spinae plane block. *Can. J. Anaesth.* **2020**, *67*, 942–948. [CrossRef] [PubMed]
13. Vidal, E.; Giménez, H.; Forero, M.; Fajardo, M. Erector spinae plane block: A cadaver study to determine its mechanism of action. Bloqueo del plano del músculo erector espinal: Estudio anatómico-cadavérico para determinar su mecanismo de acción. *Rev. Esp. Anestesiol. Reanim. Engl. Ed.* **2018**, *65*, 514–519. [CrossRef] [PubMed]
14. Temirov, T.; Ben-David, B.; Mustafin, A.; Viderman, D. Erector Spinae Plane Block in Management of Pain After Kidney Transplantation. *Pain Med.* **2019**, *20*, 1053–1054. [CrossRef] [PubMed]
15. Sharipova, V.; Alimov, A.; Siyabayev, F.; Sadikov, M. Erector Spinae Plane Block for Postoperative Analgesia After Kidney Transplant. *Transplantation* **2022**, *20* (Suppl. S1), 83–85. [CrossRef] [PubMed]
16. Vishwanath, P.; Balakundi, P.; Deo, A.S. Continuous Erector Spinae Plane Analgesia in Kidney Transplant Recipients: A Quality Improvement Project. *Cureus* **2023**, *15*, e39151. [CrossRef]
17. Macaire, P.; Ho, N.; Nguyen, V.; Van, H.P.; Thien, K.D.N.; Bringuier, S.; Capdevila, X. Bilateral ultrasound-guided thoracic erector spinae plane blocks using a programmed intermittent bolus improve opioid-sparing postoperative analgesia in pediatric patients after open cardiac surgery: A randomized, double-blind, placebo-controlled trial. *Reg. Anesthesia Pain Med.* **2020**, *45*, 805–812. [CrossRef]
18. Aksu, C.; Şen, M.C.; Akay, M.A.; Baydemir, C.; Gürkan, Y. Erector Spinae Plane Block vs Quadratus Lumborum Block for pediatric lower abdominal surgery: A double blinded, prospective, and randomized trial. *J. Clin. Anesthesia* **2019**, *57*, 24–28. [CrossRef]
19. Mostafa, S.F.; Abdelghany, M.S.; Abdelraheem, T.M.; Abu Elyazed, M.M. Ultrasound-guided erector spinae plane block for postoperative analgesia in pediatric patients undergoing splenectomy: A prospective randomized controlled trial. *Pediatr. Anesthesia* **2019**, *29*, 1201–1207. [CrossRef]
20. Singh, S.; Jha, R.K.; Sharma, M. The analgesic effect of bilateral ultrasound-guided erector spinae plane block in paediatric lower abdominal surgeries: A randomised, prospective trial. *Indian J. Anaesth.* **2020**, *64*, 762–767. [CrossRef]
21. Elsabbagh, A.M.M.; Ghoneim, I.M.; Moiz, A.; Welch, K.R.; Brown, J.S.M. Enhanced Recovery After Surgery Pathway in Kidney Transplantation: The Road Less Traveled. *Transplant. Direct* **2022**, *8*, e1333. [CrossRef]
22. Capuano, P.; Hileman, B.A.; Martucci, G.; Raffa, G.M.; Toscano, A.; Burgio, G.; Arcadipane, A.; Kowalewski, M. Erector spinae plane block versus paravertebral block for postoperative pain management in thoracic surgery: A systematic review and meta-analysis. *Minerva Anestesiol.* **2023**, *89*, 1042–1050. [CrossRef]
23. Nisi, F.; Sella, N.; DI Gregorio, G.; Lubian, M.; Giustiniano, E.; Rosboch, G.L.; Balzani, E.; Toscano, A.; Strano, G.; Rispoli, M.; et al. The safety of thoracic paravertebral block and erector spinae plane block in patients treated with anticoagulant or antiplatelet therapy. A narrative review of the evidence. *Minerva Anestesiol.* **2023**, *89*, 914–922. [CrossRef] [PubMed]
24. Tsui, B.C.H.; Kirkham, K.; Kwofie, M.K.; Tran, D.Q.; Wong, P.; Chin, K.J.; Sondekoppam, R.V. Practice advisory on the bleeding risks for peripheral nerve and interfascial plane blockade: Evidence review and expert consensus. *Can. J. Anaesth.* **2019**, *66*, 1356–1384. [CrossRef] [PubMed]

25. Das Adhikary, S.; Prasad, A.; Soleimani, B.; Chin, K.J. Continuous Erector Spinae Plane Block as an Effective Analgesic Option in Anticoagulated Patients After Left Ventricular Assist Device Implantation: A Case Series. *J. Cardiothorac. Vasc. Anesthesia* **2019**, *33*, 1063–1067. [CrossRef] [PubMed]
26. Little, C.; Rahman, S. Quadratus Lumborum Blocks in Nephrectomy: A Narrative Review. *Local Reg. Anesthesia* **2021**, *14*, 57–65. [CrossRef] [PubMed]
27. Onay, M.; Kayhan, G.E.; Özen, A.; Baş, S.; Yelken, B. Comparison of ultrasound-guided quadratus lumborum block and erector spinae plane block in terms of their effects on postoperative pain in open nephrectomy. *Minerva Anestesiol.* **2023**, *89*, 32–39. [CrossRef]

Journal of
Clinical Medicine

MDPI

Review

The Impact of Regional Anesthesia in Masking Acute Compartment Syndrome after Limb Trauma

Nicole Hilber [1,*], Anna Dodi [1], Stephan Blumenthal [1], Heinz Bruppacher [1], Alain Borgeat [2,3] and José Aguirre [1]

1 Institute of Anesthesiology, City Hospital Zurich, 8008 Zurich, Switzerland; stephan.blumenthal@stadtspital.ch (S.B.); josealejandro.aguirre@stadtspital.ch (J.A.)
2 Department of Anesthesiology, Balgrist Campus Zurich, 8008 Zurich, Switzerland; alain.borgeat@balgrist.ch
3 Department of Surgery, University of Illinois at Chicago, Chicago, IL 60607, USA
* Correspondence: nicoledominique.hilber@stadtspital.ch

Abstract: Regional anesthesia has shown to be successful in controlling major pain in trauma patients. However, the possibility of masking acute compartment syndrome (ACS) after peripheral nerve blocks for limb injuries is still controversially discussed. Therefore, we aimed to summarize the current literature regarding this topic to shed light on the impact of peripheral regional anesthesia on the diagnosis of ACS in trauma patients. We searched Pubmed, Google Scholar and the Cochrane Library for literature following the PRISMA (preferred reporting items for systematic reviews and meta-analyses) guidelines. The analysis of these reports was included in the context of the current literature concerning this topic. We found no (randomized) studies, and only six case reports dealing with the impact of peripheral nerve blocks and ACS in patients after a limb trauma met our criteria and were included in our review. Only one reported a delay in the diagnosis of ACS. In most of the cases (5 of 6), the breakthrough pain, despite the nerve block, proved to be a good indicator of a developing ACS. However, despite some narrative articles about the topic including some recommendations about the possibly safe use of regional anesthesia techniques for limb trauma, there is still no international consensus and only one national guideline focusing on the possibly safe use of peripheral nerve blocks in trauma patients at risk of ACS. After reviewing the respective literature, we consider that intra-articular analgesia, sensory blocks, fascial plane blocks and low-concentration continuous peripheral nerve blocks are effective for analgesia and a low-risk analgesia tool for trauma and postsurgical patients at risk of ACS due to the fact that they do not lead to a dense block. Finally, we summarized suggestions based on the results of the literature for the different regional anesthesia modalities in these patients in a table to facilitate the use of these techniques.

Keywords: regional anesthesia; limb trauma; compartment syndrome; anesthesia; pain management; nerve block

1. Introduction

Peripheral (continuous) regional anesthesia is considered a highly effective analgesia regimen after elective and trauma surgery [1], avoiding the complications caused by opioids such as dizziness, nausea and vomiting and urinary retention. Moreover, its positive impact on the long-term functional outcome after elective large joint replacement has also been described [2]. However, its use is controversially discussed due to anecdotal reports [3] blaming peripheral nerve blocks for masking an incipient ACS [4]. There is limited knowledge concerning the impact of regional anesthesia on the diagnosis of ACS [4–6], as highlighted by the American and European Societies of regional anesthesia (ASRA, ESRA) [7]. In fact, the American College of Surgeons National Surgical Quality Improvement Project (ACS-NSQIP) published data where no differences in postoperative complications after lower extremity fractures comparing a regional or general anesthesia regimen could be shown [8]. Moreover, Zadrazil et al. recently published a case series of

565 pediatric patients using regional anesthesia for pain treatment after extremity trauma and could not describe a single case of ACS [9].

This controversy has pushed a Working Party established by the Association of Anaesthetists of Great Britain and Ireland to publish the first Guidelines dealing with regional analgesia for lower leg trauma and the risk of ACS [10]. They offered a multi-professional, consensus opinion based on an objective, narrative review of case reports and case series, aiming to provide pragmatic guidance for optimal analgesia and highlighting the need for careful observation of ACS in any patient at risk, independent of the analgesia regimen. Based on our previous publications [5,6,11], and encouraged by the topic of this special issue, we performed a systematic review, screening all studies, case reports/series and reviews available with the aim of summarizing the literature regarding the impact of peripheral regional anesthesia of the upper and lower extremities in trauma on ACS. However, to draw a complete picture about the impact of regional anesthesia and ACS, we studied the current literature dealing with other regional anesthesia modalities and summarized all results in a final table to facilitate the use of these techniques in the trauma setting.

1.1. What Is Acute Compartment Syndrome?

The definition of ACS includes a pressure increase within a fixed osteofascial anatomic space. The high pressure leads to decreased tissue perfusion and to an impairment of the cellular function. It can end in persistent damage with considerable functional loss after muscle necrosis [12,13]. Three factors influence the outcome in the case of increased compartment pressure: the amount and the duration of the pressure as well as the severity of the soft tissue damage. Severe injuries to soft tissues and fractures are the main causes of developing ACS [4,14]. ACS is less common in women and children than in men [6,14]. In a developing ACS, pain is considered to be a clinical symptom of pivotal importance. However, muscle tenseness, paresthesia and paresis might also indicate ACS. No palpable pulses are considered a late sign and are associated with a poor functional outcome [5,6,11]. The pain increases with stretching of the involved muscle compartment and is often reported as more intense and severe than should be expected for the injury. Moreover, pain worsens with time, and does not respond to increasing doses of pain medication, including opioids and boluses of local anesthetics applied through a peripheral nerve catheter [5,6,10,11] (Table 1).

Table 1. Symptoms and signs of acute compartment syndrome.

Symptoms	Signs
• Pain is greater than expected or increasing • Paresthesia in affected extremity • Splinting or removal of casts leads to no relief • Raise in pain and analgesic demand	• Pain after passive stretching of the respective compartment • Swollen and tense compartment • Pallor • Pulselessness (late sign) • Muscle weakness • Sensory deficit of the nerves enclosed in the compartment
Note: In the early stage of ACS, pulses might be present, but they are absent in the late stage. Therefore, palpable pulses do not exclude ACS. During the early development of ACS, the capillary refill is present. ACS can occur in open fractures. Clinical signs remain unclear due to their low specificity and sensitivity. After regional anesthesia or opioid patient-controlled analgesia (PCA), probably more sensitive clinical signs of ACS: - Breakthrough pain despite well-working regional anesthesia. - Increase demand of analgesics.	

The data from the Royal Infirmary of Edinburgh report an annual incidence of 3.1 per 100,000 people (7.3 per 100,000 men and 0.7 per 100,000 women) on average [15]. ACS is commonly seen in males and in patients younger than 35 years [16]. After extremity trauma, 40% of all cases of ACS are described after tibial shaft fracture, whereas 23% are described after soft tissue tibial trauma and 18% after forearm fractures [17,18]. The incidence of ACS in children is lower despite the fact that they show a higher preexisting compartment pressure [19,20].

A crucial fact is that ACS might also be present in the absence of fractures. Different medical conditions with abnormal bleeding diatheses (clotting disorders, hemophilia, etc.), neurocognitive impairment and neurologic disorders with reduced sensitivity and sensibility of the limbs, as well as intramedullary nails, vascular injury, burns, high energy injury and the use of tourniquets are associated with an increased risk of ACS [15].

1.2. Diagnosis of Acute Compartment Syndrome

Clinical symptoms and signs are summarized in Table 1. It is important to recognize that the specificity of clinical signs is 97–98%; however, their sensitivity is as low as 13–19% [6]. In the presence of one clinical symptom, the probability of diagnosing ACS correctly is 25%. This probability increases to 93% if three clinical symptoms are present. [6].

The measurement of compartment pressure is the golden standard to determine if fasciotomy is indicated or not [11]. It is crucial that an immediate diagnosis is made, followed by surgical treatment to prevent further damage to the tissues; therefore, an objective measurement of the compartment pressure has to be performed using of the commercially available pressure devices [21]. Interestingly, there is no final consensus about the threshold value of compartmental pressure and its relation to systolic, diastolic or mean blood pressure for the diagnosis and treatment of ACS [22].

A noninvasive tool which might show an incipient ACS is near-infrared spectroscopy (NIRS), which analyzes the relative oxygen saturation ($rScO_2$) of tissue hemoglobin [23,24].

NIRS can measure changes in local muscle oxygen saturation, offering continuous, noninvasive monitoring of intra-compartmental ischemia and hypoxia [25,26].

1.3. Treatment of ACS

The only treatment to avoid permanent damage after diagnosis of ACS is a surgical decompression of the affected osteofascial compartments [27,28]. The outcome after fasciotomy actually depends on the timing and the additional injuries. A delay of surgical ACS treatment for more than 12 h impairs the outcome [29–31]. In fact, Hayakawa et al. reported that performing a fasciotomy within 6 h after ACS diagnosis showed a satisfactory outcome in 88% of cases, leading to an amputation rate of 3.2% and a mortality rate of 2%. However, a fasciotomy performed after 12 h had a satisfactory outcome in 15% of cases, leading to 14% amputations and 4.3% reported deaths [32]. However, there are reports of residual functional impairment if fasciotomy is delayed for only 2 h after ACS diagnosis [33–38]. The surgical fasciotomy can be performed safely under general or (short-acting) regional anesthesia [21].

2. Methods

Pubmed, Google Scholar and the Cochrane Library were searched for literature concerning compartment syndrome in the upper and lower extremities in combination with a peripheral nerve block (PNB) and trauma in adult patients in the time period January 1980–June 2023. We excluded articles written in any languages other than English. The use of only intravenous opioid patient-controlled analgesia (PCA) and elective surgeries was also excluded. We used keywords such as 'acute compartment syndrome', 'upper extremity', 'lower extremity', 'trauma', 'peripheral nerve block', 'nerve block', 'regional anesthesia', 'compartment syndrome', 'upper limb' and 'lower limb', in different combinations. We followed the PRISMA guidelines. Some of the articles were cross-referenced.

We also studied articles concentrating on other regional anesthesia techniques used for trauma patients, like central blocks (epidural (EDA) and spinal anesthesia), intra-articular analgesia, intravenous regional anesthesia (IVRA), wound infusion and fascial plane blocks for extremity surgery, to check the references and to summarize the data reported and offer suggestions based on the results of the literature for the different regional anesthesia modalities.

3. Results

We identified 296 citations, 90 of which were related to the topic: compartment syndrome and regional anesthesia in the reviewed time period. We excluded duplicates (n = 46), articles including only PCA and no regional anesthesia (n = 8) and articles not in English (n = 3), which gave us a total of 35 full-text articles. We further excluded from the primary analysis articles including peripheral blocks for elective surgery (6), articles including patients in a study protocol for liposomal bupivacaine (1), articles including pediatric trauma and regional anesthesia (1), articles dealing with IVRA (7) and articles including spinal/EDA (12). Therefore, we included a total of six full-text articles in the final analysis: case reports (n = 6) (Table 2) (Figure 1).

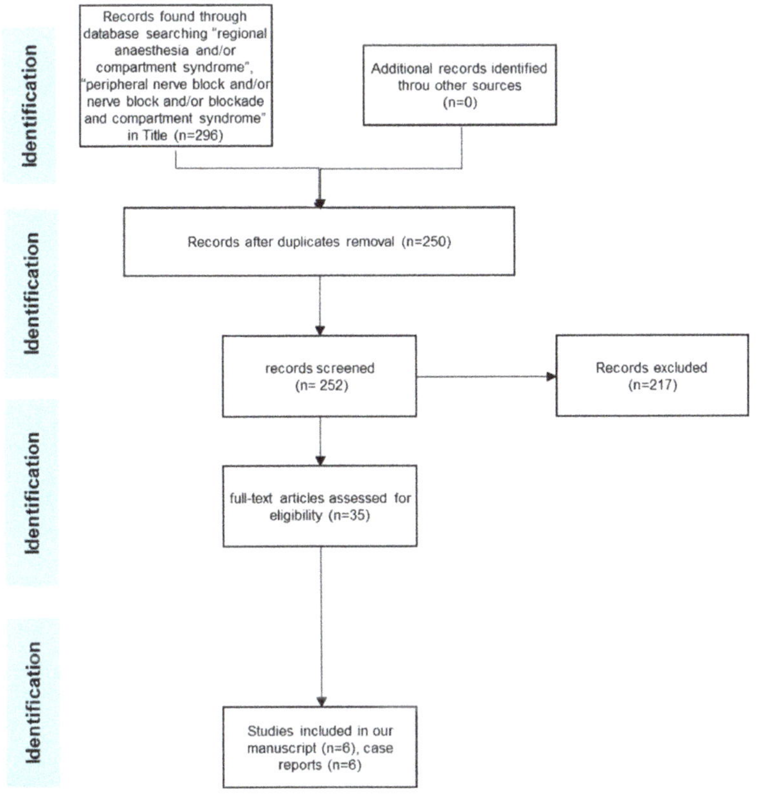

Figure 1. Data search diagram.

Only one case reported a possible delay in the diagnosis of ACS. Ganeshan et al. [39] reported a case of a 75-year-old man with a distal radius fracture. The surgery was performed after an axillary nerve block. However, the local anesthetic used, and its concentration and volume were not reported. After the failure of K-wires, a volar periarticular locking plate was put in place. After surgery, the patient was sent home. Unfortunately, the authors did not report if the patient was discharged after the block had worn off with full sensory and motor blockade. There was no documented monitoring of the patient for signs/symptoms of developing ACS in the time frame from post-surgery until block resolution. Only 24 h after surgery did the patient present to the emergency department with blisters, and loss of sensation and motor function in the fingers and wrist.

The case by Hyder et al. [3] was published in an orthopedic journal with the title "Compartment syndrome in tibial shaft fracture missed because of a local nerve block", clearly suggesting that regional anesthesia was the cause of a delayed diagnosis of ACS. In this case, a 28-year-old male received an intramedullary nailing to fix a closed tibial shaft fracture. Postoperatively, the patient received a former called 3 in 1 block (a femoral nerve with uncertain spread to the obturator and lateral cutaneous nerve or the thigh) for pain control. The patient's complaints about paresthesia of the foot were attributed to the triple nerve block. The symptoms persisted, and 48 h later, he could not flex his great toe. A fasciotomy was performed, but after surgery, the patient needed an ankle-foot orthosis for walking due to anterior tibial compartment necrosis.

Rauf et al. [40] reported a case of a young man with a mid-shaft fracture of the radius and a malalignment after ORIF (open reduction internal fixation). The patient received a supraclavicular block using a mixture of lidocaine 2%, adrenaline and bupivacaine 0.5% prior to general anesthesia. Twenty minutes after extubation, the patient complained about dull and severe pain in his forearm. Despite the administration of paracetamol, diclofenac and morphine, the pain did not resolve and a dense sensory and motor blockade was still present. No compartment pressure monitoring was performed, but after the removal of the cast, the radial pulse was absent. The wound was explored in the operating room. A bleeding vessel was identified as causing the clinical symptoms. There was no fasciotomy performed and the patient did not suffer any long-term disabilities. The patients of the other reported cases [5,39,41,42] suffered severe pain up to a visual analogue scale (VAS) 10/10, despite a functioning peripheral nerve block. All cases using peripheral nerve blocks are summarized in Table 2.

3.1. *Other Regional Anesthesia Techniques and ACS*

3.1.1. Neuraxial Blocks

We did not find a case where a single shot epidural or single shot spinal anesthesia was implicated in the delay of an ACS. However, continuous epidural analgesia has been reported to mask symptoms of ACS, delaying its diagnosis [43]. Mar and colleagues [43] reviewed 23 cases where continuous epidural analgesia (EDA) was blamed for masking ACS, and they could show that in 90% of the cases, patients showed the classical symptoms of ACS but these symptoms were not recognized in time. Breakthrough pain, a heavy clinical indicator of ACS, was ignored in most cases. However, a dense block caused by continuous EDA delayed the diagnosis of ACS in four cases.

3.1.2. Intravenous Regional Anesthesia

Different reports have implicated intravenous RA (IVRA) in causing ACS [44–50].

In the cases describing ACS after IVRA, the use of prolonged and high-pressure tourniquets as well as the extravascular or erroneous injection of a foreign substance into the forearm venous system were the most likely causes of ACS.

3.1.3. Single Shot/Continuous Intra-Articular Injection

After local infiltration analgesia (LIA) or continuous wound infusion (CWI), there is no report of a delay in diagnosis of ACS.

3.1.4. Compartment/Fascial Plane Blocks

After compartment/fascial plane block, there is no report of a delay in diagnosis of ACS.

Table 2. Cases included in this review.

Author	Gender	Age	Injury	Procedures	Nerve Block	Local Anesthetics	Symptoms of ACS	Diagnostic/ Treatment/ Time after ACS Diagnosis	Comments
Munk-Andersen [41]	Male	12 y	Distal tibia and fibula fracture	Temporary external fixation, debridement	Preop: SS distal sciatic nerve block Postop: SS distal sciatic nerve block POD 1: US-guided distal sciatic nerve catheter	Preop: Lidocaine 2%, 10 mL Postop: Ropivacaine 0.375%, 20 mL 1. postop day: Lidocaine 2% bolus, Ropivacaine 0.2% 4 mL/h	Circa 7 h after PNC, the calf muscles were tense and sore. After 8.5 h, sudden, severe pain, worsened by passive foot movement	No CP-measurement/ Fasciotomy immediate after the appearance of severe pain worsened by passive movement of the foot.	No delay due to PNB. Increased post OP myoglobine, indicated muscle ischemia. No permanent damage was reported.
Uzel [42]	Male	26 y	Third-degree, closed transverse fracture of the left femur	Splint, cen-tromedullary nailing 15 h and 15 min after the accident. The procedure took 80 min.	SS femoral block preoper-atively in combination with GA	Ropivacaine 0.75%, 20 mL	Thigh pain ca. 2 h post OP, 16 h later unusually severe pain (VAS 9/10), no sensomotor deficit, pressure in the ventral compartment 54 mmHg	No CP-measurement prior to fasciotomy. Fasciotomy of the anterior thigh compartment in SA. Apart from ventral compartment, intraoperatively, other compartments showed normal pressures.	No delay due to PNB. Severe breakthrough pain present. 16 h after FNB, probably no persistent anesthesia. No permanent damage was reported.
Ganeshan [39]	Male	75 y	Distal radius fracture	Initially K-wires placed, after 3 w, they became loose. The K-wires were removed and a plaster below elbow cast was applied. 3 w later, internal fixation with a volar peri-articular locking plate.	Axillary nerve block	Not reported	24 h after discharge, swelling of the forearm and fingers, hemorrhagic blisters, loss of sensation in the fingers, loss of active movements in the fingers and wrist. Passive movement of the fingers led to severe pain. Finger capillary refill increased to >4 s.	CP measurement: 46 mmHg and 50 mmHg in the anterior and 22 mmHg in the posterior compartment. Operation within 1 h of presentation. Fasciotomy and excision of unhealthy muscle.	LA used, neurological status at discharge, recovery time, start of symptoms after block worn off: not reported. Unlikely that an LA lasts for 24 h after an axillary block for ambulatory surgery. Discharge with risk of ACS with no telephone control of recovery and pain status to be blamed.

Table 2. *Cont.*

Author	Gender	Age	Injury	Procedures	Nerve Block	Local Anesthetics	Symptoms of ACS	Diagnostic/ Treatment/ Time after ACS Diagnosis	Comments
Aguirre [5]	Female	47 y	Complex distal humerus fracture	Open reposition, osteosynthesis of the capitulum, trochlea humeri including radial condyles and open arm splint. The procedure took 150 min.	Preop: IFC no LA administered until postoperative checking of the sensomotor function.	Initial bolus 30 mL 0.5% ropi, CI ropi 0.3% at 6 mL/h, additional bolus of 5 mL, lockout time 20 min.	Severe forearm pain (VAS 9/10) 14 h post OP. Persistent pain despite ropi 0.5% 20 mL bolus and complete motor and sensory blockade.	CP measurement of extensor compartment (40 mmHg) with fasciotomy 1 h thereafter.	No. Persistent pain despite IFC and bolus ropi. No permanent damage was reported.
Rauf [40]	Male	19 y	Mid-shaft fracture of the radius	Revision surgery because of malalignment of the radial plate 12 d earlier.	Preoperatively a SCB prior to GA.	10 mL lido 2% + adrenaline and 10 mL Bupi 0.5%	20 min after extubation, dull pain in the forearm developed during further 20 min. 2 h post block severe pain (VAS 10/10), not responsive to analgesics and despite a dense sensory and motor block. Swollen and tense forearm, no palpable radial pulse, prolonged capillary refill time after cast removal.	Immediate exploration under GA. A bleeding vessel was secured and hematoma cleared out. No fasciotomy. No wound closure, sterile occlusive dressing. 6 h after SCB, signs of block resolution. Time from clinical presentation until surgery was <30 min.	No. Breakthrough pain, which did not resolve after administration of morphine, paracetamol and diclofenac. No permanent damage was reported.
Hyder [3]	Male	28 y	Closed fracture of the tibial shaft	Intramedullary nailing, initially stabilized with a plaster cast.	After surgery: "triple nerve block" (former 3 in one block) was performed.	Bupi 0.5%	Altered sensations in his foot and leg, initially varying in areas. After 48 h, there was an inability to actively extend the big toe.	CP measurement after 48 h: 108 mmHg in the anterior compartment. Fasciotomy (timeframe unclear after diagnosis) showed dead muscles.	No. The block did not impair the sensomotor areas described (sciatic nerve). 48 h duration unlikely after Bupi. Patient walked thereafter with an orthosis.

Abbreviations: Bupi: Bupivacaine; CI: continuous infusion; CP: Compartment pressure; FNB: femoral nerve block; GA: general anesthesia; IFC: infraclavicular catheter; LA: local anesthetic; lido: lidocaine; PNB: Peripheral nerve block, PNC: peripheral nerve catheter; POD: postoperative day; Ropi: ropivacaine; SA: spinal anesthesia; SCB: supraclavicular bock; SS: single shot; VAS: visual analogue scale.

4. Discussion

Of the included six case reports dealing with peripheral nerve blocks and ACS, only one remains unclear. In the report by Ganeshan et al., without further information about the medications used for the blockade, and with unclear monitoring for ACS symptoms after the surgery, it is difficult to state that the peripheral nerve block delayed ACS diagnosis [39]. Additionally, ambulatory surgery in patients at risk of developing ACS remains controversial and close post-discharge monitoring is highly recommended [49]. The timeline remains unclear: when did the block wear off? When did pain start? Why did the patient wait for so long and present to the emergency department only the day after surgery with blisters, and motor and sensory compromise of the wrist and fingers? [39]. This patient suffered from persistent dysfunctions of the hand and wrist after surgery for ACS and is an unfortunate example of the need for some basic guidelines for this specific complication in the ambulatory surgery setting: not to be alone at home the first night after surgery, written information about postoperative care, a phone number of healthcare professionals as well as a follow-up call the day after surgery. Mobile apps and remote monitoring will possibly improve postoperative follow-up [51]. The case presented by Hyder et al. [3] is a clear misunderstanding of basic anatomy. After a femoral nerve block with or without the involvement of other nerves of the lumbar plexus, the sciatic nerve remains unblocked. Moreover, it would only cover analgesia in the area of the insertion of the medullar nail for an analgesia duration of approximately 8 h [11,52]. Despite this anatomical fact, and the clear misunderstanding of local anesthetic pharmacology, Tran et al. [53] recently blamed this block for the delay of ACS. Severe breakthrough pain reaching a VAS 10/10 shows that the peripheral nerve blockade did not impair or preclude ACS diagnosis. Such sudden and severe pain must make the attending doctor suspicious, and an incipient ACS has to be ruled out [5].

We are aware that there is not much literature concerning the question if a peripheral nerve block may delay the diagnosis of ACS. However, in most of the articles blaming regional anesthesia for masking ACS, there was an epidural analgesia (EDA) or an intravenous opioid patient-controlled analgesia (PCA) present. Actually, PCA and continuous EDA might mask the symptoms of acute compartment syndrome [4,16,19–24,31]. In fact, single shot epidural or single shot spinal anesthesia have not been associated with ACS [14,54–61].

However, continuous epidural analgesia has been reported to mask symptoms of ACS, delaying its diagnosis. In the review by Mar and colleagues [43], continuous epidural analgesia (EDA) was blamed for masking ACS in 23 cases and they could show that in 90% of the cases, patients showed the classical symptoms of ACS but these symptoms were not recognized in time. Breakthrough pain, a heavy clinical indicator of ACS, was ignored in most cases. However, a dense block caused by continuous EDA delayed the diagnosis of ACS in four cases.

In the recent Pro-Con debate about the use of PNB for trauma patients, authors highlighted the fact that a developing ACS with breakthrough pain might be more easily detected [62].

Considering other regional anesthesia techniques, intravenous RA (IVRA) has been implicated in causing ACS [44–48]. IVRA is frequently performed in trauma in different parts of the world and the concept of causing ACS performing an IVRA is not well understood [49,50]. The most controversial theories focus on the double tourniquet used for this technique and emphasize the ischemia-reperfusion injury leading to hyperemia, swelling and the additional application of high volumes of local anesthetics and adjuvants into a "newly created compartment." [45]. Additionally, other factors like inflation pressure and duration as well as the use of hypertonic saline infusion [44,47,48] have also been involved in the development of ACS. According to the literature, ACS after IVRA can be caused by (1) placing the intravenous line and injection into the radial artery, (2) an idiosyncratic allergic reaction to the local anesthetic or the preservative and (3) inadvertent injection of an inappropriate agent into the forearm venous system [44,47,48].

Continuous wound (articular) infusion (CWI) or peri-articular infiltration (local infiltration analgesia [LIA]) are effective regional analgesia techniques but have no impact on motor or major sensory block due to the lack of effect on major nerves [63,64]. The surgery most profiting from these techniques is total knee arthroplasty, whereas hip surgery and upper extremity trauma are controversially discussed [65]. Fascial plane blocks represent a modern regional analgesia approach, where high volumes of low-concentration local anesthetics are injected for analgesia, therefore avoiding central blocks or PNBs. Fascial plane blocks lead to minimal, if at all, motor block and therefore offer an underestimated alternative for patients at risk of ACS. In fact, classic perineural blocks could be replaced by techniques like midfemoral saphenous nerve blocks for medial tibia plateau fractures, supra-inguinal fascia iliaca blocks for femur neck fractures and quadratus lumborum blocks for hip fractures [66,67].

The articles we included are case reports and therefore represent only class IV evidence according to the Agency for Healthcare Research and Quality (AHRQ). This is the main limitation of this review. There are no randomized controlled studies available on this topic. There are some articles stating that regional anesthesia does not delay the diagnosis of ACS [28,29], but these studies are also based on case series, which limits the evidence. Considering the fact that even PCA has been blamed for masking ACS [16,20–22], using well-adapted regional anesthesia techniques might offer different advantages. Apart from the avoidance of opioid-related side effects, the breakthrough pain, through a functioning continuous peripheral nerve block, can be used as an early diagnostic tool, as shown in five of our included cases. In fact, breakthrough pain persisted after systemic analgesics and even after a top up of the perineural catheter. As stated by Aguirre et al., 'proper documentation and a high level of suspicion coupled with postoperative repeated clinical and, if needed, invasive monitoring are of utmost importance' [3].

5. Conclusions

Due to the low quality of data, only six case reports, it is difficult to state that regional anesthesia could routinely be used in trauma patients. Five of these case reports show that regional anesthesia did not mask the diagnosis of ACS and the sixth case report remains inconclusive due to missing data. We can state that if surgeons and anesthesiologists keep a high index of suspicion, adapt the regional anesthesia techniques and use basic clinical monitoring in patients at risk of ACS, regional anesthesia remains a valuable option for good postoperative pain management. Even though in most case reports high concentrations of local anesthetics were used when breakthrough pain was present, we recommend the use of local anesthetics, volumes and concentrations to avoid dense and long-lasting blocks. Moreover, ACS must be excluded when (breakthrough) pain cannot be managed despite a well-placed continuous regional anesthesia. Due to the unclear literature concerning IVRA and ACS, this technique should not be used in trauma surgery [3,25]. Moreover, dense motor blocks [3,32] and high-concentration epidural catheters [43] should be avoided; we recommend lower concentrations and higher flowrates to achieve that.

We summarized the Recommendations from the ESRA/ASRA Joint Committee Statement [7] and the Recommendations of the Association of Anaesthetists of Great Britain and Ireland [10] (Tables 3 and 4) to display the two existing Anesthesia Societies' recommendations on this topic. Moreover, based on the literature reported in this review and our experience [5], we summarized possible suggestions for the different regional anesthesia modalities to apply in patients at risk of ACS in a table to facilitate the use of these techniques (Table 5).

Table 3. Recommendations from the ESRA/ASRA Joint Committee Statement, modified according to Ivani G et al. [7].

All patients with regional anaesthesia/acute pain should be followed by the actue pain service.
Perform compartment pressure measurement if ACS is suspected.
If regional anesthesia is performed in patients at high risk of ACS, the dose (volume and concentration) of local anesthetics should be reduced.
Carefully evaluate the use of adjuvants due to the possible increase in block duration and block intensity.
Use bupivacaine, levobupivacaine or ropivacaine at concentraions of 0.1–0.25% for single shot peripheral nerve blocks and neuraxial blocks.
Use bupivacaine 0.125% or ropivacaine 0.1–0.2% at rates of 0.1–0.3 mg/kg/hr for continuous peripheral nerve blocks and continuous neuraxial blocks.

Table 4. Recommendations of the Association of Anaesthetists of Great Britain and Ireland, modified according to Nathanson NH et al. [10].

Manage patients at risk of ACS within agreed, multidisciplinary protocols.
Trained staff should be able to indentify signs and symptoms of ACS in the postoperative period.
The use of objective scoring charts is recommended.
All surgery or trauma patients should be offered effective analgesia after full explanation and documented informed consent.
In the case of no consensus between anesthetist and surgeon, the role of the anaesthetist as the expert on pain relief should be respected.
Avoid the use of neuraxial or peripheral regional techniques resulting in dense blocks of long duration significantly exceeding the duration of surgery.
Use lower concentrations of local anaesthetic drugs without adjuncts for single shot or continuous peripheral nerve blocks provided post-injury, and postoperative surveillance is appropriate and effective to avoid delays in diagnosis of ACS.
Due to the lack of reliable, published data on the safety and efficacy of analgesia in patients at risk of ACS and as prospective randomized trials would need to be large due to the low evidence of ACS, the Working Party recommends the conduct of prospective audits.

Table 5. Suggestions for anesthesia and postoperative analgesia in patients at high-risk of postoperative ACS.

Anesthesia Techniques	Drugs to Be Used	Duration of Action	Recommendation for Trauma
Single shot PNB (SPNB)	Lidocaine 1.5% Mepivacaine 1% Chloroprocaine 2–3%	Lidocaine: 2.5–3 h Mepivacaine: 2–4 h Chloroprocaine: 1–2 h	For low postoperative pain, adapted local anesthetics to surgery time. Consider low-dose CPNB.
Continuous PNB (CPNB)	Ropivacaine: bolus with 10–20 mL of 0.1–0.2% PCRA: ropivacaine 0.1–0.2% (0.3%) 4–6 mL/h, bolus 3–4 mL, lock out 20–30 min	While infused and 30–60 min after stopping the infusion. No motor function impairment at low dosages.	Consider if catheter placement possible without previous block (or the block is performed with short-acting LA or low-concentration LA to avoid a long-lasting, dense block)
CWI/IAI/(C)FPB	Ropivacaine 0.2–0.3% Bupivacaine 0.25%. Dexamethasone I.V. 8–12 mg for FPB	Covers pain only during infusion.	Use whenever possible: good analgesia, no case report blaming this technique for masking ACS.
Single shot spinal (SSPA)	Bupivacaine 0.5% hyperbaric/isobaric low-dose (7.5 mg–max 10 mg); if needed add fentanyl/clonidine Mepivacaine 1% (30 mg) Chloroprocaine 1% 50 mg Prilocaine 2% hyper/isobaric 30–60 mg	Bupivacaine: 3–4 h Mepivacaine: 2–3 h Chloroprocaine: 1–2 h Prilocaine: 1.5–2.5 h	Use for lower limb trauma if possible to adapt duration to surgery time. No case report blaming SSPA for masking ACS.
Continuous spinal (CSPA)	Surgery: Bupivacaine (isobaric or) hyperbaric 0.5% during surgery 0.5–2 mL initial bolus, thereafter adaptation to surgery time and sensory level. Analgesia: Bupivacaine isobaric 0.125–0.2% for 0.5–1 mL/h	Bupivacaine: 2–3.5 h	No published case blaming CSPA for masking ACS. However, dense, long-lasting motor block possible if used also after surgery. Therefore, use CSPA for longer lasting surgery and in cases GA is not the optimal choice. Avoid using CSPA for analgesia after surgery if risk of ACS due to possible dense block.
Single shot epidural (EDA)	Lidocaine 1.5% Chloroporcaine 3% (Ropivacaine 0.75%–1%)	Lidocaine: 3.5 h Chloroprocaine: 2.5 h Ropivacaine: 3–6 h	No published case blaming EDA for masking ACS. However, a dense motor block is possible. Use EDA in cases GA is not the optimal choice.
Continuous epidural (CEDA)	Ropivacaine 0.1% (−0.2%) Levobupivacaine 0.125%; if needed add sufentanil 1 μ/mL, fentanyl 1–3 μ/mL	While infused and 2–4 h after stopping the infusion. A block resolution within 60 min achieved after wash out with 30 mL saline.	Avoid if GA, SPA or CPNB possible. Different case reports blaming CEDA for masking ACS.
General anesthesia (GA)	Propofol/volatile anesthetics Low-dose long-acting opioids (fentanyl); remifentanil TCI until low-concentration CPNB start possible.	Remifentanil: 5 min after TCI is stopped.	Avoid ideally for high-risk patients. If GA, combine with CPNB for postoperative analgesia.

Abbreviations: ACS: Acute compartment syndrome, (c) FPB: (continuous) fascia plane block, CWI: continuous wound infusion, EDA: epidural anesthesia, IAI: intra-articular infusion, LA: local anesthetic, PNB: peripheral nerve block, SPA: spinal anesthesia.

Author Contributions: N.H.: This author helped summarize the included literature, and helped with the writing of the manuscript with the composition of tables and clinical suggestions for the use of regional anesthesia. A.D.: This author helped with the literature search, literature reading and correction of the manuscript. S.B.: This author helped with the literature search, literature reading and correction of the manuscript. H.B.: This author helped with the literature search, literature reading and correction of the manuscript. A.B.: This author helped overview the material, reviewed the tables and manuscript and performed the final editing. J.A.: This author had the idea of putting this literature together, helped overview the material, reviewed the tables and manuscript and performed the final editing. All authors have read and agreed to the published version of the manuscript.

Funding: This research received no external funding.

Conflicts of Interest: The authors declare no conflicts of interest.

References

1. Gadsden, J.; Warlick, A. Regional anesthesia for the trauma patient: Improving patient outcomes. *Local Reg. Anesth.* **2015**, *8*, 45–55. [CrossRef]
2. Atchabahian, A.; Schwartz, G.; Hall, C.B.; Lajam, C.M.; Andreae, M.H. Regional analgesia for improvement of long-term functional outcome after elective large joint replacement. *Cochrane Database Syst. Rev.* **2015**, *2015*, CD010278. [CrossRef]
3. Hyder, N.; Kessler, S.; Jennings, A.G.; De Boer, P.G. Compartment syndrome in tibial shaft fracture missed because of a local nerve block. *J. Bone Jt. Surg. Br.* **1996**, *78*, 499–500. [CrossRef]
4. Marhofer, P.; Halm, J.; Feigl, G.C.; Schepers, T.; Hollmann, M.W. Regional Anesthesia and Compartment Syndrome. *Anesth. Analg.* **2021**, *133*, 1348–1352. [CrossRef] [PubMed]
5. Aguirre, J.A.; Gresch, D.; Popovici, A.; Bernhard, J.; Borgeat, A. Case scenario: Compartment syndrome of the forearm in patient with an infraclavicular catheter: Breakthrough pain as indicator. *Anesthesiology* **2013**, *118*, 1198–1205. [CrossRef] [PubMed]
6. Aguirre, J.A.; Wolmarans, M.; Borgeat, A. Acute Extremity Compartment Syndrome and (Regional): Anesthesia: The Monster Under the Bed. *Anesthesiol. Clin.* **2022**, *40*, 491–509. [CrossRef] [PubMed]
7. Ivani, G.; Suresh, S.; Ecoffey, C.; Bosenberg, A.; Lonnqvist, P.A.; Krane, E.; Veyckemans, F.; Polaner, D.M.; Van de Velde, M.; Neal, J.M. The European Society of Regional Anaesthesia and Pain Therapy and the American Society of Regional Anesthesia and Pain Medicine Joint Committee Practice Advisory on Controversial Topics in Pediatric Regional Anesthesia. *Reg. Anesth. Pain Med.* **2015**, *40*, 526–532. [CrossRef] [PubMed]
8. Brovman, E.Y.; Wallace, F.C.; Weaver, M.J.; Beutler, S.S.; Urman, R.D. Anesthesia Type Is Not Associated with Postoperative Complications in the Care of Patients with Lower Extremity Traumatic Fractures. *Anesth. Analg.* **2019**, *129*, 1034–1042. [CrossRef] [PubMed]
9. Zadrazil, M.; Opfermann, P.; Marhofer, P.; Westerlund, A.I.; Haider, T. Brachial plexus block with ultrasound guidance for upper-limb trauma surgery in children: A retrospective cohort study of 565 cases. *Br. J. Anaesth.* **2020**, *125*, 104–109. [CrossRef] [PubMed]
10. Nathanson, M.H.; Harrop-Griffiths, W.; Aldington, D.J.; Forward, D.; Mannion, S.; Kinnear-Mellor, R.G.M.; Miller, K.L.; Ratnayake, B.; Wiles, M.D.; Wolmarans, M.R. Regional analgesia for lower leg trauma and the risk of acute compartment syndrome: Guideline from the Association of Anaesthetists. *Anaesthesia* **2021**, *76*, 1518–1525. [CrossRef] [PubMed]
11. Aguirre, J. The role of regional anestheisa (RA) in patients at risk for acute compartment syndrome (ACS). In *Update on Regional Anesthesia and Pain Management*; De Andrés, J., Ed.; Editorial MRA: Barcelona, Spain, 2018; Volume XXI, pp. 405–431.
12. Friedrich, J.B.; Shin, A.Y. Management of forearm compartment syndrome. *Hand Clin.* **2007**, *23*, 245–254, vii. [CrossRef]
13. Sigamoney, K.; Khincha, P.; Badge, R.; Shah, N. Compartment sydrome: Challenges and solutions. *Orthop. Res. Rev.* **2015**, *7*, 137–148.
14. Dunwoody, J.M.; Reichert, C.C.; Brown, K.L. Compartment syndrome associated with bupivacaine and fentanyl epidural analgesia in pediatric orthopaedics. *J. Pediatr. Orthop.* **1997**, *17*, 285–288. [CrossRef]
15. McQueen, M.M.; Gaston, P.; Court-Brown, C.M. Acute compartment syndrome. Who is at risk? *J. Bone Jt. Surg. Br.* **2000**, *82*, 200–203.
16. Martin, J.T. Compartment syndromes: Concepts and perspectives for the anesthesiologist. *Anesth. Analg.* **1992**, *75*, 275–283. [CrossRef]
17. Noorpuri, B.S.; Shahane, S.A.; Getty, C.J. Acute compartment syndrome following revisional arthroplasty of the forefoot: The dangers of ankle-block. *Foot Ankle Int.* **2000**, *21*, 680–682. [CrossRef] [PubMed]
18. Elliott, K.G.; Johnstone, A.J. Diagnosing acute compartment syndrome. *J. Bone Jt. Surg. Br.* **2003**, *85*, 625–632. [CrossRef]
19. Cometa, M.A.; Esch, A.T.; Boezaart, A.P. Did continuous femoral and sciatic nerve block obscure the diagnosis or delay the treatment of acute lower leg compartment syndrome? A case report. *Pain Med.* **2011**, *12*, 823–828. [CrossRef] [PubMed]
20. Klucka, J.; Stourac, P.; Stouracova, A.; Masek, M.; Repko, M. Compartment syndrome and regional anaesthesia: Critical review. *Biomed Pap. Med. Fac. Univ. Palacky Olomouc Czech Repub.* **2017**, *161*, 242–251. [CrossRef] [PubMed]
21. Murdock, M.; Murdoch, M.M. Compartment syndrome: A review of the literature. *Clin. Podiatr. Med. Surg.* **2012**, *29*, 301–310. [CrossRef]

22. Janzing, H.M. Epidemiology, Etiology, Pathophysiology and Diagnosis of the Acute Compartment Syndrome of the Extremity. *Eur. J. Trauma Emerg. Surg.* **2007**, *33*, 576–583. [CrossRef] [PubMed]
23. Arbabi, S.; Brundage, S.I.; Gentilello, L.M. Near-infrared spectroscopy: A potential method for continuous, transcutaneous monitoring for compartmental syndrome in critically injured patients. *J. Trauma* **1999**, *47*, 829–833. [CrossRef] [PubMed]
24. Shuler, M.S.; Reisman, W.M.; Kinsey, T.L.; Whitesides, T.E., Jr.; Hammerberg, E.M.; Davila, M.G.; Moore, T.J. Correlation between muscle oxygenation and compartment pressures in acute compartment syndrome of the leg. *J. Bone Jt. Surg. Am.* **2010**, *92*, 863–870. [CrossRef] [PubMed]
25. Rolfe, P. In vivo near-infrared spectroscopy. *Annu. Rev. Biomed. Eng.* **2000**, *2*, 715–754. [CrossRef] [PubMed]
26. Widder, S.; Ranson, M.K.; Zygun, D.; Knox, L.; Laupland, K.B.; Laird, P.; Ball, C.G.; Kirkpatrick, A.W. Use of near-infrared spectroscopy as a physiologic monitor for intra-abdominal hypertension. *J. Trauma* **2008**, *64*, 1165–1168. [CrossRef]
27. Shadgan, B.; Menon, M.; Sanders, D.; Berry, G.; Martin, C., Jr.; Duffy, P.; Stephen, D.; O'Brien, P.J. Current thinking about acute compartment syndrome of the lower extremity. *Can. J. Surg* **2010**, *53*, 329–334.
28. Kashuk, J.L.; Moore, E.E.; Pinski, S.; Johnson, J.L.; Moore, J.B.; Morgan, S.; Cothren, C.C.; Smith, W. Lower extremity compartment syndrome in the acute care surgery paradigm: Safety lessons learned. *Patient Saf. Surg.* **2009**, *3*, 11. [CrossRef]
29. Heckman, M.M.; Whitesides, T.E., Jr.; Grewe, S.R.; Rooks, M.D. Compartment pressure in association with closed tibial fractures. The relationship between tissue pressure, compartment, and the distance from the site of the fracture. *J. Bone Jt. Surg. Am.* **1994**, *76*, 1285–1292. [CrossRef]
30. Geary, N. Late surgical decompression for compartment syndrome of the forearm. *J. Bone Jt. Surg. Br.* **1984**, *66*, 745–748. [CrossRef]
31. Janzing, H.; Broos, P.; Rommens, P. Compartment syndrome as a complication of skin traction in children with femoral fractures. *J. Trauma* **1996**, *41*, 156–158. [CrossRef]
32. Hayakawa, H.; Aldington, D.J.; Moore, R.A. Acute traumatic compartment syndrome: A systematic review of results of fasciotomy. *Trauma* **2009**, *11*, 5–35. [CrossRef]
33. Cascio, B.M.; Pateder, D.B.; Wilckens, J.H.; Frassica, F.J. Compartment syndrome: Time from diagnosis to fasciotomy. *J. Surg. Orthop. Adv.* **2005**, *14*, 117–121; discussion 120–121.
34. Walker, B.J.; Noonan, K.J.; Bosenberg, A.T. Evolving compartment syndrome not masked by a continuous peripheral nerve block: Evidence-based case management. *Reg. Anesth. Pain Med.* **2012**, *37*, 393–397. [CrossRef]
35. Kucera, T.J.; Boezaart, A.P. Regional anesthesia does not consistently block ischemic pain: Two further cases and a review of the literature. *Pain Med.* **2014**, *15*, 316–319. [CrossRef]
36. Sermeus, L.; Boeckx, S.; Camerlynck, H.; Somville, J.; Vercauteren, M. Postsurgical compartment syndrome of the forearm diagnosed in a child receiving a continuous infra-clavicular peripheral nerve block. *Acta Anaesthesiol. Belg.* **2015**, *66*, 29–32. [PubMed]
37. Torrie, A.; Sharma, J.; Mason, M.; Cruz Eng, H. Regional anesthesia did not delay diagnosis of compartment syndrome: A case report of anterior compartment syndrome in the thigh not masked by an adductor canal catheter. *Am. J. Case Rep.* **2017**, *18*, 444–447. [CrossRef] [PubMed]
38. Camelo, C.R.; Eklund, S.E.; Brusseau, R.; Gomez-Morad, A.D. Ischemic pain not masked by regional anesthesia. *Reg. Anesth. Pain Med.* **2020**, *45*, 244–245. [CrossRef]
39. Ganeshan, R.M.; Mamoowala, N.; Ward, M.; Sochart, D. Acute compartment syndrome risk in fracture fixation with regional blocks. *BMJ Case Rep.* **2015**, *2015*, bcr2015210499. [CrossRef] [PubMed]
40. Rauf, J.; Iohom, G.; O'Donnell, B. Acute compartment syndrome and regional anaesthesia—A case report. *Rom. J. Anaesth. Intensive Care* **2015**, *22*, 51–54. [PubMed]
41. Munk-Andersen, H.; Laustrup, T.K. Compartment syndrome diagnosed in due time by breakthrough pain despite continuous peripheral nerve block. *Acta Anaesthesiol. Scand.* **2013**, *57*, 1328–1330. [CrossRef] [PubMed]
42. Uzel, A.P.; Steinmann, G. Thigh compartment syndrome after intramedullary femoral nailing: Possible femoral nerve block influence on diagnosis timing. *Orthop. Traumatol. Surg. Res.* **2009**, *95*, 309–313. [CrossRef]
43. Mar, G.J.; Barrington, M.J.; McGuirk, B.R. Acute compartment syndrome of the lower limb and the effect of postoperative analgesia on diagnosis. *Br. J. Anaesth.* **2009**, *102*, 3–11. [CrossRef]
44. Guay, J. Adverse events associated with intravenous regional anesthesia (Bier block): A systematic review of complications. *J. Clin. Anesth.* **2009**, *21*, 585–594. [CrossRef]
45. Ananthanarayan, C.; Castro, C.; McKee, N.; Sakotic, G. Compartment syndrome following intravenous regional anesthesia. *Can. J. Anaesth.* **2000**, *47*, 1094–1098. [CrossRef]
46. Maletis, G.B.; Watson, R.C.; Scott, S. Compartment syndrome. A complication of intravenous regional anesthesia in the reduction of lower leg shaft fractures. *Orthopedics* **1989**, *12*, 841–846. [CrossRef]
47. Hastings, H., 2nd; Misamore, G. Compartment syndrome resulting from intravenous regional anesthesia. *J. Hand Surg. Am.* **1987**, *12*, 559–562. [CrossRef]
48. Mabee, J.R.; Bostwick, T.L.; Burke, M.K. Iatrogenic compartment syndrome from hypertonic saline injection in Bier block. *J. Emerg. Med.* **1994**, *12*, 473–476. [CrossRef] [PubMed]
49. Luce, E.A.; Mangubat, E. Loss of hand and forearm following Bier block: A case report. *J. Hand Surg. Am.* **1983**, *8*, 280–283. [CrossRef] [PubMed]
50. Ball, C.M. Failed intravenous arm block or diagnostic test? *Anaesth. Intensive Care.* **1985**, *13*, 433–434. [CrossRef]

51. Rohi, A.; Olofsson, M.E.T.; Jakobsson, J.G. Ambulatory anesthesia and discharge: An update around guidelines and trends. *Curr. Opin. Anaesthesiol.* **2022**, *35*, 691–697. [CrossRef] [PubMed]
52. Eyres, K.S.; Hill, G.; Magides, A. Compartment syndrome in tibial shaft fracture missed because of a local nerve block. *J. Bone Jt. Surg. Br.* **1996**, *78*, 996–997. [CrossRef]
53. Tran, A.A.; Lee, D.; Fassihi, S.C.; Smith, E.; Lee, R.; Siram, G. A systematic review of the effect of regional anesthesia on diagnosis and management of acute compartment syndrome in long bone fractures. *Eur. J. Trauma Emerg. Surg.* **2020**, *46*, 1281–1290. [CrossRef]
54. Beerle, B.J.; Rose, R.J. Lower extremity compartment syndrome from prolonged lithotomy position not masked by epidural bupivacaine and fentanyl. *Reg. Anesth.* **1993**, *18*, 189–190.
55. Goldsmith, A.L.; McCallum, M.I. Compartment syndrome as a complication of the prolonged use of the Lloyd-Davies position. *Anaesthesia* **1996**, *51*, 1048–1052. [CrossRef]
56. Heyn, J.; Ladurner, R.; Ozimek, A.; Vogel, T.; Hallfeldt, K.K.; Mussack, T. Gluteal compartment syndrome after prostatectomy caused by incorrect positioning. *Eur. J. Med. Res.* **2006**, *11*, 170–173.
57. Iwasaka, H.; Itoh, K.; Miyakawa, H.; Noguchi, T.; Kitano, T.; Taniguchi, K.; Honda, N. Compartment syndrome after prolonged lithotomy position in patient receiving combined epidural and general anesthesia. *J. Anesth.* **1993**, *7*, 468–470. [CrossRef] [PubMed]
58. Llewellyn, N.; Moriarty, A. The national pediatric epidural audit. *Paediatr Anaesth.* **2007**, *17*, 520–533. [CrossRef]
59. Montgomery, C.J.; Ready, L.B. Epidural opioid analgesia does not obscure diagnosis of compartment syndrome resulting from prolonged lithotomy position. *Anesthesiology* **1991**, *75*, 541–543. [CrossRef] [PubMed]
60. Stotts, A.K.; Carroll, K.L.; Schafer, P.C.; Santora, S.D.; Branigan, T.D. Medial compartment syndrome of the foot: An unusual complication of spine surgery. *Spine* **2003**, *28*, E118–E120. [CrossRef]
61. Tuckey, J. Bilateral compartment syndrome complicating prolonged lithotomy position. *Br. J. Anaesth.* **1996**, *77*, 546–549. [CrossRef]
62. Samet, R.E.; Torrie, A.M.; Chembrovich, S.V.; Ihnatsenka, B.V. Pro-Con Debate: Peripheral Nerve Blockade Should Be Provided Routinely in Extremity Trauma, Including in Patients at Risk for Acute Compartment Syndrome. *Anesth. Analg.* **2023**, *136*, 855–860. [CrossRef]
63. Liu, S.S.; Richman, J.M.; Thirlby, R.C.; Wu, C.L. Efficacy of continuous wound catheters delivering local anesthetic for postoperative analgesia: A quantitative and qualitative systematic review of randomized controlled trials. *J. Am. Coll. Surg.* **2006**, *203*, 914–932. [CrossRef]
64. Aguirre, J.; Baulig, B.; Dora, C.; Ekatodramis, G.; Votta-Velis, G.; Ruland, P.; Borgeat, A. Continuous epicapsular ropivacaine 0.3% infusion after minimally invasive hip arthroplasty: A prospective, randomized, double-blinded, placebo-controlled study comparing continuous wound infusion with morphine patient-controlled analgesia. *Anesth. Analg.* **2012**, *114*, 456–461. [CrossRef] [PubMed]
65. Yung, E.M.; Got, T.C.; Patel, N.; Brull, R.; Abdallah, F.W. Intra-articular infiltration analgesia for arthroscopic shoulder surgery: A systematic review and meta-analysis. *Anaesthesia* **2021**, *76*, 549–558. [CrossRef] [PubMed]
66. Chin, K.J.; Lirk, P.; Hollmann, M.W.; Schwarz, S.K.W. Mechanisms of action of fascial plane blocks: A narrative review. *Reg. Anesth. Pain Med.* **2021**, *46*, 618–628. [CrossRef] [PubMed]
67. Black, N.D.; Stecco, C.; Chan, V.W.S. Fascial Plane Blocks: More Questions Than Answers? *Anesth. Analg.* **2021**, *132*, 899–905. [CrossRef]

Journal of
Clinical Medicine

MDPI

Article

Continuous Superior Trunk Block versus Single-Shot Superior Trunk Block with Intravenous Dexmedetomidine for Postoperative Analgesia in Arthroscopic Shoulder Surgery: A Prospective Randomized Controlled Trial

Bora Lee [1], Jaewon Jang [1], Joon-Ryul Lim [2], Eun Jung Kim [1], Donghu Kim [1], Yong-Min Chun [2,*,†] and Yong Seon Choi [1,*,†]

1 Department of Anesthesiology and Pain Medicine, Severance Hospital and Anesthesia and Pain Research Institute, Yonsei University College of Medicine, 50-1 Yonsei-ro, Seoul 03722, Republic of Korea
2 Department of Orthopedic Surgery, Arthroscopy and Joint Research Institute, Severance Hospital, Yonsei University College of Medicine, Seoul 03722, Republic of Korea
* Correspondence: osmin120@yuhs.ac (Y.-M.C.); yschoi@yuhs.ac (Y.S.C.)
† These authors contributed equally to this work.

Abstract: Background/Objectives: Intravenous dexmedetomidine (DEX) can increase the analgesia duration of peripheral nerve block; however, its effect in combination with superior trunk block (STB) remains unclear. We examined whether combining single-shot STB (SSTB) with intravenous DEX would provide noninferior postoperative analgesia comparable to that provided by continuous STB (CSTB). **Methods:** Ninety-two patients scheduled for elective arthroscopic rotator cuff repair were enrolled in this prospective randomized trial. Patients were randomly assigned to the CSTB or SSTB + DEX group. Postoperatively, each CSTB group patient received 15 mL of 0.5% ropivacaine and a continuous 0.2% ropivacaine infusion. Each SSTB group patient received a 15 mL postoperative bolus injection of 0.5% ropivacaine. DEX was administered at 2 mcg/kg for 30 min post anesthesia, then maintained at 0.5 mcg/kg/h till surgery ended. Pain scores were investigated every 12 h for 48 h post operation, with evaluation of rebound pain incidence and opioid consumption. **Results:** The SSTB + DEX group had significantly higher median pain scores at 12 h post operation (resting pain, 8.0 vs. 3.0; movement pain, 8.0 vs. 5.0) and a higher incidence of rebound pain (56% vs. 20%) than the CSTB group. However, no significant between-group differences were observed in pain scores postoperatively at 24, 36, or 48 h. The CSTB group required less opioids and fewer rescue analgesics within 12–24 h post operation than the SSTB + DEX group. **Conclusions:** Compared with CSTB, SSTB + DEX required additional adjuvant or multimodal analgesics to reduce the risk and intensity of postoperative rebound pain in patients who underwent arthroscopic rotator cuff repair.

Keywords: brachial plexus block; catheters; dexmedetomidine; pain; postoperative; nerve block

1. Introduction

Arthroscopic shoulder surgery involves significant pain during the early postoperative period. During this period, postoperative pain control is essential to accomplish early rehabilitation and recovery. Interscalene brachial plexus block (ISB) is the standard approach used to manage acute pain after shoulder surgery. Given that single-shot ISB can provide an analgesic effect for 8 h post operation, studies have reported strategies for optimal pain management, including local anesthetic adjuvants for single-shot or continuous ISB, to control pain beyond 12–24 h after shoulder surgery. Continuous ISB provides better pain relief and less rebound pain than single-shot ISB; however, the procedure necessitates catheter insertion, leading to additional equipment costs and requiring specialized provider training [1,2]. The benefits of ISB may be offset by the related high incidence of hemidiaphragmatic paresis. To spare the phrenic nerve, a superior trunk block (STB) can be performed immediately before the location where the suprascapular nerve branches from the superior trunk. This method provides sufficient analgesia while preserving diaphragmatic function after shoulder arthroplasty [3–5]. Most studies have investigated the combined effects of adjuvants with single-shot ISB, with only a few studies comparing the pain control effect of single-shot ISB combined with an adjuvant with that of continuous ISB. The analgesic effects of continuous superior trunk block (CSTB) compared with those of single-shot superior trunk block (SSTB) and intravenous dexmedetomidine (DEX) on pain after arthroscopic shoulder surgery remain unclear.

We hypothesized that SSTB combined with intravenous DEX would provide noninferior analgesia compared with that provided by CSTB in patients undergoing arthroscopic shoulder surgery. This study aimed to examine this hypothesis. The primary study endpoint was pain scores at 24 h post operation. Secondary endpoints included the incidence of rebound pain, opioid consumption, and pain scores at other times within the 48 h postoperative period.

2. Materials and Methods

This prospective randomized controlled study was approved by the Severance Hospital Institutional Review Board (protocol number: 4-2021-0853) on 13 August 2021, and registered at ClinicalTrials.gov (NCT05020821, principal investigator: Jaewon Jang, date of registration: 25 August 2021). This study was conducted according to the guidelines of the Declaration of Helsinki and followed the Consolidated Standards for Reporting Trials reporting guidelines for clinical trials. We enrolled 92 adult patients scheduled for elective arthroscopic rotator cuff repair between September 2021 and August 2022. The exclusion criteria were a history of shoulder surgery, contraindications to peripheral nerve block use, allergy to lidocaine or ropivacaine, heart failure, arrhythmia, preoperative bradycardia, opioid use disorder, or hepatic or renal insufficiency. All patients provided written informed consent.

2.1. Randomization and Study Protocol

Patients were randomly assigned to the CSTB or SSTB + DEX group using a computer-generated randomization sequence by an investigator not involved in intraoperative patient management. The same investigator provided two sets of solutions, namely, the experimental drug (DEX) and placebo (normal saline), which were both colorless and transparent. The attending anesthesiologists, other investigators, surgeons, and nursing staff were blinded to the group allocation assignments before the nerve block procedure.

A standard monitoring protocol was used after each patient arrived in the operating room. All patients underwent general anesthesia with tracheal intubation using propofol (1.0–2.0 mg/kg), rocuronium (0.6–0.8 mg/kg), and remifentanil (0.05–0.1 mcg/kg/min). Anesthesia was maintained using sevoflurane and remifentanil (0.01–0.1 mcg/kg/min) in an air/oxygen mixture. In the SSTB + DEX group, DEX was administered at 2 mcg/kg for 30 min after anesthesia induction, followed by the administration of the fixed maintenance dose at 0.5 mcg/kg/h until the end of surgery. In the CSTB group, an equivalent volume of the placebo solution was administered similarly. When the heart rate was <50 beats/min or the systolic pressure was <80 mmHg, the anesthesiologist administered an atropine bolus injection (0.5 mg) or a continuous infusion of norepinephrine (0.01–0.1 mcg/kg/min), respectively. Dexamethasone was not administered to exclude its effects as an adjuvant for nerve block. The same surgeon performed all surgical procedures while each patient was in a beach chair position and maintained controlled hypotension. Neuromuscular [illegible]de was reversed using neostigmine (1 mg) and glycopyrrolate (0.2 mg) after the [illegible]cedure.

[illegible]dure

[illegible]e administered postoperatively to avoid catheter dislodgement. The [illegible]s were placed in a supine position, with the head slightly turned to the contralateral side of the operative side. Subsequently, a linear ultrasound probe (6 to 13-MHz, HFL38xp, SonoSite Inc., Bothell, WA, USA) was used to perform a sequential prescan from the supraclavicular fossa to the upper part of the interscalene groove, and then in the reverse direction to the supraclavicular fossa [6]. After tracing C5 and C6 convergence, we identified the suprascapular nerve originating from the superior trunk. After sterile skin preparation, STB was performed based on the group assignment. In the CSTB group, we used an end-hole perineural catheter through a catheter-over-needle system (E-cath, PAJUNK® GmbH, Geisingen, Germany). An 18-gauge cannula with an indwelling 21-gauge needle was advanced in plane at a lateral-to-medial direction until the tip was located just deep into the superior trunk. Non-adrenalized ropivacaine (10 mL, 0.5%) was injected to facilitate hydrodissection to expose space for catheter insertion. Next, a 21-gauge end-hole E-catheter was inserted through an indwelling 18-gauge cannula. To ensure correct catheter tip placement in the medial aspect beneath the superior trunk, additional non-adrenalized ropivacaine (5 mL, 0.5%) was injected during ultrasound imaging (Figure S1). A sterile occlusive dressing and an anchoring device were used to secure the catheter. In the SSTB + DEX group, STB was performed in a similar manner using an insulated stimulating needle (22 gauge, 50 mm; UniPlex Nanoline, Pajunk, Geisingen, Germany). Local anesthetic (15 mL of 0.5% ropivacaine) with epinephrine (1:200,000) was injected to extensively surround the trunk in the lateral, inferior, and medial aspects.

2.3. Postoperative Management

In the post-surgery ward, each patient was prescribed acetaminophen (1200 mg) at 8 h intervals as required to control postoperative pain before hospital discharge. Intravenous tramadol (50 mg) was administered as rescue analgesia when the numeric rating scale pain score (NRS) was >4. No steroids were administered after surgery. In the CSTB group, patients received a continuous infusion of 0.2% ropivacaine (a total volume of 300 mL) at a basal rate of 5 mL/h, a 4 mL bolus, and a 30 min lockout time using a disposable patient-controlled infusion pump (Accufuser, Woo Young Medical, Republic of Korea). In the SSTB + DEX group, DEX was no longer administered after surgery. Based on routine clinical practice, all patients were discharged 1 day post operation. All patients received phone calls from an investigator at 36 and 48 h post operation for evaluation of pain scores and any block- or equipment-related complications. The catheters were removed at each patient's local clinic 48 h after surgery.

2.4. Outcome Assessments

The primary outcome was the 24 h postoperative resting pain score. Pain scores at other times, rebound pain incidence and opioid consumption were included as secondary endpoints. Pain intensities at rest and during activity were assessed using an 11-point numeric pain score (0, no pain, to 10, worst imaginable pain). Pain scores were recorded at five points: the preoperative baseline, and 12, 24, 36, and 48 h postoperatively. Rebound pain was defined as severe pain (NRS score ≥ 7) at the surgical site following the STB resolution. The administration of tramadol was converted to the oral morphine equivalents [7].

2.5. Statistical Analysis

The noninferiority hypothesis was used to calculate the sample size based on the primary endpoint. A pain score standard deviation of 3.2 was used for the calculation [8]. The predetermined noninferiority margin was 2 points on the 11-point pain intensity scale [9]. To achieve a significance level of 2.5% and power of 80%, 41 patients were required in each group. To account for a dropout rate of 10%, 46 patients were included in each group. The noninferiority hypothesis for the primary outcome was assessed using a one-sided t-test (between-group difference in pain score of $\geq$2 points) at a significance level of 2.5%. We performed between-group comparisons of preoperative measurements and secondary outcomes. Parametricity was confirmed using the Shapiro–Wilk and Kolmogorov–Smirnov tests. Parametric and non-parametric continuous variables were analyzed using an independent t-test and a Mann–Whitney U test, respectively. Between-group comparisons of categorical variables were conducted using Fisher's exact test or a χ^2 test, as appropriate. Parametric and non-parametric continuous variables are shown as means ± standard deviation and medians (interquartile range), respectively, while categorical variables are shown as numbers (percentages). All statistical analyses were performed using R (version 3.5.1; R Foundation for Statistical Computing, Vienna, Austria), IBM SPSS Statistics for Windows, version 23.0 (IBM Corp., Armonk, NY, USA), or MedCalc Statistical Software version 18.11.3. Statistical significance was set at $p < 0.05$.

3. Results

Among the 111 patients screened for eligibility, we enrolled 92 and allocated them to either group. One CSTB group patient was excluded because her Horner's syndrome diagnosis required catheter removal at 6 h post operation. One SSTB + DEX group patient was excluded due to changes in the surgical procedure. Accordingly, we included data from 90 patients in the final analysis. A flowchart of the study is presented in Figure 1.

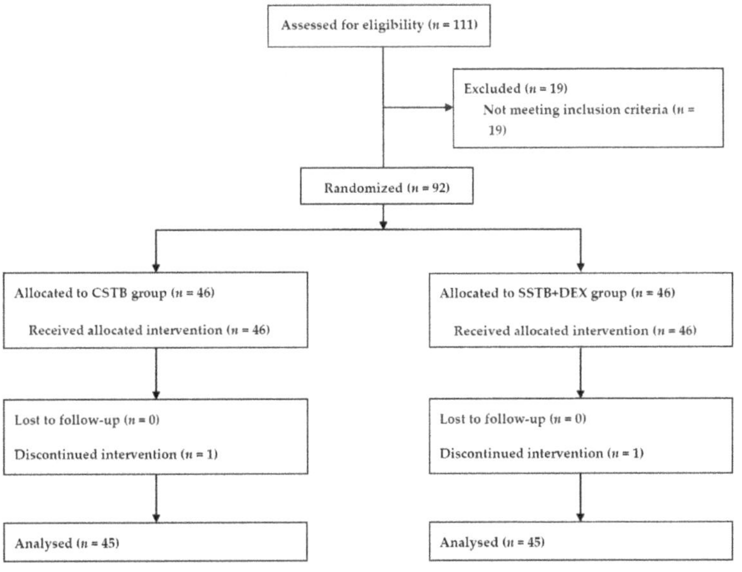

Figure 1. CONSORT study flow diagram. CONSORT, Consolidated Standards for Reporting Trials; CSTB, continuous superior trunk block; SSTB + DEX, single shot of superior trunk block with intravenous dexmedetomidine.

No significant between-group differences were observed in patient characteristics and operative data (Table 1). No significant between-group differences were found in the number of patients requiring intraoperative atropine, the fluid amount, or the minimum blood pressure; however, the minimum heart rate was significantly lower in the SSTB + DEX group than in the CSTB group (49 bpm vs. 52 bpm, $p = 0.007$). In addition, systolic, mean, and diastolic blood pressures were lower in the CSTB group compared with that of SSTB + DEX group, but without statistical significance.

Table 1. Demographic and operative data.

	CSTB Group (n = 45)	SSTB + DEX Group (n = 45)	p Value
Age (years)	65 ± 7	62 ± 8	0.126
Female/Male	20/25	19/26	>0.999
Height (cm)	160.6 ± 8.5	160.8 ± 8.9	0.931
Weight (kg)	64.5 (59.0–70.5)	62.5 (57.0–69.0)	0.345
Body mass index (kg/m^2)	24.9 (23.5–26.2)	24.6 (22.8–26.1)	0.399
ASA class (I/II/III)	22/16/7	17/25/3	0.121
Surgical procedure			
Arthroscopic rotator cuff repair	45 (100)	45 (100)	
Subpectoral biceps tenodesis	30 (67)	22 (49)	0.135
Operation time (min)	90 (70–115)	90 (70–105)	0.539
Anesthesia time (min)	148.7 ± 29.9	152.9 ± 31.4	0.515
Fluid amount (mL)	550 (450–650)	550 (450–650)	0.939
Remifentanil use (mcg)	448 (388–576)	442 (371–579)	0.473
Norepinephrine (mcg)	256 (117–336)	208 (124–293)	0.416
The number of patients who required intraoperative atropine	0	3 (7)	0.242
Minimum SBP	81 (78–83)	83 (78–85)	0.256
Minimum DBP	36 ± 6	38 ± 6	0.067
Minimum MBP	52 (49–57)	55 (51–59)	0.088
Minimum heart rate	52 (49–57)	49 (46–53)	0.007

Values are presented as median (interquartile range), mean ± standard deviation, or number of patients (%). ASA, American Society of Anesthesiologists; CSTB, continuous superior trunk block; DBP, diastolic blood pressure; MBP, mean blood pressure; SBP, systolic blood pressure; SSTB + DEX, single shot of superior trunk block with intravenous dexmedetomidine.

The mean scores for resting pain 24 h post operation were 4.4 ± 2.3 and 5.0 ± 2.0 in the CSTB and SSTB + DEX groups, respectively, and the between-group difference was 0.64 (95% confidence interval [CI], −0.25 to 1.54). Since the upper limit of the 95% CI was lower than the predefined noninferiority margin (δ = 2), noninferiority was established (Figure 2). The mean difference in the moving pain score 24 h post operation was 1.09 (95% CI, 0.21–1.97), which also indicated noninferiority. Similarly, the lack of a significant between-group difference in the resting and moving pain scores 36 and 48 h postoperatively also indicated noninferiority. However, the resting and moving pain scores at 12 h post operation were significantly higher in the STB + DEX group than in the CSTB group, with a mean between-group difference of >2 (mean difference in resting pain score, 3.31; 95% CI, 1.97 to 4.65; mean difference of moving pain score, 3; 95% CI, 1.67–4.33). The pain scores at 12 h post operation indicated that SSTB + DEX was inferior to CSTB. The resting and moving median pain scores at 12 h post operation were significantly higher in the SSTB + DEX group than in the CSTB group (resting pain, 8.0 vs. 3.0; movement pain, 8.0 vs. 5.0), with no between-group difference in the pain scores at the other time points (Figure 3).

The median between-group time difference in time to first pain was 3 h (14 h vs. 11 h, p = 0.014, Table 2). The rebound pain incidence was 20% and 56% in the CSTB and SSTB + DEX groups, respectively (p = 0.001); the overall incidence was 38%. Opioid consumption within the 12–24 h postoperative period was higher in the SSTB + DEX group than that in the CSTB group. The SSTB + DEX group had more patients requiring rescue analgesics within the 12–24 h post operation than the CSTB group. DEX use was not associated with a prolonged post-anesthesia care unit stay. No patients experienced adverse pulmonary events and, at the 48 h follow-up, no patients reported any block- or equipment-related complications.

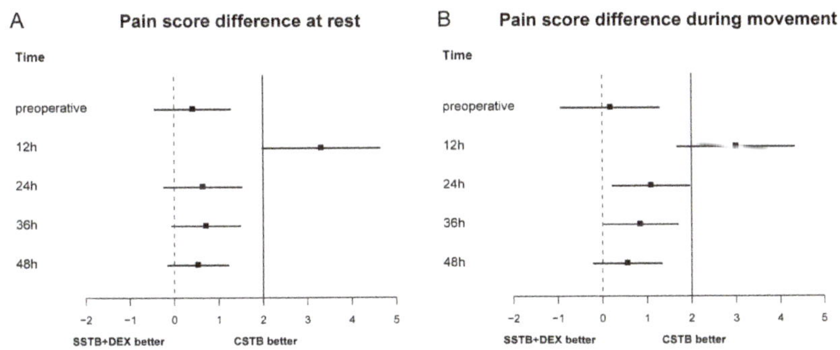

Figure 2. Noninferiority diagram of between-group differences in the numerical rating scale pain scores within 48 h post operation, both at rest (**A**) and during movement (**B**). The solid line indicates a noninferiority margin (δ) of 2. Squares indicate differences in the mean pain score, while error bars indicate the 95% CIs of the between group differences. Statistical significance was set at $p < 0.05$. CSTB, continuous superior trunk block; SSTB + DEX, single shot of superior trunk block with intravenous dexmedetomidine.

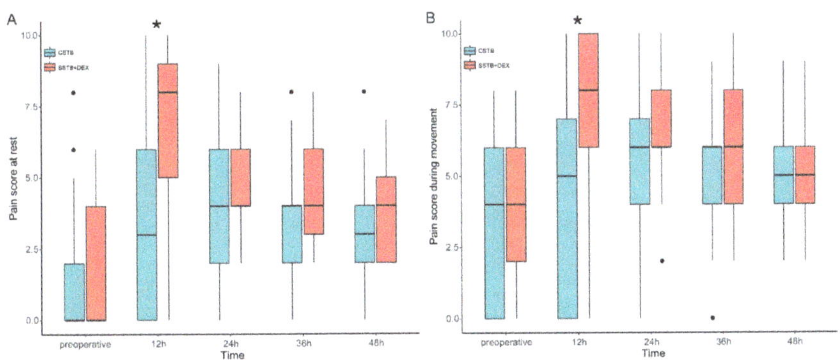

Figure 3. Pain scores at rest (**A**) and during movement (**B**). Boxplot represents the median with the 25th/75th percentile. Whiskers reveal the minimum/maximum values, excluding outliers. Points represent the outliers. CSTB, continuous superior trunk block; SSTB + DEX, single shot of superior trunk block with intravenous dexmedetomidine. * $p < 0.05$ between the CSTB and SSTB + DEX groups in the post hoc analysis.

Table 2. Postoperative variables.

	CSTB Group (n = 45)	SSTB + DEX Group (n = 45)	p Value
Time to first pain report (h)	14 (10–15)	11 (10–13)	0.014
Patients experiencing rebound pain (n)	9 (20)	25 (56)	0.001
Patients requiring rescue analgesics (n)			
0–12 h	9 (20)	9 (20)	>0.999
12–24 h	23 (51)	36 (80)	0.008
Opioid consumption (morphine equivalents)			
0–12 h	0 (0–0)	0 (0–0)	>0.999
12–24 h	10 (0–10)	20 (10–20)	<0.001
Postoperative anesthesia care unit (PACU) stay (min)	38 (30–55)	48 (35–63)	0.070

Values are presented as median (interquartile range) or number of patients (%). CSTB, continuous superior trunk block; SSTB + DEX, single shot of superior trunk block with intravenous dexmedetomidine.

4. Discussion

In our study, SSTB + DEX yielded significantly inferior analgesia at 12 h post operation than CSTB did. Furthermore, SSTB was associated with a higher rebound pain incidence than CSTB. The patients in the CSTB group required less opioid consumption and fewer rescue analgesics within the postoperative 12–24 h period than those in the SSTB + DEX group. However, SSTB + DEX yielded pain scores comparable to those of CSTB within 24–48 h post operation.

Single-injection ISB is an important component of multimodal analgesia for postoperative pain and provides effective analgesia during the early postoperative period (6–8 h postoperatively) to reduce opioid requirement [10]. Continuous ISB has been shown to lead to better analgesia, less opioid consumption, better sleep patterns, and a higher quality of recovery than single-injection ISB [11–13]. Given the difficulty and cost of catheterization, most recent studies have focused on increasing the analgesic duration of single-shot ISB by adding perineural or intravenous adjuvants [14–18]. Among the various adjuvants for local anesthetics, intravenous DEX prolongs the analgesic duration of single-shot ISB and reduces postoperative analgesic consumption [3,19,20]. However, limited studies exist on the effectiveness of intravenous administration of DEX, in addition to STB, a phrenic-sparing alternative to ISB. Therefore, this study compared the postoperative analgesic effect of CSTB with that of combined SSTB and intravenous DEX in patients undergoing arthroscopic rotator cuff repair.

DEX provides prolonged analgesia when used as a single-shot peripheral nerve block adjuvant [18–21]. In contrast, perineural DEX delays rehabilitation due to prolonged motor blockade [21]. Its use includes specific potential risks, including "off-label" use in the absence of US Food and Drug Administration approval. A recent study showed that intravenous dexamethasone and DEX notably extended the period before the first pain relief request after single-shot ISB following arthroscopic shoulder surgery [17]. Intravenous DEX (2.0 mcg/kg) significantly increases the ISB analgesia duration (median increase of 218 min, compared with the control group). It also reduces the cumulative opioid consumption within the 24 h postoperative period [14]. Kang et al. revealed that 0.5 mcg/kg or 1.0 mcg/kg of intravenous DEX did not have a clinical analgesic effect, with only 2 mcg/kg of intravenous DEX significantly increasing the duration of ISB [14]. Accordingly, we administered a 2 mcg/kg loading dose of intravenous DEX after induction, followed by continuous intravenous infusion of a maintenance dose of 0.5 mcg/kg/h until the end of surgery [18,22]. Central nerve system $\alpha 2$ receptor binding mediates the analgesic effect of intravenous DEX. Pain transmission is suppressed via subdued interneuron hyperpolarization and inhibition of nociceptive transmitter (e.g., substance P and glutamate) release [14,17,22].

Generally, pain after arthroscopy peaks on postoperative day 1, with severe postoperative pain occurring in some cases within the first 48 h post operation [23]. Here, the patients in the CSTB group had lower opioid consumption than those in the SSTB + DEX group within 12–24 h post operation, which is consistent with previous reports [8,11,13,24,25]. This could be explained by rebound pain after STB resolution. Although single-shot peripheral nerve block is an effective analgesic method, patients can experience a relatively rapid increase in severe pain following block resolution, which is referred to as rebound pain [26]. Since brachial plexus block or STB completely blocks the surgical site for shoulder surgery, there is a higher risk of rebound pain after the block wears off following shoulder surgery than following other surgeries, including total knee arthroplasty [26]. In the absence of adequate systemic analgesia after block resolution, this rebound pain can be attributed to unmasking the expected nociceptive response. Strategies for reducing rebound pain include routine prescription of a systemic multimodal analgesic regimen and extending the analgesic duration of peripheral nerve block through the continuous catheter technique or local anesthetic adjuvants [2]. The multimodal analgesic regimen frequently included acetaminophen, nonsteroidal anti-inflammatory medications, and gabapentinoids to reduce opioid consumption [27]. The rebound pain is associated with age, female sex, bone surgery, and the absence of intraoperative dexamethasone [26]. Perineural dexamethasone adjunct to single-shot ISB decreases the incidence and severity of rebound pain (37% vs. 83%), as well as sleep disturbance, compared with a placebo [15]. Here, the patients in the CSTB group exhibited a significantly lower incidence of rebound pain than those in the SSTB + DEX group (20% vs. 56%). Our study found that the rate of rebound pain within the CSTB group was markedly lower than that seen in previous research, where perineural dexamethasone was used as an adjuvant to single-shot ISB; however, the study designs of the previous and the present study were not identical and cannot be directly compared [15]. Our study revealed that patients who received SSTB + DEX required more analgesics to reduce the intensity of rebound pain within 12–24 h post operation, which implies that individuals in the SSTB + DEX group need an additional multimodal analgesic regimen to reduce the rebound pain compared to those in the CSTB group in patients undergoing arthroscopic rotator cuff repair. Most studies on single-shot ISB using DEX [14,17] assessed pain occurring within 24 h post operation while not considering the occurrence of rebound pain. Furthermore, unlike our study, the previous studies included not only rotator cuff repair but also Bankart repair, which has a lower postoperative pain intensity [14,17]. Therefore, further studies are warranted to determine whether DEX can effectively reduce rebound pain as dexamethasone can after arthroscopic rotator cuff repair. Additionally, we compared the hemodynamic differences between the two groups. The influence of DEX resulted in a statistically significantly lower minimum heart rate in the SSTB + DEX group compared with the CSTB group. Conversely, systolic, diastolic, and mean blood pressures tended to be higher in the SSTB + DEX group. Moreover, although not statistically significant, the amount of norepinephrine administered was higher in the CSTB group. This is thought to occur due to the reduced use of other anesthetics for maintaining anesthesia or biphasic blood pressure responses as a result of DEX administration [28]. The initial doses of DEX caused a 13% decrease in mean arterial pressure, while subsequent higher doses led to a gradual rise in mean arterial pressure, with peak individual increases averaging 12% above the baseline [28]. Using IV DEX as an adjuvant, considering the risk of bradycardia induced by DEX, appears necessary.

This study had some limitations. Firstly, blinding was not optimal since patients in the SSTB + DEX group were not provided with sham catheters. To avoid investigator bias, neck dressings were adequately concealed in all patients until they were discharged. Secondly, SSTB has been associated with significantly less hemidiaphragmatic paresis than single-shot ISB [3]. We did not compare whether CSTB caused more hemidiaphragmatic paresis than SSTB due to accumulated local anesthetic volume. However, none of our patients experienced postoperative dyspnea or desaturation. Thirdly, we did not use other adjuvants, including dexamethasone, to investigate the effect of DEX. Therefore, additional studies are needed to determine whether the simultaneous use of DEX and dexamethasone in addition to STB can effectively reduce rebound pain, especially after arthroscopic rotator cuff repair. Finally, the generalizability of this study to patients in clinical settings different from those in our center, such as outpatients or patients using strong opioids, may be limited.

5. Conclusions

CSTB had lower pain scores at 12 h post operation and was associated with a lower incidence of rebound pain and opioid consumption than SSTB + DEX. SSTB + DEX requires more systemic multimodal analgesics or adjuvants to reduce the risk and intensity of rebound pain within 12–24 h post operation and there was also an additional risk of DEX-induced bradycardia.

Supplementary Materials: The following supporting information can be downloaded at: https://www.mdpi.com/article/10.3390/jcm13071845/s1, Figure S1: Ultrasonographic image of the catheter for superior trunk block (blue arrowheads). ASM, anterior scalene muscle; MSM, middle scalene muscle; SA, subclavian artery; SSN, suprascapular nerve; ST, superior trunk.

Author Contributions: Conceptualization, B.L., Y.-M.C. and Y.S.C.; methodology, B.L., Y.-M.C. and Y.S.C.; software, B.L.; validation, B.L., Y.-M.C. and Y.S.C.; formal analysis, B.L.; investigation, J.J., J.-R.L., E.J.K. and D.K.; data curation, J.J. and J.-R.L.; writing—original draft preparation, B.L.; writing—review and editing, Y.-M.C. and Y.S.C.; visualization, B.L.; supervision, Y.-M.C. and Y.S.C.; project administration, B.L., Y.-M.C. and Y.S.C. All authors have read and agreed to the published version of the manuscript.

Funding: This research received no external funding.

Institutional Review Board Statement: This prospective randomized controlled study was approved by the Severance Hospital Institutional Review Board (protocol code 4-2021-0853 and date of approval 13 August 2021), and registered at ClinicalTrials.gov (NCT05020821, principal investigator: Jaewon Jang, date of registration: 25 August 2021). This study followed the Consolidated Standards for Reporting Trials reporting guidelines for clinical trials.

Informed Consent Statement: All participants provided their consent after being fully informed about the study's nature and procedures.

Data Availability Statement: The data that contribute to the findings of this study can be obtained from the corresponding author upon reasonable request.

Acknowledgments: The authors would like to thank the biostatistician (Ha Yan Kim, Biostatistics Collaboration Unit, Department of Biomedical Systems Informatics, Yonsei University College of Medicine) employed for their statistical comments and analyses.

Conflicts of Interest: The authors declare no conflicts of interest.

References

1. Vorobeichik, L.; Brull, R.; Bowry, R.; Laffey, J.G.; Abdallah, F.W. Should continuous rather than single-injection interscalene block be routinely offered for major shoulder surgery? A meta-analysis of the analgesic and side-effects profiles. *Br. J. Anaesth.* **2018**, *120*, 679–692. [CrossRef] [PubMed]
2. Muñoz-Leyva, F.; Cubillos, J.; Chin, K.J. Managing rebound pain after regional anesthesia. *Korean J. Anesthesiol.* **2020**, *73*, 372–383. [CrossRef] [PubMed]
3. Kang, R.; Jeong, J.S.; Chin, K.J.; Yoo, J.C.; Lee, J.H.; Choi, S.J.; Gwak, M.S.; Hahm, T.S.; Ko, J.S. Superior trunk block provides noninferior analgesia compared with interscalene brachial plexus block in arthroscopic shoulder surgery. *Anesthesiology* **2019**, *131*, 1316–1326. [CrossRef]
4. Kim, D.H.; Lin, Y.; Beathe, J.C.; Liu, J.; Oxendine, J.A.; Haskins, S.C.; Ho, M.C.; Wetmore, D.S.; Allen, A.A.; Wilson, L.; et al. Superior trunk block: A phrenic-sparing alternative to the interscalene block: A randomized controlled trial. *Anesthesiology* **2019**, *131*, 521–533. [CrossRef] [PubMed]
5. Robles, C.; Berardone, N.; Orebaugh, S. Effect of superior trunk block on diaphragm function and respiratory parameters after shoulder surgery. *Reg. Anesth. Pain Med.* **2022**, *47*, 167–170. [CrossRef] [PubMed]
6. Karmakar, M.K.; Pakpirom, J.; Songthamwat, B.; Areeruk, P. High definition ultrasound imaging of the individual elements of the brachial plexus above the clavicle. *Reg. Anesth. Pain Med.* **2020**, *45*, 344–350. [CrossRef]
7. Nielsen, S.; Degenhardt, L.; Hoban, B.; Gisev, N. A synthesis of oral morphine equivalents (OME) for opioid utilisation studies. *Pharmacoepidemiol. Drug Saf.* **2016**, *25*, 733–737. [CrossRef] [PubMed]
8. Bojaxhi, E.; Lumermann, L.A.; Mazer, L.S.; Howe, B.L.; Ortiguera, C.J.; Clendenen, S.R. Interscalene brachial plexus catheter versus single-shot interscalene block with periarticular local infiltration analgesia for shoulder arthroplasty. *Minerva Anestesiol.* **2019**, *85*, 840–845. [CrossRef]
9. Farrar, J.T.; Portenoy, R.K.; Berlin, J.A.; Kinman, J.L.; Strom, B.L. Defining the clinically important difference in pain outcome measures. *Pain* **2000**, *88*, 287–294. [CrossRef]
10. Abdallah, F.W.; Halpern, S.H.; Aoyama, K.; Brull, R. Will the real benefits of single-shot interscalene block please stand up? A systematic review and meta-analysis. *Anesth. Analg.* **2015**, *120*, 1114–1129. [CrossRef]
11. Yun, S.; Jo, Y.; Sim, S.; Jeong, K.; Oh, C.; Kim, B.; Lee, W.Y.; Park, S.; Kim, Y.H.; Ko, Y.; et al. Comparison of continuous and single interscalene block for quality of recovery score following arthroscopic rotator cuff repair. *J. Orthop. Surg.* **2021**, *29*, 23094990211000142. [CrossRef] [PubMed]
12. Kim, J.H.; Koh, H.J.; Kim, D.K.; Lee, H.J.; Kwon, K.H.; Lee, K.Y.; Kim, Y.S. Interscalene brachial plexus bolus block versus patient-controlled interscalene indwelling catheter analgesia for the first 48 hours after arthroscopic rotator cuff repair. *J. Shoulder Elb. Surg.* **2018**, *27*, 1243–1250. [CrossRef] [PubMed]
13. Salviz, E.A.; Xu, D.; Frulla, A.; Kwofie, K.; Shastri, U.; Chen, J.; Shariat, A.N.; Littwin, S.; Lin, E.; Choi, J.; et al. Continuous interscalene block in patients having outpatient rotator cuff repair surgery: A prospective randomized trial. *Anesth. Analg.* **2013**, *117*, 1485–1492. [CrossRef] [PubMed]

14. Kang, R.; Jeong, J.S.; Yoo, J.C.; Lee, J.H.; Choi, S.J.; Gwak, M.S.; Hahm, T.S.; Huh, J.; Ko, J.S. Effective dose of intravenous dexmedetomidine to prolong the analgesic duration of interscalene brachial plexus block: A single-center, prospective, double-blind, randomized controlled trial. *Reg. Anesth. Pain Med.* **2018**, *43*, 488–495. [CrossRef] [PubMed]
15. Woo, J.H.; Lee, H.J.; Oh, H.W.; Lee, J.W., Baik, H.J.; Kim, Y.J. Perineural dexamethasone reduces rebound pain after ropivacaine single injection interscalene block for arthroscopic shoulder surgery: A randomized controlled trial. *Reg. Anesth. Pain Med.* **2021**, *46*, 965–970. [CrossRef] [PubMed]
16. Fang, J.; Shi, Y.; Du, F.; Xue, Z.; Cang, J.; Miao, C.; Zhang, X. The effect of perineural dexamethasone on rebound pain after ropivacaine single-injection nerve block: A randomized controlled trial. *BMC Anesthesiol.* **2021**, *21*, 47. [CrossRef] [PubMed]
17. Kang, R.A.; Jeong, J.S.; Yoo, J.C.; Lee, J.H.; Gwak, M.S.; Choi, S.J.; Hahm, T.S.; Cho, H.S.; Ko, J.S. Improvement in postoperative pain control by combined use of intravenous dexamethasone with intravenous dexmedetomidine after interscalene brachial plexus block for arthroscopic shoulder surgery: A randomised controlled trial. *Eur. J. Anaesthesiol.* **2019**, *36*, 360–368. [CrossRef]
18. Abdallah, F.W.; Dwyer, T.; Chan, V.W.; Niazi, A.U.; Ogilvie-Harris, D.J.; Oldfield, S.; Patel, R.; Oh, J.; Brull, R. IV and perineural dexmedetomidine similarly prolong the duration of analgesia after interscalene brachial plexus block: A randomized, three-arm, triple-masked, placebo-controlled trial. *Anesthesiology* **2016**, *124*, 683–695. [CrossRef]
19. Kirksey, M.A.; Haskins, S.C.; Cheng, J.; Liu, S.S. Local anesthetic peripheral nerve block adjuvants for prolongation of analgesia: A systematic qualitative review. *PLoS ONE.* **2015**, *10*, e0137312. [CrossRef]
20. Hussain, N.; Grzywacz, V.P.; Ferreri, C.A.; Atrey, A.; Banfield, L.; Shaparin, N.; Vydyanathan, A. Investigating the efficacy of dexmedetomidine as an adjuvant to local anesthesia in brachial plexus block: A systematic review and meta-analysis of 18 randomized controlled trials. *Reg. Anesth. Pain Med.* **2017**, *42*, 184–196. [CrossRef]
21. Vorobeichik, L.; Brull, R.; Abdallah, F.W. Evidence basis for using perineural dexmedetomidine to enhance the quality of brachial plexus nerve blocks: A systematic review and meta-analysis of randomized controlled trials. *Br. J. Anaesth.* **2017**, *118*, 167–181. [CrossRef] [PubMed]
22. Weerink, M.A.S.; Struys, M.M.R.F.; Hannivoort, L.N.; Barends, C.R.M.; Absalom, A.R.; Colin, P. Clinical pharmacokinetics and pharmacodynamics of dexmedetomidine. *Clin. Pharmacokinet.* **2017**, *56*, 893–913. [CrossRef] [PubMed]
23. Stiglitz, Y.; Gosselin, O.; Sedaghatian, J.; Sirveaux, F.; Molé, D. Pain after shoulder arthroscopy: A prospective study on 231 cases. *Orthop. Traumatol. Surg. Res.* **2011**, *97*, 260–266. [CrossRef] [PubMed]
24. Hasan, S.S.; Rolf, R.H.; Sympson, A.N.; Eten, K.; Elsass, T.R. Single-shot versus continuous interscalene block for postoperative pain control after shoulder arthroplasty: A prospective randomized clinical trial. *J. Am. Acad. Orthop. Surg. Glob. Res. Rev.* **2019**, *3*, e014. [CrossRef] [PubMed]
25. Malik, T.; Mass, D.; Cohn, S. Postoperative analgesia in a prolonged continuous interscalene block versus single-shot block in outpatient arthroscopic rotator cuff repair: A prospective randomized study. *Arthroscopy* **2016**, *32*, 1544–1550.e1. [CrossRef] [PubMed]
26. Barry, G.S.; Bailey, J.G.; Sardinha, J.; Brousseau, P.; Uppal, V. Factors associated with rebound pain after peripheral nerve block for ambulatory surgery. *Br. J. Anaesth.* **2021**, *126*, 862–871. [CrossRef] [PubMed]
27. McLaughlin, D.C.; Cheah, J.W.; Aleshi, P.; Zhang, A.L.; Ma, C.B.; Feeley, B.T. Multimodal analgesia decreases opioid consumption after shoulder arthroplasty: A prospective cohort study. *J. Shoulder Elb. Surg.* **2018**, *27*, 686–691. [CrossRef]
28. Ebert, T.J.; Hall, J.E.; Barney, J.A.; Uhrich, T.D.; Colinco, M.D. The effects of increasing plasma concentrations of dexmedetomidine in humans. *Anesthesiology* **2000**, *93*, 382–394. [CrossRef]

Journal of
Clinical Medicine

MDPI

Article

Evaluating the Efficacy of the Erector Spinae Plane Block as a Supplementary Approach to Cardiac Anesthesia during Off-Pump Coronary Bypass Graft Surgery via Median Sternotomy: A Randomized Clinical Trial

Sujin Kim [1], Seung Woo Song [1], Yeong-Gwan Jeon [1], Sang A. Song [1], Soonchang Hong [2] and Ji-Hyoung Park [1,*]

[1] Department of Anesthesiology and Pain Medicine, Wonju College of Medicine, Yonsei University, Wonju 26426, Republic of Korea; sjkim624@yonsei.ac.kr (S.K.); yonfong@yonsei.ac.kr (S.W.S.); ygjeon@yonsei.ac.kr (Y.-G.J.); iad0506@naver.com (S.A.S.)

[2] Department of Cardiovascular Surgery, Wonju College of Medicine, Yonsei University, Wonju 26426, Republic of Korea; hongsc93@yonsei.ac.kr

* Correspondence: killerjhjh@yonsei.ac.kr; Tel.: +82-33-741-1604

Abstract: Background: Pain control after off-pump coronary artery bypass graft (OPCAB) facilitates mobilization and improves outcomes. The efficacy of the erector spinae plane block (ESPB) after cardiac surgery remains controversial. **Methods:** We aimed to investigate the analgesic effects of ESPB after OPCAB. Precisely 56 patients receiving OPCAB were randomly divided into ESPB and control groups. The primary outcome was visual analog scale (VAS) pain scores at 6, 12, 24, and 48 h postoperatively. Secondary outcomes were the dose of rescue analgesics in terms of oral morphine milligram equivalents, the dose of antiemetics, the length of intubation time, and the length of stay in the intensive care unit (ICU). **Results:** The VAS scores were similar at all time points in both groups. The incidence of severe pain (VAS score > 7) was significantly lower in the ESPB group (50% vs. 15.4%; p = 0.008). The dose of rescue analgesics was also lower in the ESPB group (19.04 ± 18.76, 9.83 ± 12.84, p = 0.044) compared with the control group. The other secondary outcomes did not differ significantly between the two groups. **Conclusions:** ESPB provides analgesic efficacy by reducing the incidence of severe pain and opioid use after OPCAB.

Keywords: coronary artery disease; cardiac surgical procedures; sternotomy; myocardial revascularization; erector spinae plane block; pain; postoperative

1. Introduction

Despite the advantages of reduced transfusion and hospital stay, off-pump coronary artery bypass grafting (OPCAB) is not preferred over on-pump coronary artery bypass grafting (CABG) because of the risk of ineffective revascularization [1]. However, contrary to these results, there are studies indicating that both CABG and OPCAB are safe options, and OPCAB is still being performed in many cases [2]. Although OPCAB does not use a cardiopulmonary bypass machine, it uses a sternal retractor, internal mammary artery harvester, and chest tube after surgery [3]. Persistent chest pain is related to the intensity of acute pain after surgery, and 22% of patients continue to experience pain 3 months after sternotomy [4]. Therefore, similar to other cardiac surgeries, pain control after OPCAB is a key factor for facilitating patient mobilization and improving recovery.

Since its introduction in 2016, the erector spinae plane block (ESPB) has been gaining popularity in various surgeries owing to its ease of implementation and low risk of adverse effects [5]. However, evidence remains insufficient to confirm the efficacy of various block techniques performed after cardiac surgery, and there is no gold standard for pain management after cardiac surgery.

This trial aimed to investigate the efficacy of ESPB after OPCAB. We hypothesize that ESPB reduces pain scores after surgery and the dose of rescue analgesics used (calculated as the oral morphine milligram equivalent, [MME]).

2. Materials and Methods

2.1. Study Design

This was a single-center, double-blind, randomized controlled trial. This study was approved by the Institutional Review Board of Yonsei University in Wonju and ensured compliance with ethical standards, patient confidentiality, and adherence to relevant regulatory guidelines (CR322089). As part of ethical practice and transparency in clinical research, all participants involved in this study were appropriately registered in Korea's Clinical Research Information Service, ensuring their inclusion and documentation in a national database (https://cris.nih.go.kr/, accessed at KCT0008781; registration date: 30 August 2023).

2.2. Study Population

We enrolled 56 patients aged 19 years or older with a diagnosis of coronary artery disease scheduled for OPCAB surgery at Severance Christian Hospital in Wonju, Korea, from December 2022 to August 2023. All the patients underwent surgery performed by one cardiovascular surgeon (S.H.). We excluded patients with contraindications to nerve block surgery (coagulopathy, infection at the procedure site, allergic reaction to local anesthetic, or refusal to undergo the procedure) from the study. Patients with comorbidities (sepsis, thoracic deformity, and increased intracranial pressure) who were excluded at the discretion of the anesthesiologist, those who had difficulty giving voluntary consent due to illiteracy or cognitive dysfunction, and those who underwent emergency surgery were also excluded from this study.

2.3. Randomization and Blinding

The patients were randomly assigned into ESPB and control groups using a computer. Except for one researcher who performed the ESPB (S.K.), the patients and other physicians participating in this study did not know to which group the patients were assigned. The assignments were secured in sequentially numbered sealed opaque envelopes. At the end of the surgery, one of the authors opened the envelope containing the study assignment and performed a pain block procedure. After the patient was transferred to the intensive care unit (ICU), the patient and researcher who participated in data collection (S.S.) were blinded.

2.4. Perioperative Management

Midazolam (0.05 mg/kg), sufentanil (1–2 mcg/kg), rocuronium (0.8 mg/kg), and sevoflurane were used to induce anesthesia. After tracheal intubation, Arrowg+ard Blu® MAC (Teleflex Inc., Limerick, Ireland) and Swan-Ganz® (Edwards Lifesciences, Irvine, CA, USA) catheters were inserted to facilitate intraoperative monitoring for right heart function (e.g., pulmonary artery pressure, central venous pressure, cardiac index of right heart, etc.). Transesophageal echocardiography was performed to monitor cardiac contractility, lusitropy, and wall motion abnormalities during surgery. Anesthesia was maintained via the inhalation of sevoflurane and infusion of sufentanil and rocuronium. The sevoflurane inhalation rate was controlled using Sedline electroencephalography guidance (Masimo, Irvine, CA, USA). The sufentanil infusion rate was adjusted according to the overall hemodynamic data by the attending anesthesiologist, who suggested that the intensity of the surgical stimuli and rocuronium be adjusted by a train of four watches within the surgical neuromuscular block range. At the end of the surgery, the patient was placed in the lateral decubitus position for ESPB. One of the authors (S.K.) performed ESPB under ultrasonographic guidance to ensure the accuracy and efficacy of the block. Subsequently, as part of the postoperative pain management strategy, an intravenous patient-controlled analgesia (PCA) regimen was prescribed by the attending anesthesiologist. This PCA system was designed to deliver analgesia tailored to individual patient needs and contained an approximate dosage of 18 mcg/kg of fentanyl, allowing for controlled and adjustable pain relief in response to patient-initiated dosing. The patients were transferred to the ICU, and the primary physician (S.H.) oversaw postoperative pain management. The dosage of postoperative analgesics was recorded in MME. Intravenous tramadol (50 mg), intramuscular or subcutaneous meperidine (25 mg), oral Ultracet® (Janssen Korea Ltd., Seoul, Republic of Korea; tramadol [37.5 mg]/acetaminophen [325 mg]), and transdermal fentanyl patches (25 mcg/h) were used postoperatively. Withdrawal from the study was considered in cases of conversion to on-pump surgery or hypersensitivity reactions during anesthetic induction.

2.5. Erector Spinae Plane Block

After the surgical procedure, the patient was placed in the lateral decubitus position for the ESPB. The skin overlying the intended block area was prepared and disinfected with betadine. Using ultrasound guidance, the anatomical structures were visualized to confirm the T5 level and relevant surrounding structures. The trapezius, rhomboid, and erector spinae muscles were visualized via an ultrasound to guide the insertion of an echogenic needle (Echoplex®; Vygon, France) into the desired plane. Using an in-plane ultrasound approach, the needle was advanced until it reached the plane of the erector spinae muscles. The needle position was confirmed by hydrodissection using 2–3 mL of saline. Once the correct placement of the needle within the erector spinae plane was confirmed, a mixture of local anesthetics was injected. The administered dose was a 20 mL mixture consisting of 0.225% ropivacaine, 1% lidocaine, and normal saline. The ESPB was performed with a total volume of 40 mL, with 20 mL on each side.

2.6. Outcome Measures

The primary outcome of this study was the assessment of postoperative pain intensity using the Visual Analog Scale (VAS) at 6, 12, 24, and 48 h postoperatively. The VAS, ranging from 0 (no pain) to 10 (worst imaginable pain), provided a quantitative measurement of the pain experienced by the patients. The highest VAS score was recorded at each time point.

Secondary outcomes measured included the dose of rescue analgesics injected into patients (in MME), the dose of antiemetics used, the length of intubation time, and the length of stay in the ICU.

2.7. Sample Size Calculation

The sample size calculation was derived from a previous study that reported a mean postoperative pain score of 5.48 $\pm$ 1.09 when utilizing opioid-based intravenous PCA following cardiac surgery [6]. Considering a clinically meaningful reduction of more than 1 point in the average pain score, with a type I error of 0.05 and a power of 0.90, a sample size of 25 individuals per group was required. Factoring in a potential dropout rate of 10%, the study aimed to include 56 participants, with 28 individuals allocated to each group.

2.8. Statistical Analysis

All statistical analyses were performed using the IBM SPSS statistical software (IBM SPSS Statistics for Windows, version 27, IBM Corporation, Armonk, NY, USA). Continuous variables were presented as the mean $\pm$ standard deviation (SD). For continuous variables such as postoperative pain intensity (measured by VAS) and time from the end of anesthesia to extubation, a comparison between the intervention and control groups was conducted using the independent samples t-test. This statistical test was used to assess whether there were significant differences in the means of the continuous variables between the two groups. The significance level was set at $p < 0.05$, and 95% confidence intervals were calculated to estimate the precision of the mean differences between the groups. The Mann–Whitney U test was performed to ensure the accuracy of the analysis. Regarding categorical variables, such as the presence or absence of perioperative complications, relevant statistical tests, such as the chi-square test, were used to evaluate the association or difference in frequency between the intervention and control groups. Repeated measurements of pain scores were corrected using post hoc Bonferroni correction.

3. Results

Initially, 72 patients were assessed for eligibility, and 16 patients were excluded for the following reasons, including surgery performed on-pump CABG (n = 7) and emergency surgery (n = 8), and the participants declined (n = 1). A total of 56 patients enrolled in this study were assigned to the intervention and control groups; 4 patients dropped out because of drowsy mental status (Figure 1). Patients' characteristics and surgery data are shown in Table 1.

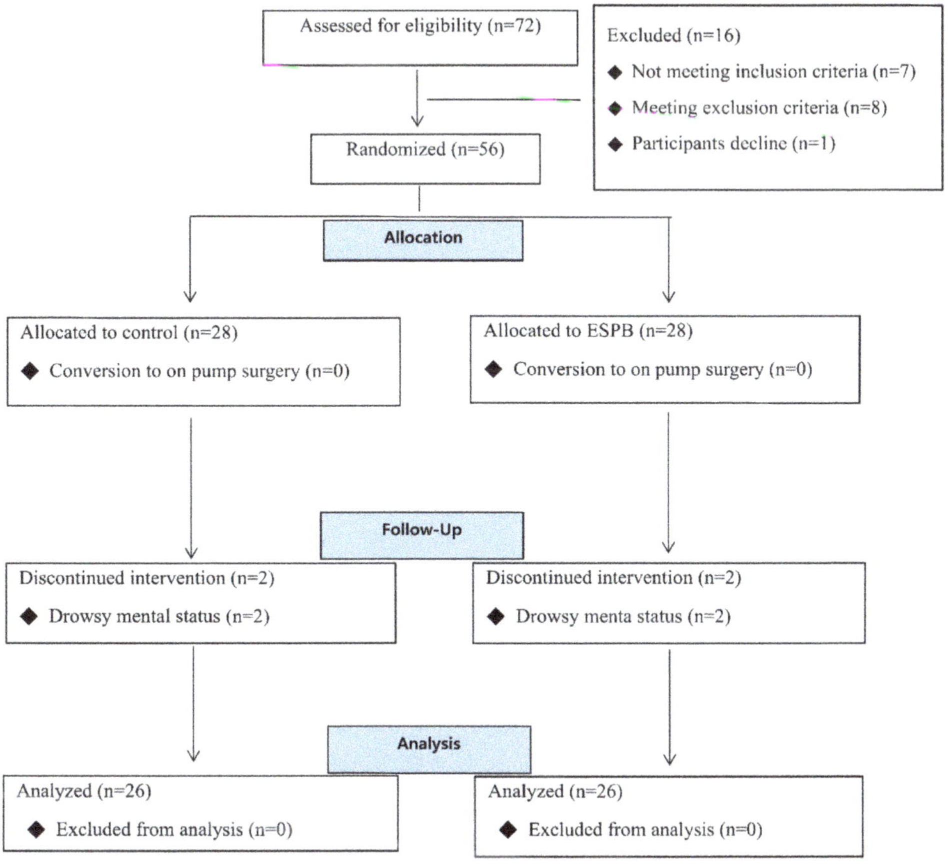

Figure 1. CONSORT flow chart.

There were no statistically significant differences in the VAS scores at 6, 12, 24, and 48 h after surgery between the two groups. Although there was no significance after repeated measurement correction, pain tended to be lower at 6 h (4.46 ± 1.98 vs. 5.96 ± 1.84, p = 0.020). However, the incidence of severe pain was significantly lower in the ESPB group than in the control group (15.4% vs. 50%, p = 0.008). Additionally, the dose of rescue analgesics was significantly reduced in the ESPB group (19.04 ± 0.49 vs. 9.83 ± 12.84, p = 0.044). The lengths of ICU and hospital stays were similar. The time to extubation did not differ between the two groups (Table 2).

Table 1. Patients' characteristics and surgery data.

	Control Group (n = 26)	ESPB Group (n = 26)	p Value
Age (years)	64.58 ± 11.07 [43, 83]	63.65 ± 10.83 [47, 85]	0.602
Female	6 (23.1)	4 (15.4)	0.482
Height (cm)	163.75 ± 9.30 [144.0, 179.1]	164.79 ± 7.97 [145.0, 183.0]	0.667
Weight (kg)	66.82 ± 13.63 [44.42, 94.40]	70.33 ± 11.11 [49.42, 90.10]	0.314
Hypertension	20 (76.9)	21 (80.8)	0.734
Diabetes mellitus	16 (61.5)	16 (61.5)	1.000
Cerebral vascular disease	5 (19.2)	2 (7.7)	0.223
Chronic kidney disease	4 (15.4)	6 (23.1)	0.482
NYHA class	2.19 ± 0.98 [1, 4]	2.00 ± 0.80 [1, 4]	0.442
CCS score	2.19 ± 0.98 [1, 4]	2.04 ± 0.72 [1, 4]	0.522
EuroSCORE	1.73 ± 1.50 [0.50, 6.29]	1.45 ± 0.73 [0.50, 3.01]	0.397
Heart failure	10 (38.5)	10 (38.5)	1.000
Ejection fraction (%)	49.19 ± 12.67 [26, 67]	49.73 ± 11.54 [27, 72]	0.873
Surgery time (min)	243.31 ± 33.27 [175, 325]	239.54 ± 31.14 [171, 315]	0.675
Anesthesia time (min)	327.31 ± 35.92 [270, 420]	331.73 ± 33.67 [250, 420]	0.649

Values are displayed as the mean ± SD [minimum, maximum] or n (%). NYHA, New York Heart Association; CCS, Canadian Cardiovascular Society.

Table 2. Outcome comparisons between the groups.

	Control Group (n = 26)	ESPB Group (n = 26)	p Value	Mean Difference (95% CI)
	Primary Outcomes			
VAS 6 h	5.96 ± 1.84 [2, 9]	4.46 ± 1.98 [0, 9]	0.020 *	−1.27 (−2.33, −0.20)
VAS 12 h	4.58 ± 2.25 [2, 9]	3.85 ± 1.87 [0, 9]	0.208	−0.73 (−1.88, 0.42)
VAS 24 h	3.73 ± 2.07 [1, 9]	3.62 ± 1.75 [1, 8]	0.829	−0.12 (−1.18, 0.95)
VAS 48 h	2.85 ± 2.39 [0, 10]	2.00 ± 1.62 [0, 6]	0.143	−0.85 (−1.99, 0.29)
VAS (7–10)	13 (50)	4 (15.4)	0.008 *	
	Secondary outcomes			
Number of rescue analgesic events	1.27 ± 1.25 [0, 4]	0.73 ± 0.92 [0, 3]	0.083	−0.54 (−1.15, 0.07)
Rescue analgesic dose (MME)	19.04 ± 18.76 [0, 60.0]	9.83 ± 12.84 [0, 45.0]	0.044 *	−9.21 (−18.16, −0.25)
Number of antiemetic agents required	0.19 ± 0.49 [0, 2]	0.15 ± 0.54 [0, 2]	0.790	−0.04 (−0.33, 0.25)
New onset atrial fibrillation, n (%)	3 (11.5)	3 (11.5)	1.000	
Pneumothorax	0 (0)	0 (0)	1.000	
Wound infection	1 (3.8)	0 (0)	0.313	
Mortality	0 (0)	0 (0)	1.000	
ICU duration (day)	1.27 ± 0.83 [1, 4]	1.12 ± 0.33 [1, 2]	0.382	−0.15 (−0.50, 0.20)
Hospital day (day)	12.50 ± 12.50 [6, 68]	9.73 ± 2.41 [7, 16]	0.277	−2.78 (−7.89, 2.36)-
Time to extubation (min)	671.15 ± 528.07 [185, 2835]	561.15 ± 263.26 [185, 1125]	0.346	−110.00 (−342.43, 122.43)

Values are displayed as the mean ± SD [minimum, maximum] or n (%). The pain score was assessed using a VAS (0 = no pain, 10 = worst imaginable pain). The rescue analgesic requirement was calculated in MME. VAS: visual analog scale; MME: morphine milligram equivalent; ICU: intensive care unit. SD: standard deviation, CI: confidence interval, * = p value < 0.05.

In the multiple regression analysis of VAS at 6 h, taking into account the influence of modifying factors, only ESPB was significantly related to the pain score (Table 3).

Table 3. Multiple regression analysis of VAS at 6 h.

Variable	Regression Coefficient	T Value	p Value
ESPB	−1.386	−2.331	0.025 *
Sex	−0.602	−0.754	0.455
Age	0.001	0.028	0.978
DM	−0.117	−0.182	0.978
EuroSCORE	−0.362	−0.182	0.856
Operation time	−0.008	−1.187	0.242
Graft number	0.084	0.170	0.866
Ejection fraction	0.021	0.712	0.481
Dose of Norepinephrine	−0.001	−0.096	0.924

ESPB is significantly related with VAS pain score at 6 h postoperatively. * = p value < 0.05.

The heart rate and mean arterial pressure (MAP) were similar between the two groups (Figure 2).

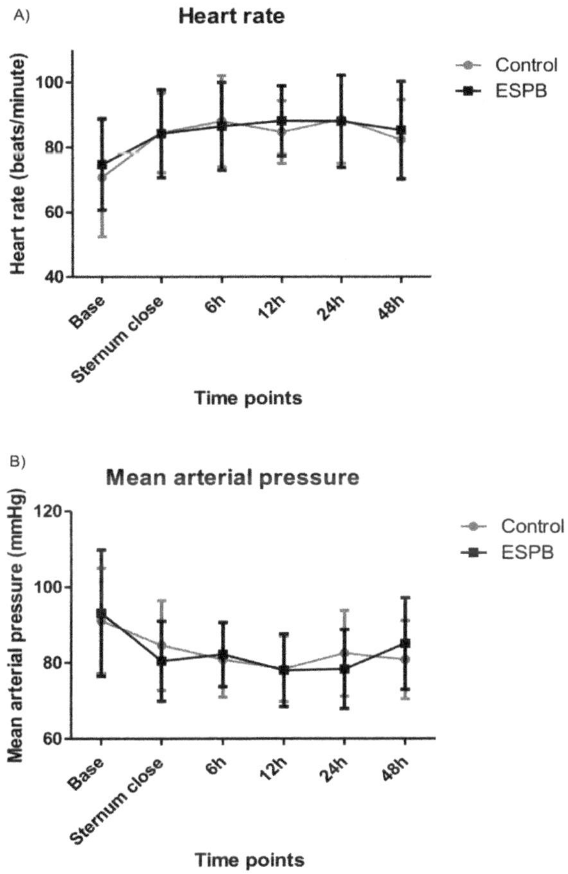

Figure 2. Hemodynamic data: (**A**) heart rate; (**B**) mean arterial pressure. Hemodynamic data did not significantly differ between the ESPB and control group.

4. Discussion

4.1. Discussion

This trial demonstrated that ESPB did not reduce pain scores, which was the primary outcome. However, the incidence of severe pain (VAS score, 7–10) and the dose of rescue analgesics were significantly reduced compared to those in the control group. Although the ESPB did not reduce the pain score, the VAS score at six hours postoperatively showed a statistically significant correlation with ESPB, considering the modifying factors.

In a previous prospective cohort study on 213 patients who underwent CABG surgery, 78% of patients experienced severe pain during coughing, and 49% experienced severe pain at rest [7]. Acute postoperative pain reduces pulmonary function parameters such as tidal volume, vital capacity, functional residual capacity, and pulmonary compliance [8]. The continuous stimulation of the sympathetic nervous system causes an oxygen supply-demand mismatch in the myocardium and dysfunction of the gastrointestinal and urinary systems. Prolonged nociceptor stimulation suppresses the immune system, leading to the infection or inhibition of wound healing [9]. Additionally, severe immediate postoperative pain is associated with the incidence of chronic pain [10].

Despite the cardioprotective function of opioids, it is recommended that their use is limited to anesthetic practice using a multimodal approach. Opioid-induced hyperalgesia and chronic neuropathic pain require another approach to replace opioids from a patient-centered care perspective after cardiac surgery [11]. Additionally, 21.7% of patients continue to use opioids for 3 months after CABG, and the global crisis of opioid dependency has become a major healthcare issue [12]. Various regional block techniques have been investigated; however, evidence supporting their use as standard treatments is lacking [13]. ESPB is a myofascial block similar to the effect of local anesthetics but spreads to the paravertebral and epidural spaces, affecting the dorsal and ventral rami of the spinal nerves [5]. Although its exact mechanism is not well understood, it is a clinical option widely used in various surgeries [14]. OPCAB does not use a cardiopulmonary bypass, and systemic inflammation is less than that in CABG; therefore, the intensity and incidence of pain are lower [15]. Pain after OPCAB occurs because of prolonged sternal retraction and the presence of chest tubes. Rib fractures, costochondritis, rib joint dislocation, left internal mammary artery harvesting, or nerve injury may occur due to sternal retraction. The presence of a chest tube may irritate the parietal pleura or pericardium [16]. The sternum is mainly innervated by spinal nerves T2–T6; however, pain is perceived in a wide area beyond the dermatome because of secondary tissue injury from distant sites [16]. In a previous systematic review, a thoracic epidural block (TEB) reduced the risk of mortality, and the number of patients treated for hematoma was 1:3552, which is very rare [17]. Nevertheless, because of the severity of the complications, there are limited works in the literature guaranteeing the efficacy of TEB in cardiac surgeries, even in OPCAB surgery, which maintains a relatively low anticoagulation time. Therefore, more superficial techniques with a lower risk of complications should be considered [18].

Our results indicated that patients who underwent ESPB experienced less severe pain despite using a lower dose of rescue analgesics after OPCAB surgery. Lower pain scores were observed in the ESPB group than in the control. This beneficial effect is in line with a previous study showing that ESPB reduced pain scores and rescue analgesics after cardiac surgery using CABG [19]. In a previous prospective observational study that investigated the intensity and location after cardiac surgery, the most painful area was the incisional site, and pain intensity diminished from postoperative day 2 [20]. Therefore, controlling acute pain by targeting the intercostal nerve distributed to the sternum is key to analgesia after OPCAB surgery. When performing ESPB, the spread of local anesthetics into the paravertebral space acting on the intercostal nerve, as well as its craniocaudal spread, may be responsible for pain reduction [5].

Regarding the reduction in rescue opioid use, we did not observe significant additional benefits such as shorter extubation time, length of stay, or reduction in the dose of antiemetics. The rescue analgesic doses (19.04 $\pm$ 0.49 vs. 9.83 $\pm$ 12.84, $p = 0.044$) used in this study were similar to a previous study (19.0 $\pm$ 2.6 vs. 11.2 $\pm$ 1.6, $p < 0.001$) comparing ESPB to intravenous PCA after CABG [21]. Despite this significant difference, the rescue doses of opioids used in both groups were too small to confirm the additional benefits.

Adverse effects related to ESPB were similar between the two groups. No significant differences were observed in the incidences of hypotension, bradycardia, or pneumothorax. In a previous review, ESPB-related complications were rare, and the procedure could be safely performed [14].

4.2. Strengths and Limitations

Since it was first described in 2016, publications relating to ESPB have increased remarkably, more than any other block technique [22]. However, there are only a limited number of RCTs [23]. To the best of the authors' knowledge, there are two studies evaluating the effectiveness of ESPB in patients undergoing OPCAB [24,25]. Both studies showed that ESPB was effective. However, one study was retrospective [24], and the other was an observational study [25]. The current trial is a high-quality RCT; therefore, it provides primary evidence that performing ESPB in OPCAB patients may be a safe analgesic option for the primary care physician. In addition, the greatest strength of ESPB is the ease of implementation. In a previous study, the success rate of ESPB and the paravertebral block performed by residents was significantly higher in the ESPB group (100% vs. 77.8%,

p = 0.002), and the duration to a performed block was short (4.39 ± 1.20 min vs. 8.18 ± 2.42 min, p < 0.001) [26]. Under ultrasound guidance, the transverse process can be easily distinguished and distanced from prominent structures, such as the pleura and vessels, as a skill that could be easily acquired.

This trial had several limitations. First, we used a large amount (18 mcg/kg of fentanyl) of opioid-based PCA in both groups. This may be a confounding factor in guaranteeing the block's efficacy. An opioid-based analgesic regimen has been used and adjusted at our institution over the past decade to provide acceptable pain relief. Nevertheless, additional ESPB reduces the need for rescue analgesics, and the incidence of severe pain would be meaningful as a multimodal approach. Second, we only assessed pain scores for up to 48 h. The effectiveness of ESPB would have been more certain if we had evaluated the incidence of chronic pain or changes in the location and intensity of pain over time. However, we already know that pain decreases after 3 days [20] and that the severity of acute pain is a major factor in the transition to chronic pain. Therefore, pain for up to 48 h may be the most important assessment criterion. Third, the sample size may be insufficient for validating the incidence of severe pain, and the dose of analgesic rescues and clinical application may be limited because of the small number of participants. Fourth, we assessed the efficacy of ESPB in a single shot. If we used a continuous block with a catheter or a longer-acting local anesthetics, the analgesic efficacy of ESPB would have been better exhibited. Finally, we performed ESPB with the patient sedated; therefore, block failure might not have been recognized.

4.3. Conclusions

In conclusion, OPCAB requires proper analgesic pain relief without adverse effects such as hematoma or pneumothorax. In line with these needs, the present trial demonstrates that ESPB lowers the incidence of severe pain and reduces the dose of opioids required.

Author Contributions: Conceptualization, S.K. and J.-H.P.; methodology, S.W.S. and S.A.S.; software, S.K. and J.-H.P.; validation, S.K., Y.-G.J. and J.-H.P.; formal analysis, S.K., S.W.S. and Y.-G.J.; investigation, S.K. and S.A.S.; resources, J.-H.P.; data curation, S.W.S., S.A.S. and J.-H.P.; writing—original draft preparation, S.K.; writing—review and editing, Y.-G.J., S.H. and J.-H.P.; visualization, S.K. and J.-H.P.; supervision, S.H. and J.-H.P.; project administration, S.K., S.H. and J.-H.P.; funding acquisition, Y.-G.J. All authors have read and agreed to the published version of the manuscript.

Funding: This research received no external funding.

Institutional Review Board Statement: This study was conducted in accordance with the Declaration of Helsinki and approved by the Institutional Review Board of Yonsei University Wonju College of Medicine (IRB No. CR322089 on 1 November 2022).

Informed Consent Statement: Informed consent was obtained from all subjects involved in this study.

Data Availability Statement: The data presented in this study are available upon request from the corresponding author.

Conflicts of Interest: The authors declare no conflicts of interest.

References

1. Shaefi, S.; Mittel, A.; Loberman, D.; Ramakrishna, H. Off-pump versus on-pump coronary artery bypass grafting-a systematic review and analysis of clinical outcomes. *J. Cardiothorac. Vasc. Anesth.* **2019**, *33*, 232–244. [CrossRef] [PubMed]
2. Ofoegbu, C.K.P.; Manganyi, R.M. Off-Pump Coronary Artery Bypass Grafting; is it Still Relevant? *Curr. Cardiol. Rev.* **2022**, *18*, e271021197431. [CrossRef] [PubMed]
3. Cogan, J. Pain management after cardiac surgery. *Semin. Cardiothorac. Vasc. Anesth.* **2010**, *14*, 201–204. [CrossRef]
4. Korsik, E.; Meineri, M.; Zakhary, W.Z.A.; Balga, I.; Jawad, K.; Ender, J.; Flo Forner, A. Persistent and acute postoperative pain after cardiac surgery with anterolateral thoracotomy or median sternotomy: A prospective observational study. *J. Clin. Anesth.* **2022**, *77*, 110577. [CrossRef]
5. Chin, K.J.; El-Boghdadly, K. Mechanisms of action of the erector spinae plane (ESP) block: A narrative review. *Can. J. Anaesth.* **2021**, *68*, 387–408. [CrossRef]

6. Imantalab, V.; Mirmansouri, A.; Mohammadzadeh Jouryabi, A.; Naderi Nabi, B.; Kanani, G.; Nassiri Sheikhani, N.; Atrkarroushan, Z.; Ghazanfar Tehran, S.; Samadpour, N. Comparing the Effectiveness of Patient Control Analgesia Pump and Bolus Morphine in Controlling Pain After Cardiopulmonary Bypass Graft Surgery. *Anesth. Pain Med.* **2017**, *7*, e12756. [CrossRef] [PubMed]
7. Lahtinen, P.; Kokki, H.; Hynynen, M. Pain after cardiac surgery: A prospective cohort study of 1-year incidence and intensity. *Anesthesiology* **2006**, *105*, 794–800. [CrossRef]
8. Roncada, G.; Dendale, P.; Linsen, L.; Hendrikx, M.; Hansen, D. Reduction in pulmonary function after CABG surgery is related to postoperative inflammation and hypercortisolemia. *Int. J. Clin. Exp. Med.* **2015**, *8*, 10938–10946.
9. Zubrzycki, M.; Liebold, A.; Skrabal, C.; Reinelt, H.; Ziegler, M.; Perdas, E.; Zubrzycka, M. Assessment and pathophysiology of pain in cardiac surgery. *J. Pain Res.* **2018**, *11*, 1599–1611. [CrossRef] [PubMed]
10. Kalso, E.; Mennander, S.; Tasmuth, T.; Nilsson, E. Chronic post-sternotomy pain. *Acta Anaesthesiol. Scand.* **2001**, *45*, 935–939. [CrossRef]
11. Kwanten, L.E.; O'Brien, B.; Anwar, S. Opioid-Based Anesthesia and Analgesia for Adult Cardiac Surgery: History and Narrative Review of the Literature. *J. Cardiothorac. Vasc. Anesth.* **2019**, *33*, 808–816. [CrossRef] [PubMed]
12. Hirji, S.A.; Landino, S.; Cote, C.; Lee, J.; Orhurhu, V.; Shah, R.M.; McGurk, S.; Kaneko, T.; Shekar, P.; Pelletier, M.P. Chronic opioid use after coronary bypass surgery. *J. Card. Surg.* **2019**, *34*, 67–73. [CrossRef]
13. Maeßen, T.; Korir, N.; Van de Velde, M.; Kennes, J.; Pogatzki-Zahn, E.; Joshi, G.P. Pain management after cardiac surgery via median sternotomy: A systematic review with procedure-specific postoperative pain management (PROSPECT) recommendations. *Eur. J. Anaesthesiol.* **2023**, *40*, 758–768. [CrossRef] [PubMed]
14. De Cassai, A.; Bonvicini, D.; Correale, C.; Sandei, L.; Tulgar, S.; Tonetti, T. Erector spinae plane block: A systematic qualitative review. *Minerva Anestesiol.* **2019**, *85*, 308–319. [CrossRef]
15. Saha, S.K.; Ranjan, R.; Adhikary, A.B. Comparison of traditional and upper thoracic epidural analgesia after off-pump coronary artery bypass graft surgery: A Quasi-experimental study. *Health Sci. Rep.* **2022**, *5*, e774. [CrossRef] [PubMed]
16. Mazzeffi, M.; Khelemsky, Y. Poststernotomy pain: A clinical review. *J. Cardiothorac. Vasc. Anesth.* **2011**, *25*, 1163–1178. [CrossRef]
17. Landoni, G.; Isella, F.; Greco, M.; Zangrillo, A.; Royse, C.F. Benefits and risks of epidural analgesia in cardiac surgery. *Br. J. Anaesth.* **2015**, *115*, 25–32. [CrossRef]
18. Caruso, T.J.; Lawrence, K.; Tsui, B.C.H. Regional anesthesia for cardiac surgery. *Curr. Opin. Anaesthesiol.* **2019**, *32*, 674–682. [CrossRef] [PubMed]
19. Krishna, S.N.; Chauhan, S.; Bhoi, D.; Kaushal, B.; Hasija, S.; Sangdup, T.; Bisoi, A.K. Bilateral Erector Spinae Plane Block for Acute Post-Surgical Pain in Adult Cardiac Surgical Patients: A Randomized Controlled Trial. *J. Cardiothorac. Vasc. Anesth.* **2019**, *33*, 368–375. [CrossRef] [PubMed]
20. Mueller, X.M.; Tinguely, F.; Tevaearai, H.T.; Revelly, J.P.; Chioléro, R.; von Segesser, L.K. Pain location, distribution, and intensity after cardiac surgery. *Chest* **2000**, *118*, 391–396. [CrossRef]
21. Oğur, L.; Akesen, S.; Gören, S.; Kan, İ.; Başağan Moğol, E.; Gurbet, A. Comparison of Intra- and postoperative effectiveness of erector spinae plane block and patient controlled analgesia in patients undergoing coronary artery bypass grafting surgery. *Am. J. Transl. Res.* **2022**, *14*, 2469–2479. [PubMed]
22. Saadawi, M.; Layera, S.; Aliste, J.; Bravo, D.; Leurcharusmee, P.; Tran, Q. Erector spinae plane block: A narrative review with systematic analysis of the evidence pertaining to clinical indications and alternative truncal blocks. *J. Clin. Anesth.* **2021**, *68*, 110063. [CrossRef]
23. Pawa, A.; King, C.; Thang, C.; White, L. Erector spinae plane block: The ultimate 'plan A' block? *Br. J. Anaesth.* **2023**, *130*, 497–502. [CrossRef] [PubMed]
24. Coşarcan, S.K.; Doğan, A.T.; Gurkan, Y.; Erçelen, Ö. Analgesic Effect of Dual Injection Technique for the Erector Spinae Plane Block in Beating Heart Coronary By-Pass Surgeries. *Cureus* **2021**, *13*, e14122. [CrossRef]
25. Wiech, M.; Żurek, S.; Kurowicki, A.; Horeczy, B.; Czuczwar, M.; Piwowarczyk, P.; Widenka, K.; Borys, M. Erector Spinae Plane Block Decreases Chronic Postoperative Pain Severity in Patients Undergoing Coronary Artery Bypass Grafting. *J. Clin. Med.* **2022**, *11*, 5949. [CrossRef] [PubMed]
26. Moustafa, M.A.; Alabd, A.S.; Ahmed, A.M.M.; Deghidy, E.A. Erector spinae versus paravertebral plane blocks in modified radical mastectomy: Randomised comparative study of the technique success rate among novice anaesthesiologists. *Indian J. Anaesth.* **2020**, *64*, 49–54. [CrossRef] [PubMed]

Journal of
Clinical Medicine

MDPI

Article

The Anterior Branch of the Medial Femoral Cutaneous Nerve Innervates Cutaneous and Deep Surgical Incisions in Total Knee Arthroplasty

Siska Bjørn [1,2,*], Thomas Dahl Nielsen [2], Anne Errboe Jensen [1], Christian Jessen [1,3], Jens Aage Kolsen-Petersen [1,2], Bernhard Moriggl [4], Romed Hoermann [4] and Thomas Fichtner Bendtsen [1,2]

1 Department of Clinical Medicine, Faculty of Health, Aarhus University, 8200 Aarhus, Denmark; anneerrboejensen@gmail.com (A.E.J.); chijss@rm.dk (C.J.); jenspete@rm.dk (J.A.K.-P.); tfb@dadlnet.dk (T.F.B.)
2 Department of Anesthesiology, Aarhus University Hospital, 8200 Aarhus, Denmark; mail@thomasdahl.eu
3 Department of Anesthesiology, Horsens Regional Hospital, 8700 Horsens, Denmark
4 Institute of Clinical and Functional Anatomy, Department of Anatomy, Histology and Embryology, Medical University of Innsbruck, 6020 Innsbruck, Austria; bernhard.moriggl@i-med.ac.at (B.M.); romed.hoermann@i-med.ac.at (R.H.)
* Correspondence: siskabjoern@clin.au.dk

Abstract: Background/Objectives: The intermediate femoral cutaneous nerve (IFCN), the saphenous nerve, and the medial femoral cutaneous nerve (MFCN) innervate the skin of the anteromedial knee region. However, it is unknown whether the MFCN has a deeper innervation. This would be relevant for total knee arthroplasty (TKA) that intersects deeper anteromedial genicular tissue layers. Primary aim: to investigate deeper innervation of the anterior and posterior MFCN branches (MFCN-A and MFCN-P). Secondary aim: to investigate MFCN innervation of the skin covering the anteromedial knee area and medial parapatellar arthrotomy used for TKA. **Methods:** This study consists of (1) a dissection study and (2) unpublished data and post hoc analysis from a randomized controlled double-blinded volunteer trial (EudraCT number: 2020-004942-12). All volunteers received bilateral active IFCN blocks (nerve block round 1) and saphenous nerve blocks (nerve block round 2). In nerve block round 3, all volunteers were allocated to a selective MFCN-A block. **Results:** (1) The MFCN-A consistently innervated deeper structures in the anteromedial knee region in all dissected specimens. No deep innervation from the MFCN-P was observed. (2) Sixteen out of nineteen volunteers had an unanesthetized skin gap in the anteromedial knee area and eleven out of the nineteen volunteers had an unanesthetized gap on the skin covering the medial parapatellar arthrotomy before the active MFCN-A block. The anteromedial knee area and medial parapatellar arthrotomy was completely anesthetized after the MFCN-A block in 75% and 82% of cases, respectively. **Conclusions:** The MFCN-A shows consistent deep innervation in the anteromedial knee region and the area of MFCN-A innervation overlaps the skin area covering the medial parapatellar arthrotomy. Further trials are mandated to investigate whether an MFCN-A block translates into a clinical effect on postoperative pain after total knee arthroplasty or can be used for diagnosis and interventional pain management for chronic neuropathic pain due to damage to the MFCN-A during surgery.

Keywords: medial femoral cutaneous nerve; total knee arthroplasty; postoperative pain; chronic neuropathic pain

1. Introduction

The medial femoral cutaneous nerve (MFCN) plays a major role in the skin innervation of the anteromedial knee region [1–4]. The MFCN originates from the femoral nerve along with the intermediate femoral cutaneous nerve branches, and together they constitute the anterior femoral cutaneous nerve branches [1,5]. The MFCN divides into an anterior

(MFCN-A) and a posterior branch (MFCN-P) at the apex of the femoral triangle or more proximally [4,6,7]. A recent study focusing on the midline skin incision for total knee arthroplasty showed that the MFCN-A innervated the skin incision in approximately half of the cases, and the MFCN-P innervated the midline incision in zero cases [4]. This knowledge is important because branches from the MFCN-A may be damaged during the surgical skin incision, potentially causing chronic neuropathic pain. The study presented a novel selective block of the MFCN-A, which could be used as a target for both diagnosis and interventional treatment of chronic neuropathic pain [4].

The MFCN is described as a 'skin' nerve in the literature apart from an older dissection study by Horner and Dellon, who briefly mention that the MFCN innervates the medial retinaculum [8]. However, it is not described how this observation was verified or whether it was consistent [8]. For total knee arthroplasty, the currently most common surgical approach is a midline skin incision followed by a medial parapatellar arthrotomy through the deeper tissue layers [9,10]. Our clinical observation is that a subgroup of patients after total knee arthroplasty complain of pain in the anteromedial knee region despite a distal femoral triangle block in the midthigh anesthetizing the saphenous nerve and the medial vastus nerve. This residual pain could be caused solely by insufficient anesthesia of the midline skin incision or because the MFCN has a deeper innervation in the anteromedial knee region including the medial retinaculum.

We hypothesized that the MFCN-A innervates deeper structures in the anteromedial knee region and that the MFCN-A is the main contributor to the innervation of the area covering the medial parapatellar arthrotomy.

Our objective was to investigate whether the MFCN-A and MFCN-P are solely skin nerve branches as indicated by the name and the literature, or if they have a consistent deeper innervation in the anteromedial knee region. A secondary aim was to investigate the contribution from the MFCN to the innervation of the skin area covering the medial parapatellar arthrotomy used for total knee arthroplasty and to the entire anteromedial knee area.

2. Materials and Methods

This study consists of a dissection study and unpublished data from a randomized controlled double-blinded volunteer trial (EudraCT number: 2020-004942-12) and a post hoc analysis performed on data from this trial.

2.1. Ultrasound-Guided MFCN-A Block

Block technique for the selective MFCN-A block was originally described by Bjørn et al. [4]. The subject is placed supine and the femoral artery identified at the level of the inguinal crease and followed distally. The needle insertion point for the selective MFCN-A block is approximately at the level of the apex of the femoral triangle. Depending on the level of optimal visualization the block can be performed where the MFCN-A is centered on top of the sartorius in cross-sectional view or slightly more distal towards the anterolateral border of the muscle. The MFCN-A descends across the anterior side of the sartorius muscle embedded in a duplicature of the fascia lata (Figure 1) [4].

In the dissection study, the selective MFCN-A block was performed at a more distal level [11]. The MFCN-A is often more easily seen approximately at the level of the base of the patella, and therefore this distal approach was used in cadavers where ultrasound visualization is notoriously difficult (Figure 2). In the volunteer study, the more proximal approach described above was applied in order to anesthetize all branches from the MFCN-A [4].

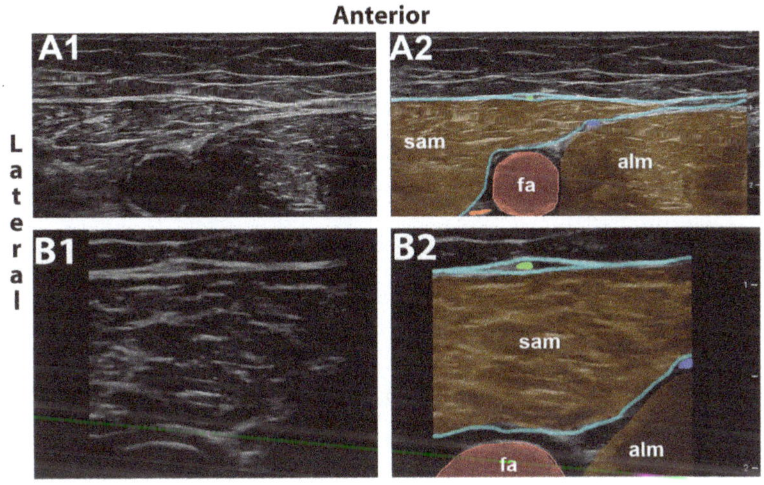

Figure 1. MFCN-A block used in volunteers. Ultrasound images showing the level of injection for the MFCN-A block without (**A1**) and with (**A2**) color overlay using 15 MHz. (**B1**) and (**B2**) is a 19 MHz image without and with color overlay corresponding to (**A1**) and (**A2**). MFCN-A (green dot) can be approached selectively in a duplicature of the fascia lata anterior to the sartorius muscle (sam). Adductor longus muscle, alm; posterior branch of medial femoral cutaneous nerve, blue dot; saphenous nerve, orange dot.

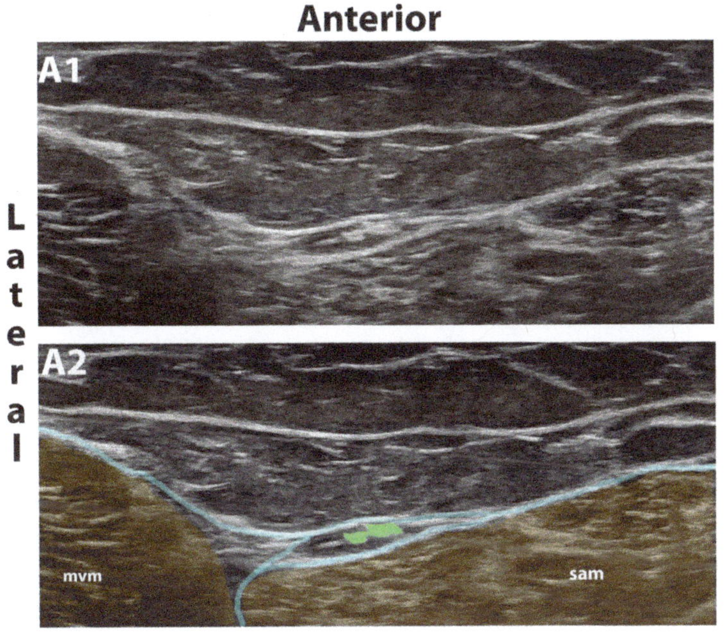

Figure 2. Distal MFCN-A block used in cadavers. Ultrasound image without (**A1**) and with (**A2**) color overlay showing a more distal approach to the selective MFCN-A block compared to Figure 1. The MFCN-A (green dots) is often more easily seen at this distal level approximately at the level of the base of the patella and was therefore used in cadavers where visualization was difficult. The distal approach is not advisable in patients because the MFCN-A has often split into several branches at this level. Mvm, medial vastus muscle; sam, sartorius muscle; fascia lata, cyan lines.

2.2. Dissection Study

The dissection study was performed on 16 intact cadaver sides from 8 cadavers donated to the Institute of Clinical and Functional Anatomy of the Medical University of Innsbruck for scientific and educational purposes. In the supine cadaver, the MFCN-A was identified using ultrasound (Figure 2) and marked by injection of 0.1 mL high viscosity special dye.

All injections were performed by the authors Nielsen and Bendtsen. Subsequently, standardized dissections were performed by two other authors, Moriggl and Hoermann. The outcomes of the dissection study were (A) correct identification of the MFCN-A by ultrasound (see below) and (B) MFCN-A and MFCN-P innervation of deeper structures (i.e., deep to the fascia lata) in the anteromedial knee region by dissection. (A): Decision of 'Correct identification of the MFCN-A by ultrasound' required that the MFCN-A was correctly stained by injected dye, and that correct identity of the stained MFCN-A was verified by tracing it back to the origin from the MFCN and further to the origin from the femoral nerve during dissection. Meticulous care was taken to separate the MFCN-A from the intermediate femoral cutaneous nerve during dissection. (B): Verification of innervation from the MFCN-A and MFCN-P to deeper structures (i.e., deep to the fascia lata) required that terminal branches from the MFCN-A and MFNC-P could be followed distally and seen to dive into the medial retinaculum.

2.3. Volunteer Study

The trial included 20 healthy volunteers of 18 years or older and American Society of Anesthesiology (ASA) I and II classification. Exclusion criteria were inability to cooperate, weight < 60 kg (to avoid local anesthetic systemic toxicity), body mass index > 28, pregnancy, allergy towards local anesthetics, daily use of medicine except oral contraceptives, infection around injection sites and lower limb neuropathy. Lower limb neuropathy was excluded if the volunteer reported no chronic pain in the lower limb and demonstrated normal sensation to pinprick in the dermatomes L2, L3, L4, L5 and S1. The study was conducted on the 12 and 13 December 2020 at the Department of Day Surgery, Aarhus University Hospital.

With a skin marker, a standard midline skin incision and a medial parapatellar arthrotomy were drawn bilaterally in all volunteers (Figure 3). Of note, the medial parapatellar arthrotomy exclusively transects tissue layers deep to the skin, but it was drawn on the skin as a visual proxy marker (Figure 3).

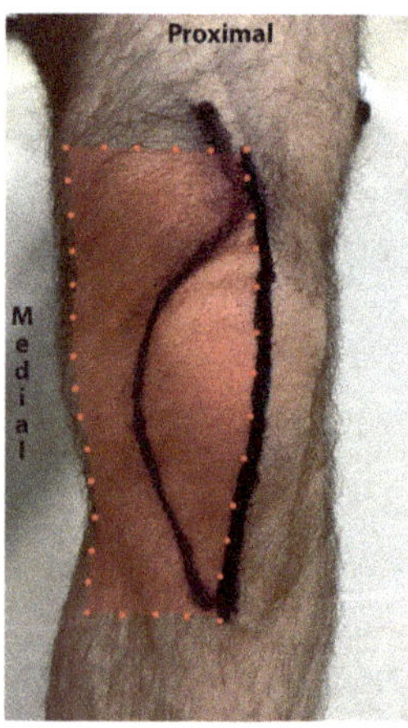

Figure 3. The figure shows a left leg where the midline skin incision and a curved line corresponding to a parapatellar arthrotomy are drawn on the skin. Of note, the parapatellar arthrotomy extends proximal to the midline incision and therefore proximal to the border of the anteromedial knee area shown in red. The anteromedial knee area is defined by the midline skin incision and a vertical line through the medial epicondyle (vertical red stippled line). Note that the parapatellar arthrotomy was drawn per protocol whereas the anteromedial knee area was estimated as a post hoc analysis.

Drawing of the parapatellar arthrotomy was described per protocol in the original study; however, these data have not been published previously [4]. In the volunteer trial, active nerve blocks were performed with 0.25% bupivacaine with 1:200,000 epinephrine [4]. All volunteers received bilateral active intermediate femoral cutaneous nerve blocks in the first block round (7 mL) and active bilateral distal femoral triangle blocks in the second block round (10 mL) (Figure 4).

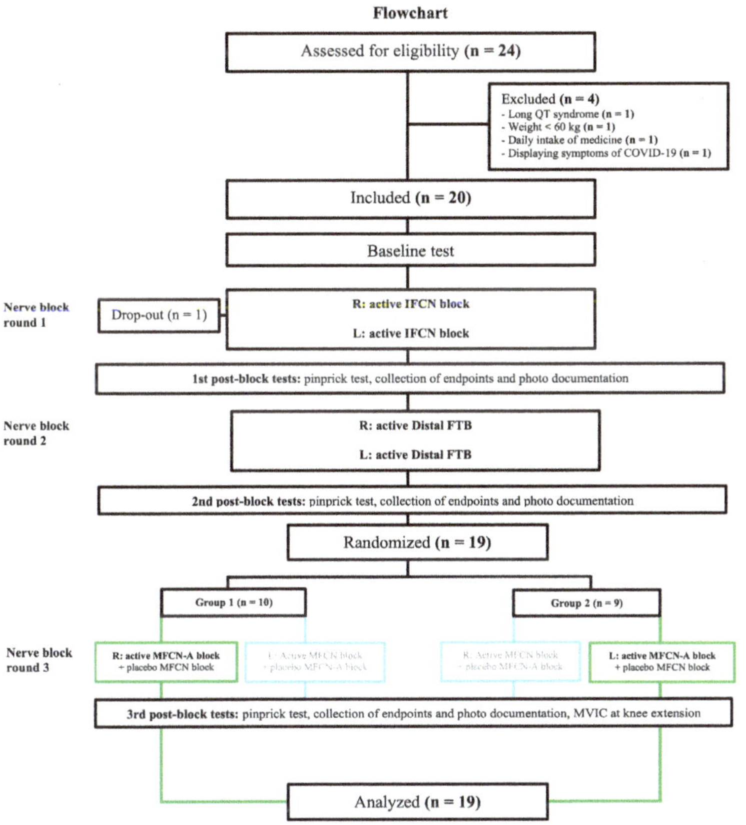

Figure 4. Flowchart. This flowchart presents the design of the nerve block rounds 1, 2 and 3. The original study included a fourth nerve block round, which is not relevant for the present study and not shown [4]. Nerve block rounds 1 and 2 only include active bilateral blocks, as the purpose was to find the subgroup with a non-anesthetized anteromedial skin gap after intermediate femoral cutaneous nerve and saphenous nerve blocks. In nerve block round 3, volunteers received an active block of the MFCN-A on one side (green boxes, bold text). This enabled analysis of how often the MFCN-A anesthetized the skin gap on the anteromedial knee area including the skin area corresponding to the parapatellar arthrotomy. Therefore, this side was the only relevant side for the present post hoc analysis (green boxes, bold text). In the original study the active block of the MFCN-A was combined with a placebo block of both the anterior and posterior branches from the MFCN on the same side (MFCN block) and vice versa on the other side (blue boxes, faded text); however, this was not relevant for the present post hoc analysis. Active indicates bupivacaine 0.25% with epinephrine 1:200,000; placebo indicates saline. FTB: femoral triangle block; IFCN block: intermediate femoral cutaneous nerve block; L: left leg; MFCN block: medial femoral cutaneous nerve block (block of both the anterior and posterior branch); MFCN-A block: selective block of the anterior branch from the MFCN; R: right leg.

For the intermediate femoral cutaneous nerve block (nerve block round 1) the transducer was placed transversely on the proximal anterior thigh. The intermediate femoral cutaneous nerves (typically two main branches) were targeted where they pierce the fascia lata. They are seen ultrasonographically in a duplicature of the fascia lata or in the subcutis [4]. This is the level of the proximal femoral triangle where the femoral artery has just dived deep to the medial border of the sartorius muscle.

The distal femoral triangle block (nerve block round 2) was performed as previously described [1,4]. The apex of the femoral triangle was identified ultrasonographically where the medial border of the sartorius muscle crosses the medial border of the adductor longus muscle. The needle insertion point was approximately 3–5 cm proximal to the apex of the femoral triangle and the target was the saphenous nerve located anterolateral to the femoral artery.

The intermediate femoral cutaneous nerves innervate the skin covering the anteromedial aspect of the proximal two-thirds of the thigh [1,2]. The infrapatellar branch of the saphenous nerve typically innervates the proximal anteromedial aspect of the lower leg. A distal femoral triangle block at the midthigh level anesthetizes the saphenous nerve including its infrapatellar branch [1,4]. Therefore, the purpose of the first two nerve block rounds was to identify the subgroup of volunteers with a non-anesthetized gap on the parapatellar arthrotomy and in the anteromedial knee area after combined intermediate femoral cutaneous nerve and saphenous nerve blocks.

Subsequently, in the third block round, all volunteers were randomly allocated to an active selective block of MFCN-A (5 mL) on one side (right or left leg) and a placebo MFCN-A block on the contralateral leg (Figure 4). This allowed for estimation of how often the MFCN-A anesthetizes the gap. The randomization only served the purpose of blinding the investigators with no intention of intergroup comparisons.

Thirty minutes after each block round, pinprick tests were performed using a sterile neurological examination pen (Neuropen, Owen Mumford, Woodstock, UK) to define the anesthetized areas on the skin. The first points where the volunteer felt normal, sharp sensation were marked as the circumference of the anesthetized area. All examinations were performed under strict blinding marking the anesthetized areas on the skin with ink only visible in ultraviolet light (i.e., ultraviolet pens), ensuring blinding of the investigator performing the next sensory test [4].

The 'anteromedial knee area' was defined as the area between the midline skin incision and a parallel line through the medial femoral epicondyle. The proximal and distal borders was defined by horizontal lines through the most proximal and distal points on the midline skin incision (Figure 3) [1].

The primary study group for outcomes A and C (see below) was the subgroup of volunteers who had a non-anesthetized gap in the anteromedial knee area after intermediate femoral cutaneous nerve and distal femoral triangle blocks (i.e., after the first two block rounds).

The outcomes were as follows: (A) Anesthesia of the medial parapatellar arthrotomy after MFCN-A block; (B) Frequencies of contribution to anesthesia of the medial parapatellar arthrotomy by MFCN-A block, distal femoral triangle block, and intermediate femoral cutaneous nerve block; (C) Anesthesia of the anteromedial knee area after MFCN-A block.

2.4. Statistics

Only descriptive statistics were applied for this analysis.

3. Results

3.1. Dissection Study

In three out of sixteen cadaver sides, dissection of the terminal part of the MFCN-A was not possible due to the condition of the cadaver. In all 13 dissected specimens, it was verified that the MFCN-A had been correctly identified sonographically and marked by ultrasound-guided injection of a special dye.

In 100% of specimens (13/13), it was verified that the MFCN-A branches innervated deeper structures (i.e., deep to the fascia lata) including the medial retinaculum in the anteromedial knee region (Figure 5(A2,B)). The MFCN-P exclusively innervated the skin in the most postero-medial part of the anteromedial knee area or posterior to this area in all 13 specimens with no deep innervation observed.

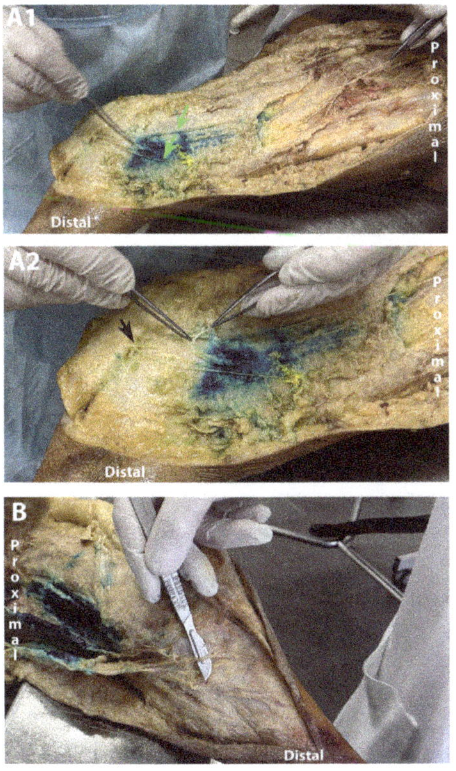

Figure 5. Dissection of the anteromedial knee region. (**A1**,**A2**) show the right side from the same cadaver. In (**A1**), the MFCN-A (lifted by tweezers) gives off minor nerve twigs before splitting into two major branches (green arrows). One of these branches is marked by special dye injection (yellow). The reason that all branches were not targeted was due to the more distal approach used in cadavers (Figure 2). In (**A2**), deep branches from MFCN-A are lifted by tweezers. MFCN-A is also seen to give cutaneous branches (**A2**, black arrow). (**B**) shows the left side from a different cadaver where deep branches from the MFCN-A are indicated by the scalpel. The injection of methylene blue was part of another dissection study and is not related to data captured for the present study.

In eleven specimens, the point of injection was proximal to any major bifurcations of the MFCN-A. In two cases, the MFCN-A bifurcated into two large branches proximal to the point of injection, and only one of the two branches was marked by special dye (Figure 5(A1)). In all 13 specimens, several branches from the MFCN-A were consistently seen to branch off proximal to the point of injection.

3.2. Volunteer Study

Twenty volunteers were enrolled, and nineteen volunteers completed the study [4]. Demographics are depicted in Table 1.

An example of a typical innervation pattern can be seen in Figure 6.

Table 1. Demographics of the volunteers who completed the study.

Number of volunteers	19
Age, mean (SD)	23.6 (2.8) years
Sex, n (%)	
Male	13 (68%)
Female	6 (32%)
ASA status, n (%)	
ASA I	19 (100%)
ASA II	0 (0%)
Height, mean (SD)	180.0 (9.2) cm
Weight, mean (SD)	75.3 (9.5) kg
BMI, mean (SD)	23.2 (1.9)

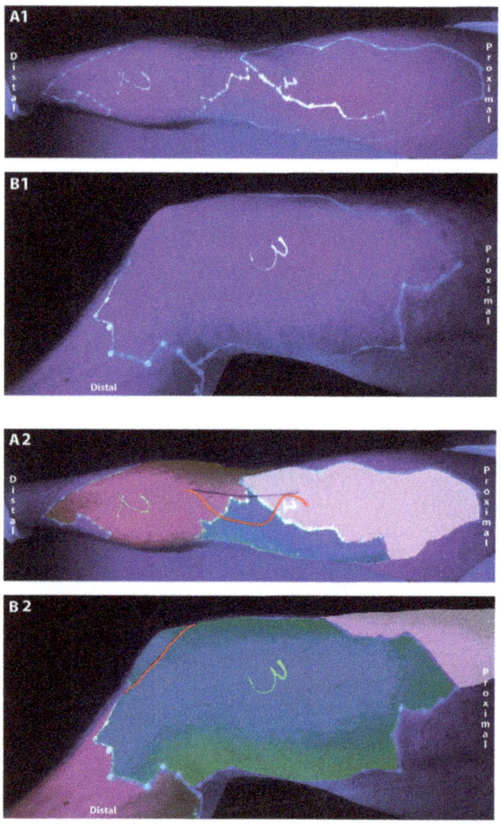

Figure 6. Cutaneous innervation areas. The figure shows a typical example of the cutaneous innervation of the anteromedial knee region in a volunteer seen in anterior (**A1**,**A2**) and medial view (**B1**,**B2**) without (**A1**,**B1**) and with color overlay (**A2**,**B2**). The picture is taken under ultraviolet light because the anesthetized areas were drawn with UV pens invisible to the naked eye. The anesthetized areas after intermediate femoral cutaneous nerve block (light lilac area, #1), distal femoral triangle block (saphenous nerve territory, orange area, #2) and MFCN-A block (green area, #3) are seen in both views. The midline skin incision and medial parapatellar arthrotomy are seen as a black and a red line, respectively (**A2**).

A non-anesthetized gap of the skin covering the medial parapatellar arthrotomy was present after intermediate femoral cutaneous nerve and saphenous nerve blocks in 11 out of the 19 volunteer legs (58%) allocated to receive an active MFCN-A block in block round 3 (Figure 4). The frequency of complete anesthesia of the gap after the MFCN-A block was 9 out of 11 (82%).

The frequencies of contribution to the innervation of the skin covering the medial parapatellar arthrotomy were as follows: MFCN-A 9/19 cases (47%), intermediate femoral cutaneous nerve 19/19 cases (100%), and saphenous nerve 16/19 cases (84%).

A non-anesthetized gap of the skin in the anteromedial knee region was present after intermediate femoral cutaneous nerve and saphenous nerve blocks in 16 out of the 19 volunteer legs (84%) allocated to receive an active MFCN-A block in block round 3 (Figure 4). The frequency of complete anesthesia of the gap after the MFCN-A block was 12 out of 16 (75%).

4. Discussion

The results from the dissection study show that the MFCN-A consistently innervates genicular layers deep to the skin in the anteromedial knee region including the medial retinaculum. This is an interesting finding because the MFCN-A is described as an exclusively cutaneous nerve in the literature apart from a brief mentioning of an innervation to the medial retinaculum by Horner and Dellon [8]. The deep innervation from the MFCN-A makes it relevant in relation to medial parapatellar arthrotomy. The fact that the MFCN-A is not only a cutaneous nerve but also innervates deeper structures in a large area of the anteromedial knee region makes it potentially interesting in relation to acute postoperative pain in the anteromedial knee area. Furthermore, deep branches from the MFCN-A may be injured during medial parapatellar arthrotomy and could therefore potentially cause neuropathic pain after total knee arthroplasty.

No deep innervation by the MFCN-P in the anteromedial knee region was observed during dissection in any cadavers. Thus, MFCN-P innervation of the skin covering the medial parapatellar arthrotomy is not a relevant proxy marker of deep innervation, and no risk of intersection of MFCN-P branches during a medial parapatellar arthrotomy would be present.

The results from the volunteer trial show a high frequency of incomplete anesthesia of the anteromedial knee region including the medial parapatellar arthrotomy after an intermediate femoral cutaneous nerve block and a distal femoral triangle (i.e., saphenous nerve) block. The addition of an MFCN-A block in the third block round effectively anesthetized the skin in the anteromedial knee region including the skin over the medial parapatellar arthrotomy in most cases. The fact that the success rate of complete cutaneous coverage of the gap after a selective MFCN-A block is high shows that the MFCN-A and not the MFCN-P is the important branch for complete cutaneous anesthesia of medial parapatellar arthrotomy and the anteromedial knee area. The dissection showed a consistent deep innervation from the MFCN-A and not the MFCN-P in the anteromedial knee area in all cadavers. This suggests that the MFCN-A could potentially be accountable for acute nociceptive pain and chronic neuropathic pain in the anteromedial knee region after total knee arthroplasty including the area of the medial parapatellar arthrotomy.

Based on our results from dissection and a volunteer trial, it is not possible to assess whether the deep MFCN-A innervation of the anteromedial knee region translates into a clinical effect in relation to acute pain after total knee arthroplasty. Very few studies have investigated the effect of a selective block of the MFCN on acute pain after total knee arthroplasty. Kampitak et al. showed that a selective block of the anterior femoral cutaneous nerve branches (i.e., an intermediate femoral cutaneous nerve block and MFCN block) combined with a distal femoral triangle block significantly improved acute pain relief after total knee arthroplasty compared to a standalone distal femoral triangle block [12,13]. Furthermore, several clinical studies have compared an injection lateral to the femoral artery at the level where the medial border of the sartorius muscle first covers the femoral artery (i.e., in the proximal femoral triangle) to an injection at the midthigh level midway between the anterior superior iliac spine and the base of the patella (distal femoral triangle block) [14–17]. The difference between the proximal and distal approach to the femoral triangle block is that the MFCN may be anesthetized by the proximal approach. Two of the studies observed superior pain relief in the group receiving a proximal femoral triangle block after total knee arthroplasty and anterior cruciate ligament reconstruction, respectively [16,17]. The studies detecting no difference between a proximal and distal femoral triangle block in relation to acute pain after total knee arthroplasty were powered to detect only very large reductions in opioid consumption [16,17]. The results showed a clear tendency of improved pain relief in the proximal group compared to the distal; however, the difference did not reach statistical significance [16,17]. Importantly, the MFCN was not specifically targeted during the proximal approach in any of the cited studies which may also have reduced the intergroup difference in postoperative pain [14–17]. Thus, clinical trials investigating the effect of supplemental anesthesia of the MFCN-A on pain after total knee arthroplasty are needed. In our clinical experience, a large subgroup of patients complains of acute pain in the anteromedial knee region after total knee arthroplasty despite a successful combined femoral triangle block and intermediate femoral cutaneous nerve block. This residual pain is typically relieved by the selective MFCN-A block. In addition, we have identified a large group of patients with chronic neuropathic pain in the anteromedial knee region allocated to our outpatient nerve injury clinic. This chronic neuropathic pain is often relieved by a diagnostic selective MFCN-A block, which identifies MFCN-A as a target of interventional pain management.

The main limitation of this study is that it is primarily based on cadaver dissection and healthy volunteers, and therefore the relevance in the clinical setting remains to be clarified. Future studies on patients undergoing total knee arthroplasty are needed to investigate the importance of the MFCN-A in the clinical setting. Another limitation is that part of the volunteer study is a post hoc analysis. Two of the outcomes (A and B) were, however, prospectively planned per protocol. Furthermore, it is a limitation that the anesthesia of the medial parapatellar arthrotomy was assessed by anesthesia of the congruent skin territory as a proxy marker in the healthy volunteers. However, the dissection study demonstrated consistent MFCN-A innervation to the deep layers in the anteromedial knee region.

5. Conclusions

In conclusion, our results from the dissection showed that the MFCN-A consistently innervates deeper structures in the anteromedial knee region including the medial retinaculum. Furthermore, results from our volunteer study showed that the anteromedial knee region including the skin area covering the medial parapatellar arthrotomy for total knee arthroplasty is incompletely anesthetized by the combined intermediate femoral cutaneous nerve and saphenous nerve blocks in the majority of cases. An additional MFCN-A block anesthetizes this area with a high success rate. Future clinical trials are needed to investigate whether anesthesia of the MFCN-A is important for relief of acute pain after total knee arthroplasty. Furthermore, the MFCN-A is at high risk of transection not only during the midline skin incision, but also during the parapatellar arthrotomy used for total knee arthroplasty due to the deep innervation. The MFCN-A may therefore potentially be involved in the development of chronic neuropathic pain after total knee arthroplasty.

Author Contributions: Conceptualization, S.B., T.D.N. and T.F.B.; Data curation, S.B.; Formal analysis, S.B., T.D.N., J.A.K.-P. and T.F.B.; Funding acquisition, T.F.B.; Investigation, S.B., T.D.N., A.E.J., C.J., B.M., R.H. and T.F.B.; Methodology, S.B., T.D.N. and T.F.B.; Resources, T.F.B.; Supervision, J.A.K.-P., T.D.N. and T.F.B.; Validation, S.B., T.D.N., A.E.J., C.J., J.A.K.-P., B.M., R.H. and T.F.B.; Writing—original draft, S.B.; Writing—review and editing, S.B., T.D.N., A.E.J., C.J., J.A.K.-P., B.M., R.H. and T.F.B. All authors have read and agreed to the published version of the manuscript.

Funding: This study was funded by the Salling Foundation (grant number 68670) and Aarhus University Research Foundation (Research training supplement). The content is solely the responsibility of the authors.

Institutional Review Board Statement: This study contains unpublished data and a post hoc analysis from a randomized, controlled double-blinded trial involving healthy subjects. The unpublished data and post hoc analysis are from a trial approved by the Danish Medicines Agency, the Central Denmark Region Committee on Health Research Ethics (date of approval 30 November 2020; Ethics Committee number: 1-10-72-266-20) and prospectively registered in the EudraCT database (EudraCT number: 2020-004942-12) [4]. The Good Clinical Practice Unit at Aalborg and Aarhus University Hospitals monitored the trial and written, informed consent was obtained from all subjects prior to inclusion

Informed Consent Statement: Informed consent was obtained from all subjects involved in the study.

Data Availability Statement: The data presented in this study are available on request from the corresponding author. The data are not publicly available in order to maintain participant privacy.

Conflicts of Interest: Thomas F. Bendtsen has obtained funding from the Sailing Foundation. The Sailing Foundation played no role in the data collection or analysis of data.

References

1. Bjørn, S.; Nielsen, T.D.; Moriggl, B.; Hoermann, R.; Bendtsen, T.F. Anesthesia of the femoral cutaneous nerves for total knee arthroplasty incision: Randomized volunteer trial. *Reg. Anesth. Pain. Med.* **2020**, *45*, 107–116. [CrossRef] [PubMed]
2. Riegler, G.; Pivec, C.; Jengojan, S.; Mayer, J.A.; Schellen, C.; Trattnig, S.; Bodner, G. Cutaneous nerve fields of the anteromedial lower limb—Determination with selective ultrasound-guided nerve blockade. *Clin. Anat.* **2021**, *34*, 11–18. [CrossRef] [PubMed]
3. Monahan, A.M.; Sztain, J.F.; Khatibi, B.; Furnish, T.J.; Jæger, P.; Sessler, D.I.; Mascha, E.J.; You, J.; Wen, C.H.; Nakanote, K.A.; et al. Continuous Adductor Canal Blocks: Does Varying Local Anesthetic Delivery Method (Automatic Repeated Bolus Doses Versus Continuous Basal Infusion) Influence Cutaneous Analgesia and Quadriceps Femoris Strength? A Randomized, Double-Masked, Controlled, Split-Body Volunteer Study. *Anesth. Analg.* **2016**, *122*, 1681–1688. [PubMed]
4. Bjørn, S.; Nielsen, T.D.; Jensen, A.E.; Jessen, C.; Kolsen-Petersen, J.A.; Moriggl, B.; Hoermann, R.; Nyengaard, J.R.; Bendtsen, T.F. The anterior branch of the medial femoral cutaneous nerve innervates the anterior knee: A randomized volunteer trial. *Minerva Anestesiol.* **2023**, *89*, 643–652. [CrossRef] [PubMed]
5. Romanes, G.J. *Cunningham's Text-Book of Anatomy*, 12th ed.; Oxford University Press: Oxford, UK, 1981; pp. 794–795.
6. Standring, S. (Ed.) *Gray's Anatomy*, 39th ed.; Elsevier Limited: Amsterdam, The Netherlands, 2005; p. 1470.
7. Lee, H.J.; Bach, J.R.; DeLisa, J.A. Medial femoral cutaneous nerve conduction. *Am. J. Phys. Med. Rehabil.* **1995**, *74*, 305–307. [CrossRef]
8. Horner, G.; Dellon, A.L. Innervation of the human knee joint and implications for surgery. *Clin. Orthop. Relat. Res.* **1994**, *301*, 221–226. [CrossRef]
9. Sanna, M.; Sanna, C.; Caputo, F.; Piu, G.; Salvi, M. Surgical approaches in total knee arthroplasty. *Joints* **2013**, *1*, 34–44. [PubMed]
10. Scott, W.N. (Ed.) *Insall & Scott. Surgery of the Knee*, 6th ed.; Elsevier: Amsterdam, The Netherlands, 2018; pp. 1653–1664.
11. Gong, W.Y.; Li, C.G.; Fan, K. A novel ultrasound-guided anterior branch of medial femoral cutaneous nerve block. *Minerva Anestesiol.* **2021**, *87*, 1387–1388. [CrossRef]
12. Kampitak, W.; Tanavalee, A.; Tansatit, T.; Ngarmukos, S.; Songborassamee, N.; Vichainarong, C. The analgesic efficacy of anterior femoral cutaneous nerve block in combination with femoral triangle block in total knee arthroplasty: A randomized controlled trial. *Korean J. Anesthesiol.* **2021**, *74*, 496–505. [CrossRef] [PubMed]
13. Johnston, D.F.; Sondekoppam, R.V.; Uppal, V.; Howard, J.L.; Ganapathy, S. Hybrid Blocks for Total Knee Arthroplasty: A Technical Description. *Clin. J. Pain.* **2018**, *34*, 222–230. [CrossRef] [PubMed]
14. Romano, C.; Lloyd, A.; Nair, S.; Wang, J.Y.; Viswanathan, S.; Vydyanathan, A.; Gritsenko, K.; Shaparin, N.; Kosharskyy, B. A Randomized Comparison of Pain Control and Functional Mobility between Proximal and Distal Adductor Canal Blocks for Total Knee Replacement. *Anesth. Essays Res.* **2018**, *12*, 452–458. [CrossRef] [PubMed]
15. Meier, A.W.; Auyong, D.B.; Yuan, S.C.; Lin, S.E.; Flaherty, J.M.; Hanson, N.A. Comparison of Continuous Proximal Versus Distal Adductor Canal Blocks for Total Knee Arthroplasty: A Randomized, Double-Blind, Noninferiority Trial. *Reg. Anesth. Pain. Med.* **2018**, *43*, 36–42. [CrossRef] [PubMed]
16. Mariano, E.R.; Kim, T.E.; Wagner, M.J.; Funck, N.; Harrison, T.K.; Walters, T.; Giori, N.; Woolson, S.; Ganaway, T.; Howard, S.K. A randomized comparison of proximal and distal ultrasound-guided adductor canal catheter insertion sites for knee arthroplasty. *J. Ultrasound Med.* **2014**, *33*, 1653–1662. [CrossRef] [PubMed]
17. Abdallah, F.W.; Mejia, J.; Prasad, G.A.; Moga, R.; Chahal, J.; Theodoropulos, J.; Dwyer, T.; Brull, R. Opioid- and Motor-sparing with Proximal, Mid-, and Distal Locations for Adductor Canal Block in Anterior Cruciate Ligament Reconstruction: A Randomized Clinical Trial. *Anesthesiology* **2019**, *131*, 619–629. [CrossRef] [PubMed]

Journal of
Clinical Medicine

MDPI

Review

Peripheral Nerve Blocks for Hip Fractures

Iyabo O. Muse [1,*], Brittany Deiling [1], Leon Grinman [1], Michael M. Hadeed [2] and Nabil Elkassabany [1]

[1] Department of Anesthesiology, University of Virginia Health System, Charlottesville, VA 22908, USA; bd8hp@uvahealth.org (B.D.); hzg6vu@uvahealth.org (L.G.); ekq8wm@uvahealth.org (N.E.)

[2] Department of Orthopedic Surgery, University of Virginia Health System, Charlottesville, VA 22903, USA; mmh2j@uvahealth.org

* Correspondence: uks9ne@uvahealth.org

Abstract: The incidence of hip fractures has continued to increase as life expectancy increases. Hip fracture is one of the leading causes of increased morbidity and mortality in the geriatric population. Early surgical treatment (<48 h) is often recommended to reduce morbidity/mortality. In addition, adequate pain management is crucial to optimize functional recovery and early mobilization. Pain management often consists of multimodal therapy which includes non-opioids, opioids, and regional anesthesia techniques. In this review, we describe the anatomical innervation of the hip joint and summarize the commonly used peripheral nerve blocks to provide pain relief for hip fractures. We also outline literature evidence that shows each block's efficacy in providing adequate pain relief. The recent discovery of a nerve block that may provide adequate sensory blockade of the posterior capsule of the hip is also described. Finally, we report a surgeon's perspective on nerve blocks for hip fractures.

Keywords: fascia iliaca block; pericapsular nerve group (PENG) block; lateral femoral cutaneous nerve

1. Introduction

Hip fracture is common among the elderly population (age > 65 yrs.) and is one of the leading causes of increased morbidity and mortality in the geriatric population. Surgical treatment within 48 h is often recommended to decrease perioperative morbidity [1]. There are several surgical procedures indicated based on the specific type of fracture and patient characteristics including open reduction internal fixation, hip hemiarthroplasty, and/or total hip arthroplasty. For optimal recovery, decreased postoperative delirium, and the early mobilization of patients, an effective pain management protocol is necessary. Pain management often consists of multimodal therapy which includes non-opioids, opioids, and regional anesthesia techniques. Peripheral nerve blocks, a component of regional anesthesia, have been shown to improve postoperative pain, reduce morphine consumption, and increase patient satisfaction after hip surgery [2]. Studies show that the use of peripheral nerve blocks and multimodal analgesia techniques may reduce the incidence of delirium and facilitate early mobilization, thus ultimately reducing morbidity and post-op 1-year mortality after hip surgery [3,4]. In this article, peripheral nerve blocks used to provide analgesia for hip fractures and their efficacy are discussed.

2. Anatomic Innervation of Hip Joint

The target nerves of the hip joint arise from the lumbar plexus (L1–L4), the lumbosacral trunk of the sacral plexus (L4–L5), and the sacral spinal nerves (S1–S4). The femoral nerve, obturator nerve, and the accessory obturator nerve supply the anterior capsule of the hip; the sciatic nerve and the nerve to the quadratus femoris mostly supply the articular branches to the posterior capsule of the hip joint. It is understood that the anterior capsule supplied by the femoral nerve, accessory obturator nerve, and the superior labrum are the predominant causes of pain in the hip joint [5,6] (Figure 1A,B). However, the site of pain is determined by the area of the femur where the fracture occurred. Most hip fractures occur in the femoral neck or intertrochanteric area (Figure 2) [7].

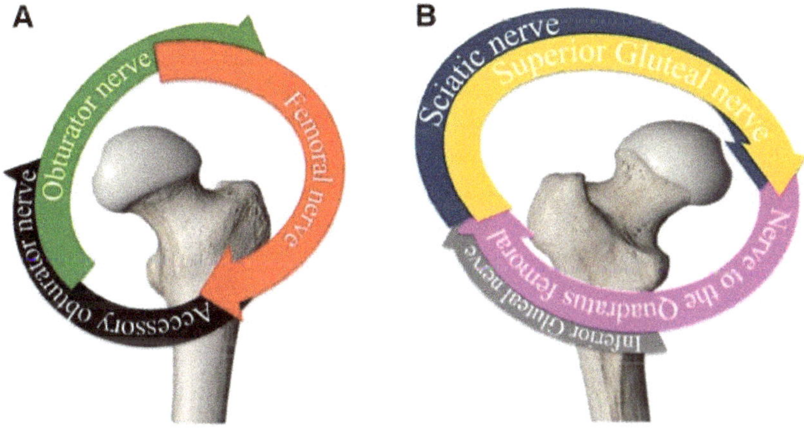

Figure 1. Schematic diagram of the nerve supply of quadrants of the hip joint: (**A**) anterior and (**B**) posterior views. Reproduced with permission from Laumonerie et al., Pain Medicine; published by Oxford University Press, 2021 [6].

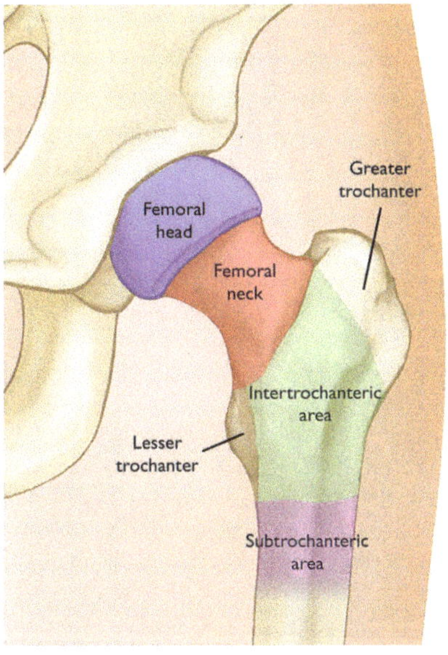

Figure 2. The areas of the femur. Most hip fractures occur in the femoral neck or intertrochanteric area. Reproduced with permission from Fischer, S and Gray, J, OrthoInfo; published by American Academy of Orthopedic Surgeons, 2020 [7].

3. Peripheral Nerve Blocks

There are several peripheral nerve blocks that can provide analgesia to the hip joint. These nerve blocks include the fascia iliaca block (FICB, supra-inguinal/infra-inguinal), femoral nerve block, lateral femoral cutaneous nerve block (LFCN), Pericapsular Nerve Group (PENG) block, quadratus lumborum block (transmuscular–anterior), lumbar plexus nerve block, sciatic nerve block, and the newly explained posterior pericapsular deep-gluteal (PPD) block.

3.1. Fascia Iliaca Block (FICB)

The fascia iliaca block (FICB) is an injection of local anesthetic into the fascia iliaca compartment and targets the femoral nerve (FN), obturator (OBN), and lateral femoral cutaneous nerve (LFCN) between the fascia iliaca and underlying iliacus muscle [8]. However, it is important to note that the FN and the LFCN is more reliably blocked by FICB, while the OBN block requires a larger volume to be blocked. Traditionally, the fascia iliaca block is performed inferior to the inguinal ligament using a landmark-based technique [9]. This technique involves drawing a line between the pubic tubercle to the anterior superior iliac spine (ASIS) and dividing this line into three sections spaced equally apart. The point of entry of the block needle is 1 cm caudal to the point dividing the lateral third and medial two-thirds of the line. The needle is then inserted perpendicular until two loss of resistances are appreciated, the first being the fascia lata and the second loss of resistance being the fascia iliaca. After a negative aspiration, local anesthesia is injected into this space under the fascia iliaca [10].

A double-blind randomized control trial demonstrated superior pain relief, less opioid consumption, and less opioid-related sedation when the conventional infra-inguinal fascia iliaca block was compared to standardized systemic morphine analgesia for the management of acute hip fracture pain [10]. A systematic review found the loss-of-resistance-technique fascia iliaca compartment block to be an effective and safe tool for preoperative pain management in patients with hip fractures [11]. With the movement away from landmark-based techniques, an ultrasound-guided technique of the FICB, called a supra-inguinal fascia iliaca block (SIFI), was described and demonstrated to be a more reliable block of the target nerves [12]. This novel approach was created by Hebbard et al. with cadaveric models that showed extensive injectate spread throughout the iliac fossa when using an ultrasound-guided supra-inguinal approach [13]. They describe using a high-frequency probe placed parasagittally over the inguinal ligament close to the ASIS with an in-plane technique and needle entry point 2–4 cm below the inguinal ligament. The needle is advanced through the fascia iliaca at the level of the inguinal ligament, and through hydrodissection, local anesthetic is deposited between the iliacus muscle and the fascia iliaca and superiorly into the iliac fossa, using approximately 30–40 mL (Figure 3) [13]. An important landmark for SIFI is the deep circumflex iliac artery which lies laterally on top of the fascia iliaca. The artery serves as a landmark to confirm adequate local anesthetic spread between the fascia planes. A randomized control trial concluded that for total hip arthroplasty, the supra-inguinal fascia iliaca block provides superior analgesia in the first six hours postoperatively and significantly less morphine consumption in the first 24 h compared to the infra-inguinal approach [14]. Specifically for hip fractures, a retrospective study found the SIFIB group had statistically significantly lower postoperative 24 h opioid consumption compared to the control group, and thus reduced opioid-related respiratory depression after hip fracture surgery in older-old patients (over 80 years old) [15].

The fascia iliaca block provides good analgesia for the hip joint and improves patient satisfaction, regardless of which approach is used. A retrospective study showed a significantly shorter length of stay and lower pain scores on postoperative days 2 and 3 in hip fracture patients who had an ultrasound-guided SIFI catheter compared to the no-block group [16]. However, a possible complication to FICB is quadricep weakness from the spread of local anesthetic to the femoral nerve. Thus, caution should be taken if ambulation is wanted on the day of surgery.

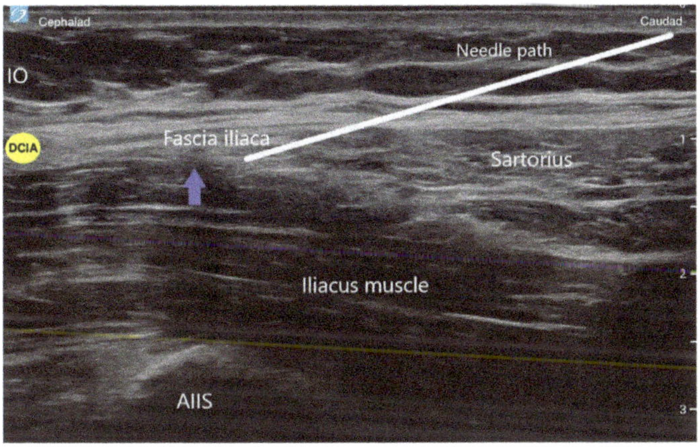

Figure 3. This is an ultrasound image of a supra-inguinal fascia iliaca (SIFI) block. The white line represents the direction of the needle. The blue arrow represents the location of local anesthetic injection. IO (internal oblique muscle); AIIS (anterior inferior iliac spine); DCIA (deep circumflex iliac artery).

3.2. Femoral Nerve Block

The femoral nerve block (FNB) continues to be one of the mainstays of regional techniques for pain management after hip fracture. Its ease of performance lends itself to accessible mastery and applicability. The femoral nerve supplies sensory fibers to the hip joint in addition to motor and sensory supply to the thigh. It arises from lumbar spinal roots L2-L4. The nerve is commonly blocked posterior to the inguinal ligament where it lies lateral to the femoral artery. An FNB is often conducted with ultrasound guidance using a high-frequency linear probe at the femoral crease with the patient lying supine. A lateral approach using an in-plane needle technique is used to inject local anesthetic (15–20 mL) either above or below the nerve (Figure 4). A continuous nerve catheter can also be placed using ultrasound guidance for prolonged analgesia.

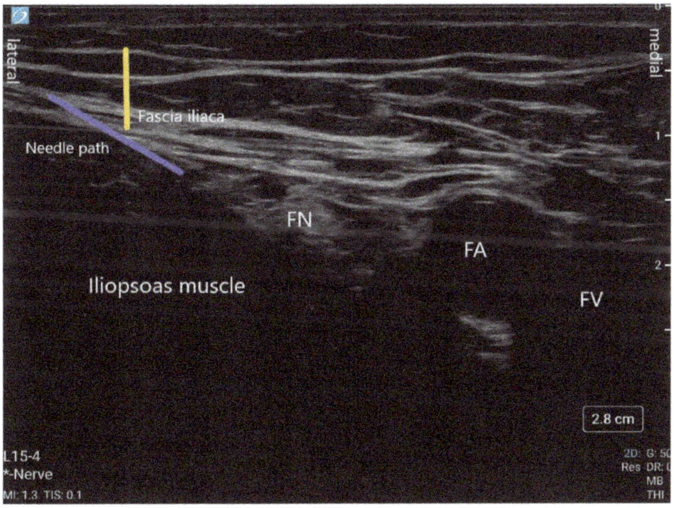

Figure 4. This is an ultrasound image of a femoral nerve block. The yellow line indicates the fascia iliaca plane. The blue line represents the needle trajectory. Local anesthetic is deposited below the nerve and above the nerve. FN (femoral nerve); FA (femoral artery); FV (femoral vein); * Nerve (ultrasound setting is in Nerve mode).

There have been several studies in the past five years relating to the femoral nerve block's pain-modulating effectiveness, its tendency to decrease VAS pain scores, its effect on early post-op mobility, and low evidence of reducing delirium in a highly susceptible population [5,17–19]. More recent randomized controlled trials (RCTs) continue to show a benefit in terms of pain control. An RCT of 110 patients in Turkey showed that when comparing patients with femoral blocks to patients just receiving acetaminophen IV, the patients with FNBs had lower VAS pain scores during positioning for intra-op spinal anesthesia [18]. A study of 407 elderly patients in Switzerland with hip fractures showed a significant reduction in the amount of post-op opioid usage as compared to those that did not receive blocks [19].

In all, the FNB continues to be a powerhouse of the regional world in terms of regional techniques for hip fracture patients. Some of our strongest evidence, the Cochrane review by Guay et al., leans heavily on the FNB, though it includes data of patients being administered other types of blocks [5]. As ultrasound techniques continue to improve, the literature will start to reflect whether there is even more benefit being gleaned than is currently reported.

3.3. Lateral Femoral Cutaneous Nerve (LFCN) Block

The lateral femoral cutaneous nerve (LFCN) block is a useful adjunct to the other nerves (femoral nerve, FICB) commonly blocked for hip fracture surgery. Its distribution at the lateral side of the leg allows for easier blockade in the context of a lateral surgical incision. The LFCN is indicated for analgesia for surgery of the anterolateral thigh, i.e., open reduction internal fixation of the hip, hip arthroplasty and/or hemiarthroplasty, muscle biopsy, and to treat meralgia paresthetica. The block is performed using a high-frequency linear ultrasound probe placed in a transverse position just distal to the anterior superior iliac spine (ASIS). The nerve can be identified as a hyperechoic structure superficially and between the sartorius and tensor fascia latae muscles (Figure 5). Depositing 3–5 mL of local anesthetic by inserting a needle using an in-plane approach and deep to the fascia lata should provide good analgesic coverage of the lateral thigh.

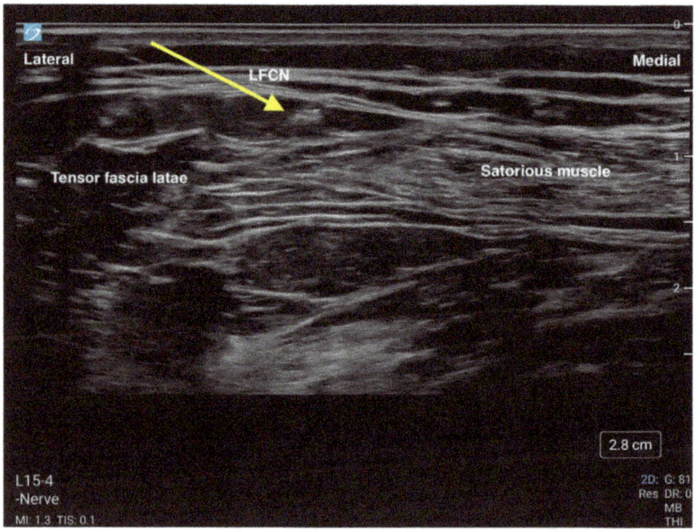

Figure 5. This is an ultrasound image of the lateral femoral cutaneous nerve (LFCN). The yellow arrow is pointing to the nerve. The nerve is blocked with a needle in the direction from lateral to medial.

Most recent studies of the LFCN occur in the context of another block such as the PENG block or the fascia iliaca block. In that context, it has been shown to be beneficial toward overall pain control and opioid sparing effect. One RCT from South Korea in 2024 placed patients into two groups, one receiving local infiltration by the surgeon (LIA) and the other with LIA + PENG and LFCN. This study showed significant reductions in pain scores and opioid consumption [20]. Another study combining PENG and LFCN evaluated whether this combination could be used as a primary block in patients. They compared three groups of patients (120 total) undergoing hip fracture surgery: GA, spinal, and RA. They found numerous benefits in the regional-only group and they concluded that PENG and LFCN may decrease postoperative pain and the length of hospital stay and allow for greater ambulation in the early postoperative period for patients with hip fractures [21]. The LFCN block was again studied as a part of a primary anesthetic, this time with the FNB as the other half, in hip fracture patients with a high co-morbidity load. The authors found the combination of blocks to be sufficient to get the patient through intramedullary nail placement as a salvage anesthetic when spinal or GA is not appropriate [22].

As the above literature shows, the LFCN block continues to serve as an important supplemental block for patients experiencing hip fracture pain. Though not utilized in isolation, its anatomic distribution makes it ideal as a rescue block for patients who have had lateral/ posterolateral hip incisions, especially in combination with blocks that are known to affect the anterior capsule.

3.4. Pericapsular Nerve Group (PENG) Block

The Pericapsular Nerve Group (PENG) block is a fascial plane block that was developed by Giron-Arango et al. at Toronto Western Hospital and the University of Toronto to block the high articular branches of the femoral (FN), obturator (ON), and accessory obturator nerves (AON) to the hip joint [23]. These branches are mostly responsible for the nociceptive pain in the anterior and superolateral capsule of the hip joint. The FN and AON are often found between the anterior inferior iliac spine (AIIS) and the iliopubic eminence (IPE), thus making it easier to target both nerves. The block is performed with the patient in the supine position. Local anesthetic is deposited using a curvilinear low-frequency ultrasound probe with an in-plane technique from lateral to medial. The needle tip is placed in the fascial plane between the psoas tendon and the ilium (Figure 6) [23,24]. As described by Giron-Arango and colleagues, an optimal ultrasound image should include the AIIS, IPE, psoas tendon, iliopsoas muscle, and more superficially, the femoral neurovascular bundle [23]. Typically, 10–20 mL of local anesthetic is adequate to provide effective analgesia if there is fluid spread along the plane displacing the psoas muscle tendon.

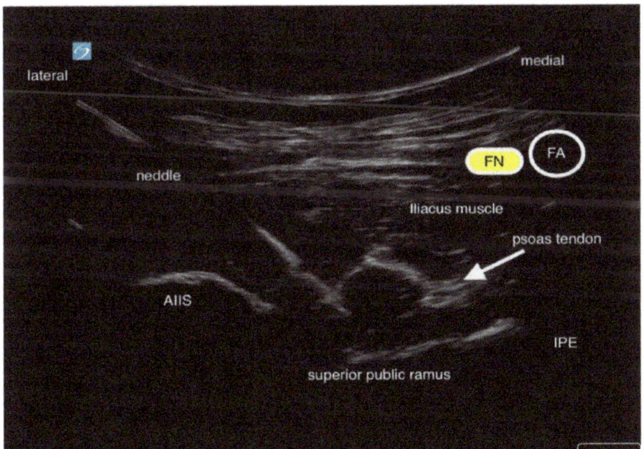

Figure 6. This is an ultrasound image of the Pericapsular Nerve Group Block (PENG). Local anesthetic is injected below the psoas tendon. The needle approach is from lateral to medial. The femoral nerve (FN) and femoral artery (FA) is seen medially.

The utilization of the PENG block in various studies has shown its superior analgesic effectiveness in lowering opioid consumption, decreasing the incidence of motor blockade, and shortening discharge time as compared to patients with no nerve block, a femoral nerve block, and an infra-inguinal fascia iliaca block with hip fractures [23,25–27]. In a single-center, double-blind, randomized controlled trial performed by Lin, Xufeng et al. in Singapore General Hospital, they found that the PENG block was superior to a sham block at reducing acute traumatic pain at 30 min ($p < 0.01$) and 3 h post block ($p < 0.05$) and reducing opioid consumption ($p < 0.05$) following hip fracture [28]. Although a PENG block is good at providing analgesia, it cannot be used as the sole anesthetic for hip surgery. It is often combined with LFCN, FICB, or FNB to provide more comprehensive analgesia for hip surgery.

3.5. Lumbar Plexus Nerve Block

The sensory innervation of the hip involves branches of both the lumbar and sacral plexus. The lumbar plexus is composed of L1–L4 nerve roots, which enter the psoas major muscle after they exit the intervertebral foramina [29]. These lumbar roots terminate as the femoral, lateral femoral cutaneous, obturator, genitofemoral, iliohypogastric, and ilioinguinal nerves as they pass through the psoas major muscle. Cadaveric studies have concluded that the lumbar plexus lies within the psoas major muscle, but the location of the obturator nerve within the psoas major muscle may vary [30].

The lumbar plexus block, also known as the psoas compartment block, targets the fascial plane within the posterior aspect of the psoas major muscle. The anterior approach to the lumbar plexus block is known as the three-in-one block (it blocks the femoral, obturator, and LFCN nerves), and many different approaches to the posterior approach have been described [31]. Winnie et al. first described the posterior approach to the lumbar plexus block, but the inadvertent neuraxial spread causing bilateral anesthesia has led to concerns with its usage [32,33]. The lumbar plexus can be blocked within the psoas major muscle using different techniques including paraesthesia, loss of resistance, nerve stimulation to elicit quadricep muscle contraction, and, in more recent years, ultrasound guidance. The adequate volume of local anesthetic is between 20 and 25 mL [34].

In addition to its analgesic benefits in hip fracture patients, the lumbar plexus block can also be used as the primary anesthetic. In comparing a single-shot lumbar plexus block as the primary anesthetic to a subarachnoid block, one study showed the lumbar plexus blockade to provide more stable intraoperative hemodynamics and a longer duration of postoperative analgesia in patients undergoing intertrochanteric hip fracture repair [35]. Even if not used as the primary anesthetic, a lumbar plexus block as an adjunct to general anesthesia compared to general anesthesia alone for hip fracture repair has been shown to improve intraoperative hemodynamics in addition to facilitating lower postoperative pain scores (1, 3, and 6 h), faster recovery times, and the decreased incidence of adverse events [36]. Although the lumbar plexus block is a great block, due to its level of difficulty and higher complication risks, its utilization has significantly dropped due to the availability of safer alternatives such as the FICB and FNB.

3.6. Erector Spinae Plane (ESP) Block and Quadratus Lumborum (QLB)

Erector spinae plane (ESP) block targets the dorsal roots of the spinal nerves as they travel in the fascial plane between the transverse processes and the erector spinae muscle. The adequate volume of local anesthetic is approximately 30 mL. ESP blocks have been reported to be used with variable degrees of effectiveness for analgesia after hip surgery in general and specifically in the setting of hip fracture surgery [37]. One report described the use of a large volume of local anesthetic mixture (40 mL) to produce surgical anesthesia in 15 patients without the need to convert to general anesthesia or add more local infiltration by the surgeon [38] MRI examination of the lumbar spine after ESP block revealed a significant contrast spread between the T12 and L5 transverse process and erector spinae muscle. Contrast material spread to the paravertebral, foraminal, and partially epidural area/spaces and in the areas where the lumbar nerves enter the psoas muscle which may hint at the mechanism of analgesia of the block [38]. The lumbar ESP block has shown similar analgesia to the infra-inguinal fascial iliaca block after elective hip arthroplasty with the potential for motor sparing of the quadriceps muscle [39]. A recent meta-analysis concluded that the use of the lumbar ESP block resulted in reduced opioid consumption in the first 24 h after surgery with significantly lower pain scores in the first 8 h after surgery [40].

The quadratus lumborum (QL) block is another relatively novel fascial plane block that aims to deposit local anesthetic in different locations relative to the muscle (anterior, lateral, or posterior) under the thoracolumbar fascia where the spinal nerves and their branches will travel. Research investigating the efficacy of the QL blocks in hip fracture surgery is still evolving. Different approaches to the QL blocks using approximately 30 mL of local anesthesia have shown reduced pain scores, reduced opioid consumption, and improved patient satisfaction when used for analgesia after hip surgery [41]. One study compared lumbar ESP and QL blocks to control groups in hip and proximal femoral surgery. This study showed improved analgesic quality in patients receiving ESPBs and QLBs [42]. When the QL block was compared to the SIFI block, the latter was found to result in prolonged analgesia and less pain during positioning for spinal anesthesia [43]. However, more research is needed to understand the benefits of ESP and QL blocks, especially in the context of more powerful blocks such as SIFI, the FNB, and PENG.

3.7. Sciatic Nerve Block (SNB)

The hip capsule is commonly split into the anterior and posterior capsule for the purposes of exploring its nociceptive innervation. The sciatic nerve is the major nerve that supplies the posterior capsule of the hip with some contribution from the nerve to quadratus femoris and superior gluteal nerve [44]. Thus, without anesthetizing this target, it is very difficult to manage posterior hip capsule pain. The transgluteal approach was the original approach described by Labat et al. However, currently, the subgluteal approach to the nerve is more common and can be blocked using ultrasound guidance. The nerve is located in the subgluteal fascial plane above the quadratus femoris muscle between the greater trochanter and ischial tuberosity [45].

Studies exploring the sciatic nerve block for hip fracture in isolation are few, and none from the last 5 years were found. More commonly, the sciatic nerve is blocked in concert with other targets that innervate the anterior capsule. In a Chinese study, the authors compared inflammatory markers of patients split in two groups: one receiving combined spinal–epidural anesthesia and the other receiving combined the lumbar plexus–sciatic nerve block as the primary block. They showed marked reductions in the inflammatory markers studied in their population, which included 62 elderly patients [46]. As seen here, the sciatic nerve was an adjunctive portion of the total regional anesthetic. Another study showed the effect of combining lumbar plexus and sciatic nerve blocks for hip fracture surgery by comparing them to spinal anesthesia, wherein they showed that a combined lumbar plexus–sciatic nerve block was equivalent to spinal anesthesia in terms of adequate anesthesia for surgery. Their study population showed a bias toward using the regional block as the primary block for sicker patients, which is their institutional norm, and providing spinal anesthesia for those deemed healthier [47].

Like the LFCN block, the sciatic nerve block is not useful as a sole anesthetic for hip fracture surgery but can be part of a holistic approach to the hip, especially when coverage to the posterior capsule is required.

3.8. Superior Gluteal Nerve (SGN) and Nerve to Quadratus Femoris Muscle

The predominant approach to pain management for hip fractures is anterior capsule coverage; however, some patients still experience significant residual posterior hip pain. The superior gluteal nerve (SGN) and the nerve to the quadratus femoris muscle are nerves that supply the posterior capsule of the hip [6,48]. The superior gluteal nerve emerges cranially to the piriformis muscle and deep to the gluteus maximus muscle and craniodorsal to the triceps coxae [48]. The nerve runs along with the superior gluteal artery and then divides into two branches covering the gluteus medius and gluteus minimus muscle, thus supplying innervation for the posterior capsule of the hip. The nerve to the quadratus femoris muscle also provides sensory innervation to the posteroinferior capsule. It arises from the upper part of the sciatic nerve.

Vermeylen et al. from Turnhout, Belgium, developed a new ultrasound-guided technique to block the nerves to the posterior capsule called the posterior pericapsular deep-gluteal (PPD) block [48]. The block is performed with the patient positioned in the lateral decubitus position with both their knee and hip flexed at 90 degrees (Figure 7a). A low-frequency curved probe is placed on the greater trochanter and aligned parallel with the long femoral axis. The probe is then moved slightly dorsal to visualize the bony landmarks: the greater trochanter, the femoral neck and head, and the posterior acetabular rim (Figure 7b) [48]. Superficial to the bony landmarks, the piriformis muscle is identified, deep to the gluteus maximus muscle. The needle is introduced in-plane from lateral to medial until the tip contacts the posterior acetabular rim near the attachment of the ischiofemoral ligament. After negative aspiration, 20 mL of local anesthetic is injected with fluid spread over the posterior acetabular rim, the posterior hip capsule, and under the piriformis muscle (Figure 7c) [48]. With this volume, the superior gluteal nerve and the nerve to the quadratus femoris muscle is expected to be covered.

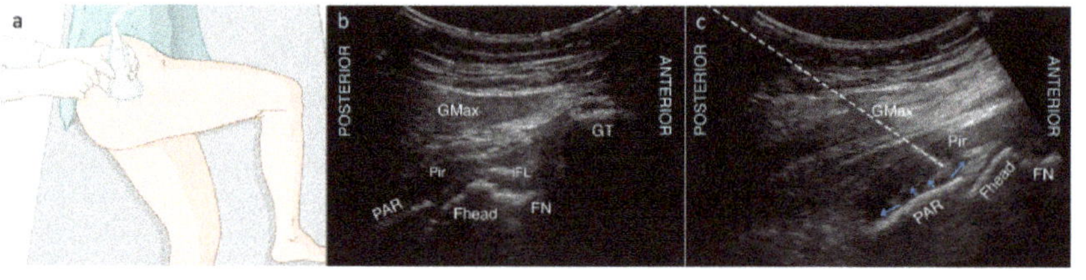

Figure 7. (**a**) Position of the patient during the posterior pericapsular deep-gluteal block. The ultrasound probe and needle are in line with the axis of the femur, with in-plane needle puncture from the posterior aspect. (**b**) Corresponding ultrasound image showing the gluteal muscles covering the bony landmarks: Fhead, femoral head; FN, femoral neck; GMax, gluteus maximus; GT, greater trochanter; IFL, ischiofemoral ligament as part of the posterior hip capsule; PAR, posterior acetabular rim; Pir, piriformis muscle. (**c**) Ultrasound image of the needle trajectory. Dashed line: needle trajectory; Blue arrows: spread of local anesthetic over the posterior acetabular rim and posterior hip capsule, deep to the piriformis muscle. Reproduced with permission from Vermeylen K et al., BJA Open; published by Elsevier, 2023 [48].

Like LFCN and PENG blocks, the SGN and nerve to the quadratus femoris muscle blocks are not useful as a sole anesthetic for hip fracture surgery but can be part of a comprehensive approach to pain management.

4. Surgeon's Perspective on Nerve Blocks for Hip Fracture

While 'hip fractures' are often grouped together, when considering the treatment options and optimal management, there are many different pathways.

Extracapsular hip fractures, including those in the intertrochanteric region and basicervical neck fractures, are treated with reduction and fixation. However, within this category, there are several implant options to choose from. Based on the implant (and difficulty of reduction), a patient may have only a small lateral approach below the vastus ridge, several smaller incisions spread from proximal to the hip joint all the way to the distal femur, or a combination of smaller and larger incisions.

Intracapsular hip fractures can be treated with open reduction and internal fixation (in young patients), which could have one or multiple approaches, including anterior and lateral. They can also be treated with fixation in situ, which would be performed from the lateral femur below the vastus ridge. Finally, they can be treated with an arthroplasty procedure—either a hemiarthroplasty or total hip arthroplasty. These procedures can be performed through many different approaches including posterior, lateral, anterolateral, or direct anterior.

In addition to knowing what type of fracture a patient has, an essential part of assessing a hip fracture patient is to determine if there are other acute illness that led to the fall. For example, illness such as anemia, heart failure, stroke, arrhythmias, and/or a myocardial infarction will need to be treated prior to a patient undergoing surgery. A preoperative assessment involving an anesthesia and medicine team is crucial for optimal outcomes. With the variability in treatment, including the surgical approach and the invasiveness of procedure, the ultimate goal is to have patients bear weight straight after surgery. Thus, it is important to have an effective postoperative analgesia which will encourage early mobilization and rehabilitation by the physical therapist. Overall, it is critical for the surgical and anesthesia team to have excellent communication to optimize care for patients.

5. Conclusions

Hip fracture is a painful injury that significantly limits mobility, thus increasing morbidity, especially in the elderly population. Early surgical treatment and the use of peripheral nerve blocks have been shown to reduce morbidity and mortality. Peripheral nerve blocks such FICB, FNB, LFCN, and PENG blocks are currently the most used blocks for hip fractures (Table 1). However, other blocks like ESP, QLB, sciatic nerve, and lumbar plexus blocks can be beneficial in certain hip fractures and surgical procedures such as hip arthroplasty or hip hemiarthroplasty. In addition to traditional blocks, we may now have a new block that anesthetizes nerves to the posterior capsule, superior gluteal nerve (SGN), and the nerve to the quadratus femoris muscle called the posterior pericapsular deep-gluteal (PPD) block. With all these peripheral nerve blocks, complete analgesia of the hip is possible, thus optimizing perioperative pain management.

Table 1. Peripheral nerve blocks with their advantages and disadvantages.

Peripheral Nerve Block	Advantages	Disadvantages
* Fascia Iliaca (FICB)	1. Blocks LFCN and FN reliably. Blocks obturator nerve more reliably with higher volume of injection. 2. Effective analgesia, supported by several RCTs. 3. Low risk of intravascular injection. 4. Good for all approaches to hip surgery.	1. High risk of quadricep weakness due to spread to femoral nerve, especially with infra-inguinal approach. 2. Requires larger volume (30–40 mL).
* Femoral Nerve (FNB)	1. Effective coverage of anterior hip joint. 2. Effective analgesia, supported by several RCTs. 3. Superficial and simple to perform. 4. Moderate risk of intravascular injection.	1. High risk of quadricep weakness. 2. High risk of nerve injury due to proximity to nerve on injection. 3. May spare LFCN depending on volume.
* Lateral Femoral Cutaneous Nerve (LFCN)	1. Low risk of nerve injury. 2. Low risk of intravascular injection. 3. Good for lateral or posterior lateral approach to hip.	1. Need to block FN separately.
* Pericapsular Nerve Group (PENG)	1. Low risk of quadricep weakness. 2. Low risk of nerve injury as it is a fascia plane block. 3. Effective analgesia, supported by some RCTs.	1. Spares LFCN and femoral nerves, thus necessitating separate blocking.

Table 1. *Cont.*

Peripheral Nerve Block	Advantages	Disadvantages
Lumbar Plexus Nerve (LP)	1. Blocks femoral, LFCN, and obturator nerves reliably. 2. Good for all approaches to hip surgery.	1. High risk of quadricep weakness. 2. High risk of nerve injury if performed without nerve stimulator or ultrasound. 3. Risk of bilateral and epidural spread. 4. Higher risk of local toxicity due to absorption. 5. Deep block; use with care in anticoagulated patients (increase peritoneum hematoma).
Quadratus Lumborum (QL)	1. Low risk of quadricep weakness if performed appropriately using both ultrasound and nerve stimulation.	1. Variable degree of evidence regarding efficacy. 2. Requires larger volume (≅30 mL). 3. Deep block (posterior/anterior); use with care in anticoagulated patients.
Erector Spinae Plane (ESP)	1. Low risk of quadricep weakness.	1. Variable degree of evidence regarding efficacy. 2. Requires larger volume (≅30–40 mL).
Sciatic Nerve (SNB)	1. No quadricep weakness. 2. Blocks posterior capsule of hip.	1. Only blocks sciatic nerve. Will need to add other blocks, i.e., FICB, FN, or LFCN, for adequate coverage of hip joint. 2. May be uncomfortable for patients; requires premedication due to positioning.
Superior Gluteal Nerve Nerve to Quadratus Femoris Muscle	1. Blocks posteroinferior capsule of hip.	1. Not useful as sole anesthetic. Will need to block with FICB and PENG.

* Commonly used for hip fracture surgery.

Author Contributions: Conceptualization, I.O.M. and N.E.; writing—original draft preparation, I.O.M., B.D., L.G., M.M.H. and N.E.; writing—review and editing, I.O.M. and N.E.; visualization, L.G. and I.O.M.; supervision, I.O.M.; literature search, N.E., I.O.M., B.D. and L.G. All authors have read and agreed to the published version of the manuscript.

Funding: This research received no external funding.

Institutional Review Board Statement: Not applicable.

Acknowledgments: The authors would like to thank Kenneth Mullen for helping to obtain an image of a PENG block.

Conflicts of Interest: The authors declare no conflicts of interest.

References

1. Roberts, K.C.; Brox, W.T.; Jevsevar, D.S.; Sevarino, K. Management of hip fractures in the elderly. *J. Am. Acad. Orthop. Surg.* **2015**, *23*, 131–137. [CrossRef]
2. Dixon, J.; Ashton, F.; Baker, P.; Charlton, K.; Bates, C.; Eardley, W. Assessment and Early Management of Pain in Hip Fractures: The Impact of Paracetamol. *Geriatr. Orthop. Surg. Rehabil.* **2018**, *9*, 2151459318806443. [CrossRef]
3. Ackermann, L.; Schwenk, E.S.; Lev, Y.; Weitz, H. Update on medical management of acute hip fracture. *Clevel. Clin. J. Med.* **2021**, *88*, 237–247. [CrossRef]
4. Downey, C.; Kelly, M.; Quinlan, J.F. Changing trends in the mortality rate at 1-year post hip fracture—A systematic review. *World J. Orthop.* **2019**, *10*, 166–175. [CrossRef] [PubMed]
5. Guay, J.; Kopp, S. Peripheral Nerve Blocks for Hip Fractures in Adults. *Cochrane Database Syst. Rev.* **2020**, *11*, CD001159. [CrossRef] [PubMed]
6. Laumonerie, P.; Dalmas, Y.; E Tibbo, M.; Robert, S.; Durant, T.; Caste, T.; Vialla, T.; Tiercelin, J.; Gracia, G.; Chaynes, P. Sensory Innervation of the Hip Joint and Referred Pain: A Systematic Review of the Literature. *Pain Med.* **2021**, *22*, 1149–1157. [CrossRef]
7. Orthoinfo and American Academy of Orthopedic Surgeons. Fischer, Stuart and Gray Joshua. "Hip Fractures". 2020. Available online: https://orthoinfo.aaos.org/en/diseases--conditions/hip-fractures (accessed on 10 May 2024).

8. Jones, M.R.; Novitch, M.B.; Hall, O.M.; Bourgeois, A.P.; Jeha, G.M.; Kaye, R.J.; Orhurhu, V.; Orhurhu, M.S.; Eng, M.; Cornett, E.M.; et al. Fascia iliaca block, history, technique, and efficacy in clinical practice. *Best Pract. Res. Clin. Anaesthesiol.* **2019**, *33*, 407–413. [CrossRef]
9. Dalens, B.; Vanneuville, G.; Tanguy, A. Comparison of the fascia iliaca compartment block with the 3-in-1 block in children. *Anesth. Analg.* **1989**, *69*, 705–713, Erratum in *Anesth. Analg.* **1990**, *70*, 474.
10. Foss, N.B.; Kristensen, B.B.; Bundgaard, M.; Bak, M.; Heiring, C.; Virkelyst, C.; Hougaard, S.; Kehlet, H. Fascia iliaca compartment blockade for acute pain control in hip fracture patients: A randomized, placebo-controlled trial. *Anesthesiology* **2007**, *106*, 773–778. [CrossRef]
11. Steenberg, J.; Møller, A. Systematic review of the effects of fascia iliaca compartment block on hip fracture patients before operation. *Br. J. Anaesth.* **2018**, *120*, 1368–1380. [CrossRef]
12. Desmet, M.; Balocco, A.L.; Van Belleghem, V. Fascia iliaca compartment blocks: Different techniques and review of the literature. *Best Pract. Res. Clin. Anaesthesiol.* **2019**, *33*, 57–66. [CrossRef]
13. Hebbard, P.; Ivanusic, J.; Sha, S. Ultrasound-guided supra-inguinal fascia iliaca block: A cadaveric evaluation of a novel approach. *Anaesthesia* **2011**, *66*, 300–305. [CrossRef] [PubMed]
14. Kumar, K.; Pandey, R.K.; Bhalla, A.P.; Kashyap, L.; Garg, R.; Darlong, V.; Malhotra, R.; Yadav, C.S. Comparison of conventional infrainguinal versus modified proximal suprainguinal approach of Fascia Iliaca Compartment Block for postoperative analgesia in Total Hip Arthroplasty. A prospective randomized study. *Acta Anaesthesiol. Belg.* **2015**, *66*, 95–100.
15. Bali, C.; Ozmete, O. Supra-inguinal fascia iliaca block in older-old patients for hip fractures: A retrospective study. *Braz. J. Anesthesiol.* **2023**, *73*, 711–717. [CrossRef]
16. Houserman, D.J.; Raszewski, J.A.; Palmer, B.; Chavan, B.; Sferrella, A.; Campbell, M.; Santanello, S. The Impact of the Fascia Iliaca Block Beyond Perioperative Pain Control in Hip Fractures: A Retrospective Review. *Geriatr. Orthop. Surg. Rehabil.* **2022**, *13*, 21514593221099107. [CrossRef]
17. Skjold, C.; Møller, A.M.; Wildgaard, K. Pre-operative femoral nerve block for hip fracture—A systematic review with meta-analysis. *Acta Anaesthesiol. Scand.* **2020**, *64*, 23–33. [CrossRef]
18. Uysal, A.İ.; Altıparmak, B.; Yaşar, E.; Turan, M.; Canbek, U.; Yılmaz, N.; Gümüş Demirbilek, S. The effects of early femoral nerve block intervention on preoperative pain management and incidence of postoperative delirium geriatric patients undergoing trochanteric femur fracture surgery: A randomized controlled trial. *Ulus. Travma Acil Cerrahi Derg.* **2020**, *25*, 109–114. [CrossRef]
19. Häusler, G.; van der Vet, P.C.R.; Beeres, F.J.P.; Kaufman, T.; Kusen, J.Q.; Poblete, B. The impact of loco-regional anaesthesia on postoperative opioid use in elderly hip fracture patients: An observational study. *Eur. J. Trauma Emerg. Surg.* **2021**, *48*, 2943–2952. [CrossRef]
20. Yoo, S.-H.; Lee, M.-J.; Beak, M.-H.; Kim, W.-J. Efficacy of Supplemental Ultrasound-Guided Pericapsular Nerve Group (PENG) Block Combined with Lateral Femoral Cutaneous Nerve Block in Patients Receiving Local Infiltration Analgesia after Hip Fracture Surgery: A Prospective Randomized Controlled Trial. *Medicina* **2024**, *60*, 315. [CrossRef] [PubMed]
21. Deemer, A.R.B.; Furgiuele, D.L.; Ganta, A.; Leucht, P.; Konda, S.; Tejwani, N.C.; Egol, K.A. The Lateral Femoral Cutaneous and Over the Hip (LOH) Block for the Surgical Management of Hip Fractures: A Safe and Effective Anesthetic Strategy. *J. Orthop. Trauma* **2023**, *37*, 135–141. [CrossRef]
22. Klimkiewicz, J.; Klimkiewicz, A.; Gutowski, M.; Rustecki, B.; Kochanowski, D.; Ryczek, R.; Lubas, A. Femoral and Lateral Femoral Cutaneous Nerve Block as Anesthesia for High-Risk Intertrochanteric Fracture Repair Patients. *J. Clin. Med.* **2022**, *11*, 3708. [CrossRef] [PubMed]
23. Girón-Arango, L.; Peng, P.W.; Chin, K.J.; Brull, R.; Perlas, A. Pericapsular nerve group (PENG) block for hip fracture. *Reg. Anesth. Pain Med.* **2018**, *43*, 859–863. [CrossRef] [PubMed]
24. Kolli, S.; Nimma, S.; Kukreja, P.; Peng, P. How I do it: Pericapsular nerve group (PENG) block. *ASRA Pain Med. News* **2023**, *48*. [CrossRef]
25. Lin, D.-Y.; Morrison, C.; Brown, B.; Saies, A.A.; Pawar, R.; Vermeulen, M.; Anderson, S.R.; Lee, T.S.; Doornberg, J.; Kroon, H.M.; et al. Pericapsular nerve group (PENG) block provides improved short-term analgesia compared with the femoral nerve block in hip fracture surgery: A single-center double-blinded randomized comparative trial. *Reg. Anesth. Pain Med.* **2021**, *46*, 398–403. [CrossRef] [PubMed]
26. Lin, D.-Y.; Brown, B.; Morrison, C.; Kroon, H.M.; Jaarsma, R.L. Pericapsular nerve group block results in a longer analgesic effect and shorter time to discharge than femoral nerve block in patients after hip fracture surgery: A single-center double-blinded randomized trial. *J. Int. Med. Res.* **2022**, *50*, 3000605221085073. [CrossRef] [PubMed]
27. Mosaffa, F.; Taheri, M.; Rasi, A.M.; Samadpour, H.; Memary, E.; Mirkheshti, A. Comparison of pericapsular nerve group (PENG) block with fascia iliaca compartment block (FICB) for pain control in hip fractures: A double-blind prospective randomized controlled clinical trial. *Orthop. Traumatol. Surg. Res.* **2022**, *108*, 103135. [CrossRef] [PubMed]
28. Lin, X.; Liu, C.W.; Goh, Q.Y.; Sim, E.Y.; Chan, S.K.T.; Lim, Z.W.; Chan, D.X.H. Pericapsular nerve group (PENG) block for early pain management of elderly patients with hip fracture: A single-center double-blind randomized controlled trial. *Reg. Anesth. Pain Med.* **2023**, *48*, 535–539. [CrossRef] [PubMed]
29. Sim, I.W.; Webb, T. Anatomy and Anaesthesia of the Lumbar Somatic Plexus. *Anaesth. Intensive Care* **2004**, *32*, 178–187. [CrossRef] [PubMed]

30. Farny, J.; Drolet, P.; Girard, M. Anatomy of the posterior approach to the lumbar plexus block. *Can. J. Anaesth.* **1994**, *41*, 480–485. [CrossRef]
31. Stevens, R.D.; Van Gessel, E.; Flory, N.; Fournier, R.; Gamulin, Z. Lumbar plexus block reduces pain and blood loss associated with total hip arthroplasty. *Anesthesiology* **2000**, *93*, 115–121. [CrossRef]
32. Winnie, A.P.; Ramamurthy, S.; Durrani, Z. The inguinal paravascular technic of lumbar plexus anesthesia: The "3-in-1 block". *Anesth. Analg.* **1973**, *52*, 989–996. [CrossRef] [PubMed]
33. Gentili, M.; Aveline, C.; Bonnet, F. Rachianesthésie totale après bloc du plexus lombaire par voie postérieure [Total spinal anes-thesia after posterior lumbar plexus block]. *Ann. Fr. D'anesth. Réanim.* **1998**, *17*, 740–742. [CrossRef] [PubMed]
34. Bendtsen, T.F.; Soeballe, K.; Petersen, E.; Moriggl, B.; Sauter, A.; Strid, J.; Boerglum, J. Ultrasound Guided Single Injection Lumbosacral Plexus Blockade for Hip Surgery Anaesthesia. *Br. J. Anaesth.* **2013**, *111*. [CrossRef]
35. Sreejit, M.S.; Ahamed, Z.A. Lumbar Plexus Block as an Effective Alternative to Subarachnoid Block for Intertrochanteric Hip fracture Surgeries in the Elderly. *Anesth. Essays Res.* **2019**, *13*, 264–268. [CrossRef]
36. Feng, J.; Tang, G.; Shui, Y.; Xiang, J.; Qin, Z. Effects of ultrasound-guided lumbar plexus and sacral plexus block combined with general anesthesia on the anesthetic efficacy and surgical outcomes in elderly patients undergoing intertrochanteric fracture surgery: A randomized controlled trial. *J. Orthop. Surg. Res.* **2024**, *19*, 171. [CrossRef] [PubMed]
37. Townsend, D.; Siddique, N.; Kimura, A.; Chein, Y.; Kamara, E.; Pope, J.; Weiser, M.; Nair, S.; Muse, I. Lumbar Erector Spinae Plane Block for Total Hip Arthroplasty Comparing 24-Hour Opioid Requirements: A Randomized Controlled Study. *Anesthesiol. Res. Pract.* **2022**, *2022*, 9826638. [CrossRef] [PubMed]
38. Ahiskalioglu, A.; Tulgar, S.; Celik, M.; Ozer, Z.; Alici, H.A.; Aydin, M.E. Lumbar Erector Spinae Plane Block as a Main Anesthetic Method for Hip Surgery in High Risk Elderly Patients: Initial Experience with a Magnetic Resonance Imaging. *Eurasian J. Med.* **2020**, *52*, 16–20. [CrossRef] [PubMed]
39. Flaviano, E.; Bettinelli, S.; Assandri, M.; Muhammad, H.; Benigni, A.; Cappelleri, G.; Mariano, E.R.; Lorini, L.F.; Bugada, D. Erector spinae plane versus fascia iliaca block after total hip arthroplasty: A randomized clinical trial comparing analgesic effectiveness and motor block. *Korean J. Anesthesiol.* **2023**, *76*, 326–335. [CrossRef]
40. Huda, A.U.; Ghafoor, H. The Use of Erector Spinae Plane Block Reduces Opioid Consumption and Pain Score in Postoperative Period After Hip Surgery: A Meta-Analysis. *Cureus* **2023**, *15*, e47477. [CrossRef]
41. Huda, A.U.; Minhas, R. Quadratus Lumborum Block Reduces Postoperative Pain Scores and Opioids Consumption in Total Hip Arthroplasty: A Meta-Analysis. *Cureus* **2022**, *14*, e22287. [CrossRef]
42. Tulgar, S.; Kose, H.C.; Selvi, O.; Senturk, O.; Thomas, D.T.; Ermis, M.N.; Ozer, Z. Comparison of Ultrasound-Guided Lumbar Erector Spinae Plane Block and Transmuscular Quadratus Lumborum Block for Postoperative Analgesia in Hip and Proximal Femur Surgery: A Prospective Randomized Feasibility Study. *Anesth. Essays Res.* **2018**, *12*, 825–831. [CrossRef] [PubMed]
43. Refaat, S.; Ali, M.M.; Elsherief, I.M.; Mohamed, M.M. Ultrasound-guided fascia iliaca block versus quadratus lumborum block for perioperative analgesia in patients undergoing hip surgery. A randomised controlled trial. *Anaesthesiol. Intensiv. Ther.* **2023**, *55*, 212–217. [CrossRef] [PubMed]
44. Birnbaum, K.; Prescher, A.; Hessler, S.; Heller, K.D. The sensory innervation of the hip joint—An anatomical study. *Surg. Radiol. Anat.* **1997**, *19*, 371–375. [CrossRef] [PubMed]
45. Nwawka, O.K.; Meyer, R.; Miller, T.T. Ultrasound-Guided Subgluteal Sciatic Nerve Perineural Injection: Report on Safety and Efficacy at a Single Institution. *J. Ultrasound Med.* **2017**, *36*, 2319–2324. [CrossRef] [PubMed]
46. Zhang, Y.; Jiang, L.; Han, Y. Reduced Concentrations of NSE, S100β, Aβ, and Proinflammatory Cytokines in Elderly Patients Receiving Ultrasound-Guided Combined Lumbar Plexus-Sciatic Nerve Block during Hip Replacement. *Genet. Res.* **2022**, *2022*, 1384609. [CrossRef] [PubMed]
47. Kaçmaz, M.; Turhan, Z.Y. Spinal anesthesia versus combined sciatic nerve/lumbar plexus nerve block in elderly patients undergoing total hip arthroplasty: A retrospective study. *Ann. Saudi Med.* **2022**, *42*, 174–180. [CrossRef]
48. Vermeylen, K.; Van Aken, D.; Versyck, B.; Casaer, S.; Bleys, R.; Bracke, P.; Groen, G. Deep posterior gluteal compartment block for regional anaesthesia of the posterior hip: A proof-of-concept pilot study. *BJA Open* **2023**, *5*, 100127. [CrossRef]

Journal of
Clinical Medicine

MDPI

Systematic Review

The Impact of Gabapentinoids on Pain-Related Outcomes after Knee and Hip Surgery: A Systematic Review with Meta-Analysis of Randomized Controlled Trials

Dmitriy Viderman [1,2,*], Mina Aubakirova [1], Azamat Salamat [3], Dastan Kaldybayev [3], Nurzhamal Sadir [1], Ramil Tankacheyev [4] and Yerkin G. Abdildin [3]

1 Department of Surgery, School of Medicine, Nazarbayev University, Astana 020000, Kazakhstan; mina.aubakirova@nu.edu.kz (M.A.)
2 Department of Anesthesiology and Intensive Care, National Research Oncology Center, Astana 010000, Kazakhstan
3 Department of Mechanical and Aerospace Engineering, School of Engineering and Digital Sciences, Nazarbayev University, Astana 010000, Kazakhstan; yerkin.abdildin@nu.edu.kz (Y.G.A.)
4 Department of Spinal Surgery, National Research Neurosurgery Center, Astana 010000, Kazakhstan
* Correspondence: drviderman@gmail.com

Abstract: Background: Postoperative pain remains a significant challenge after knee and hip surgeries, two of the most frequently performed procedures, preventing patients from seeking timely surgical help. Gabapentinoids, gabapentin, and pregabalin, have been gaining attention in postoperative pain management. **Methods:** We conducted a meta-analysis to evaluate the efficacy of gabapentinoids in pain management after knee and hip surgery. PubMed, Scopus, and Cochrane Library were searched for relevant randomized controlled trials (RCTs) published before January 2023. **Results:** Fifteen articles reporting 1320 patients were analyzed. Cumulative pain intensity at rest and on movement was lower in the experimental group with the mean difference (MD) = −0.30 [−0.55,−0.05], p-value = 0.02, and MD = −0.41 [−0.68,−0.13], p-value = 0.004, respectively. However, the difference was not clinically meaningful and lacked statistical significance at each time period. The gabapentinoid group required less opioid consumption in morphine equivalents (MD = −6.42 [−9.07, −3.78] mg, p-value < 0.001). There was a lower incidence of postoperative nausea in the experimental group with a risk ratio (RR) of 0.69 [0.55, 0.86], p-value < 0.001. A subgroup analysis showed that gabapentinoids reduced pain on movement on postoperative day two after total knee arthroplasty but not hip arthroplasty. There was insufficient data to examine the efficacy of gabapentinoids in the reduction of chronic postoperative pain in knee/hip surgery. **Conclusions:** Thus, gabapentinoids were associated with a reduction in postoperative pain intensity at rest and on movement, morphine consumption, and the incidence of postoperative nausea in the early postoperative period following knee and hip surgeries. However, pain reduction was not clinically relevant. Sedation has not been evaluated in this work and, if performed, this may have influenced the conclusions. An important limitation of this study is that different gabapentinoids, their administration times and dosages, as well as varying intraoperative management protocols, were pooled together.

Keywords: pregabalin; gabapentin; gabapentinoids; knee surgery; hip surgery; acute pain

1. Introduction

Knee and hip surgeries are one of the most frequently performed operating room procedures in clinical practice [1]. However, postoperative pain remains a significant challenge after both surgeries. Postsurgical pain is one of the major reasons patients are unwilling to undergo total hip arthroplasty (THA) or total knee arthroplasty (TKA) [2]. During joint replacement surgeries, tissue damage and postoperative inflammation serve as noxious stimuli, detected by nociceptors in the peripheral nervous system, which are transmitted to the spinal cord and then to the central nervous system through action potentials [3]. Additionally, postoperative inflammation leads to the release of inflammatory substances and cytokines, intensifying the pain experience [3]. Eventually, acute pain may potentially evolve into chronic pain [4].

General anesthesia and systemic opioids, while commonly used, cannot completely prevent central sensitization [5]. Moreover, opioids are associated with multiple complications and adverse effects [6,7]. Regional anesthetic methods provide partial relief but come with limitations [8]. Therefore, gabapentinoids, gabapentin, and pregabalin have been gaining attention in postoperative pain management as they inhibit neuronal excitation in the central nervous system, reduce hyperexcitation of dorsal horn neurons, and release excitatory neurotransmitters [9]. Moreover, the side effects of gabapentin are usually mild [9].

Kremer and colleagues summarized the analgesic mechanisms of gabapentinoids [10]. Although gabapentinoids are structurally related to GABA, their analgesic effects are primarily a result of binding to the $\alpha2\delta$ subunit of voltage-dependent calcium channels. This binding reduces calcium influx into neurons, decreasing excitatory neurotransmitter release and dampening neuronal hyperexcitability, which is crucial in neuropathic pain. It is suggested that neuropathic pain often involves an increased expression of the $\alpha2\delta$ subunit in the dorsal root ganglia and dorsal horn of the spinal cord. However, this increase is not consistent across all neuropathic conditions. Gabapentin and pregabalin normalize these elevated $\alpha2\delta$ levels caused by nerve damage, likely by inhibiting their trafficking to presynaptic terminals rather than altering their overall expression. Furthermore, gabapentinoids influence central sensitization by reducing the excitability of dorsal horn neurons and affecting supraspinal regions involved in pain processing. They modulate neuroimmune responses by reducing pro-inflammatory cytokine expression and microglial activation. Gabapentinoids also appear to reverse central hypersensitivity and suppress the hyperactivity of neurons in brain regions associated with pain. Thus, these mechanisms collectively contribute to gabapentinoids' effectiveness in managing neuropathic pain, despite not directly interacting with GABA receptors.

Pregabalin and gabapentin have been extensively studied for their antinociceptive effects; however, their efficacy in preventing or reducing acute and chronic postoperative pain remains debatable [11]. Although various systematic reviews attempted to establish their analgesic effects in hip and knee surgeries [12–14], these have produced varying results.

Therefore, the current meta-analysis aimed to synthesize existing studies to evaluate the efficacy of gabapentinoids for pain management in knee and hip surgery. Specifically, we aimed to assess gabapentinoids' effect on pain scores, opioid consumption, postoperative nausea and vomiting, and, potentially, on chronic postoperative pain.

2. Materials and Methods

2.1. Protocol

We developed the protocol for this meta-analysis for relevant articles. The protocol and methods were arranged and approved by all authors. It is publicly available at https://doi.org/10.17605/OSF.IO/SJ92M (accessed on 10 July 2024). We used the "Preferred Reporting Items for Systematic Reviews and Meta-Analyses (PRISMA)" guidelines [15].

2.2. Search Strategy and Criteria

We searched for RCTs, which studied the analgesic effects of gabapentinoids in the adult population. We searched for relevant articles in the standard databases, such as PubMed and Scopus, as well as the Cochrane Library, published before January 2023 (Figure 1). The following search terms or their combination were used during the search: "pregabalin", "gabapentin", "gabapentinoids", "knee surgery", "knee arthroplasty", "knee replacement", "arthroscopy", "hip surgery", "hip replacement", "hip arthroplasty", "acute pain", and "chronic pain". Two authors independently screened the articles. In case of disagreements, a third author was consulted.

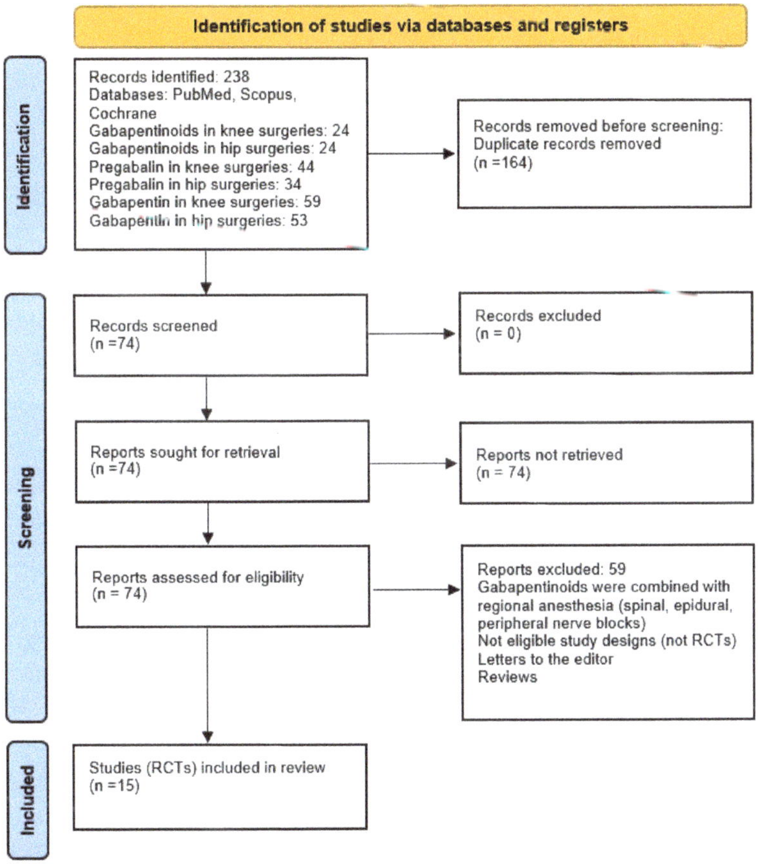

Figure 1. PRISMA diagram. The study selection process.

2.3. Screening

Screening of the articles was conducted by two authors in an independent manner. In case of disagreements, a third author was consulted. The studies were screened based on titles, then abstracts, and finally, by full texts.

2.3.1. Inclusion Criteria

The inclusion criteria were as follows:

- Patients: Patients aged 18 years old and older undergoing knee or hip surgery (knee arthroplasty, total knee replacement, ligament repair; hip arthroplasty, hip replacement);
- Intervention: Analgesic use of gabapentinoids (pregabalin or gabapentin);
- Control: Placebo;
- Outcomes: Primary—acute postoperative pain intensity at rest and on movement; secondary—postoperative morphine consumption (mg), postoperative nausea and vomiting, chronic postoperative pain;
- Study design: Randomized controlled trials (RCTs).

2.3.2. Exclusion Criteria

The exclusion criteria were as follows:

- Pediatric studies;
- Other comparators;

- Non-RCTs: retrospective studies, case reports, case series, editorials, cadaver studies, and technical reports;
- Not properly described study methodology, assessment, and/or reporting methods;
- Inability to retract the full text.

2.4. Assessment of Methodologic Quality

Two authors (MA and NS) independently appraised the quality of each study using the Cochrane risk of bias 2 tool [16] and each outcome using GRADE [17]. Discrepancies were resolved by discussion until reaching a consensus or with the involvement of a third author (DV) if required. The Cochrane risk of bias 2 tool assessed studies as having "low risk", "some concerns" or "high risk" of bias based on the "randomization process", "deviations from intended interventions", "missing outcome", "measurement of the outcome data", and "selection of the reported results". An overall risk of bias was then determined based on these five domains. A GRADE evaluation was performed for the main cumulative outcomes. Each was assessed based on the "risk of bias", "inconsistency", "imprecision", and "indirectness". Based on these, the outcomes were downgraded or upgraded to a "high", "moderate", "low", or "very low" certainty of evidence.

2.5. Data Extraction and Statistical Methods

We extracted and entered qualitative data describing the studies in a data table. Specifically, the following rubrics were used: study reference, 1st author followed by year of publication and country, design, goals (objectives) of the study, age of participants, surgery type, sample size, physical status of patients based on "American Society of Anesthesiologists" (ASA), pharmacological agents (analgesics, hypnotics, adjuvants), and observed side effects. Numeric data for statistical analysis were extracted in a spreadsheet. Some missing statistics were calculated using the methods developed by Luo et al. [18] and by Wan et al. [19]. The meta-analysis was conducted in the "Review Manager software (RevMan, version 5.4)". Since the studies reported values from different populations, we used the random effects model. The mean difference or risk ratio was used for the examination of the effect size. Forest plots were built for each outcome. Statistical heterogeneity was estimated by the I^2 statistic.

3. Results

3.1. Included Studies

The systematic search retrieved 238 original articles (Figure 1). After duplicate removal, 74 articles were screened and 15 articles [9,20–32] comprising 1320 patients (gabapentinoids—659, controls—661) matched the criteria and were analyzed (Figure 1, Table 1).

Table 1. Characteristics of the included studies. Abbreviations: A, analyzed; ASA, American Society of Anesthesiologists; N, number; NRS, Numeric Rating Scale; PCA, patient-controlled analgesia; PONV, postoperative nausea and vomiting; R, randomized; RCTs, randomized controlled trials; ROM, range of motion; TKA, total knee arthroplasty; THA, total hip arthroplasty; VAS, Visual Analogue Scale; and VRS, Verbal Rating Scale.

Author, Year, Country, Study Design	Study Goals	Age	N of Patients: Total (Intervention/Control)	Surgery; Groups	Type of Pain; ASA Status	Dose Regiment	Study Conclusions
Buvanendran et al., 2010 [31] USA, RCT	To determine if pregabalin has analgesic effects given preoperatively	64 (8.3), 63.3 (8.9)	240 (120/120)	TKA; pregabalin, placebo	Neuropathic pain; I, II, III	Pregabalin 300 mg orally	Perioperative pregabalin reduces the incidence of chronic neuropathic pain
Carmichael et al., 2013 [21], Canada, RCT	To assess pain (VAS, 0–10), morphine use, physical function, adverse events	18–80 pregabalin: 59.1 (10.1) placebo: 61.3 (15.1)	R: 47 (23/24) A: 31 (15/16)	THA; pregabalin, placebo	I–III	Pregabalin 75 mg twice daily, celecoxib 100 mg twice daily, 14 d preop, 2 h preop, during hospitalization, and 3 w after discharge	Pregabalin and celecoxib improves pain and physical function
Clarke et al., 2009 [5], Canada, RCT	To determine if gabapentin reduces pain and opioid use and find the efficient time of consumption	61.3 (10.7), 58.9 (9.4), 60.4 (8.1)	126 (42/42/42)	THA; gabapentin 600 mg/placebo, placebo/gabapentin 600 mg, placebo/placebo	Neuropathic pain	Gabapentin before surgery 19.06 ± 19.9 mg, after surgery 34.8 ± 13.1 mg in the first 24 h	No effect from gabapentin on morphine consumption or pain scores preoperatively/postoperatively

Table 1. *Cont.*

Author, Year, Country, Study Design	Study Goals	Age	N of Patients: Total (Intervention/Control)	Surgery; Groups	Type of Pain; ASA Status	Dose Regiment	Study Conclusions
Clarke et al., 2015 [32], Canada, RCT	To study the effects of pregabalin on pain and functional outcomes	60.1 (8.8), 60.2 (9.5)	184 (92/92)	THA; pregabalin, placebo	Neuropathic pain; I, II, III	Pregabalin 150 mg p.o	No improvement in physical function
Jain et al., 2012 [26], India, RCT	To evaluate pain at rest and on movement (VRS, 0–10), morphine use, rescue analgesic use, patient satisfaction, sedation, adverse events	18–75 pregabalin: 59.7 (8.63) placebo: 57.1 (8.81)	40 (20/20)	TKA; pregabalin, placebo	I, II	Pregabalin 75 mg twice a day 2 h preop; 2 d postop	Pregabalin reduces opioid use, improves postop analgesia, and yields higher patient satisfaction
Martinez et al., 2014 [27], France, RCT	To assess pain at rest and on movement (NRS, 0–10), morphine use, side effects, pressure pain thresholds, secondary hyperalgesia	18–80 placebo: 64 (11) ketamine: 60 (17) pregabalin: 64 (9) ketamine + pregabalin: 59 (12)	142 (38/34/35/35) (placebo/ketamine/ pregabalin/ketamine + pregabalin)	THA; placebo; ketamine; pregabalin; ketamine + pregabalin	I–III	Pregabalin 150 mg preop	The combination of pregabalin and ketamine has a small, beneficial clinical effect
Mathiesen et al., 2008 [24], Denmark, RCT	To examine morphine use, pain at rest and during mobilization (VAS, 0–100), PONV, sedation, dizziness, and ondansetron use	55–75 placebo: 66 (63–71) pregabalin: 67 (62–71) pregabalin + dexamethasone: 68 (64–71) median (range)	R: 126 (42/42/42) A: 120 (38/40/42) (placebo/pregabalin/ pregabalin + dexamethasone)	THA; placebo, pregabalin, pregabalin + dexamethasone	I–III	Pregabalin 300 mg 1 h preop	Pregabalin reduced postop morphine use. This was not associated with a reduced PONV. Pregabalin resulted in increased sedation. Pregabalin and dexamethasone provided no effects on pain or opioid use
Lee et al., 2015 [9], Korea, RCT	To study the postoperative pain, analgesic drug consumption, and functional outcomes after pregabalin	Pregabalin: 63.38 (10.71), placebo: 67.60 (8.98)	87 (45/42)	TKA; pregabalin, control	Neuropathic pain; I, II, III	400 mg celecoxib plus 150 mg pregabalin—1 h prior to the operation	No difference between the two groups in functional recovery
Paul et al., 2013 [20], Canada, RCT	To assess morphine use, pain (NRS, 0–10) at rest and movement, side effects, patient satisfaction, knee ROM, hemodynamics	19–90 gabapentin: 62.1 (6.4) placebo: 63.5 (6.7)	101 (52/49)	TKA; gabapentin, placebo	I–IV	600 mg gabapentin 2 h preop; 8 h for 2 postop days	No effect on postoperative morphine consumption, pain, patient satisfaction, or length of hospital stay
Paul et al., 2015 [22], Canada, RCT	To determine if gabapentin preoperatively or postoperatively would decrease postoperative morphine consumption	60.9 (9.1), 60.5 (8.5)	102 (48/54)	THA; gabapentin, placebo	Neuropathic pain	600 mg of gabapentin	No difference between placebo in morphine consumption, side effects, or pain scores
Rasmussen et al., 2010 [25], Denmark, RCT	To assess morphine use, pain at rest and during mobilization (VAS, 0–100), PONV, sedation, dizziness, hallucination, and ondansetron use	55–85 gabapentin: 72 (68–77) placebo: 70 (67–75) median (IQR)	42 (24/18)	THA; gabapentin, placebo	I–III	1200 mg gabapentin preop	Preop gabapentin, reduced pain, but not morphine use
Singla et al., 2014 [29], USA, RCT	To assess pain (0–10), knee ROM, opioid use, safety	18–80 150 mg: 63 (8.5) 300 mg: 63.7 (8.3) placebo: 63.3 (9.5)	292 (98/96/98) (150 mg/300 mg/placebo)	TKA; pregabalin 150, pregabalin 300, placebo		150 mg pregabalin (75 mg bid) or 300 mg pregabalin (150 mg bid) 12 h and 2 h preop, 6 w postop	No significant differences between pregabalin and placebo
Tobias et al., 2019 [23], Brazil, RCT	To determine if preoperative and postoperative pregabalin is associated with a reduction in postoperative pain episodes	Pregabalin: 31 (7), placebo: 30 (7)	50 (25/25)	Knee ligament repair; pregabalin, control	Neuropathic pain; I or II	Pregabalin, 75 mg/d 7 days before and 7 days after surgery	Pregabalin decreased the consumption of analgesics with side effects of dizziness
Yadeau et al., 2015 [30], USA, RCT	To determine if postoperative pain could be reduced and to determine the side effects	66 (34–79)	120 (30/30/30/30)	TKA; placebo, pregabalin 50 mg, pregabalin 100 mg, pregabalin 150 mg	Neuropathic pain; I–III	0, 50, 100, and 150 mg pregabalin	No analgesic effect of pregabalin; side effects—reduced satisfaction with analgesia and increased drowsiness
Yik et al., 2019 [28], Singapore, RCT	To determine if pregabalin preoperatively with PCA morphine, paracetamol, and etoricoxib is effective for decreasing the morphine and if it decreases the pain scores	Pregabalin: 65.1 (50–80), placebo: 66.6 (50–83)	87 (45/42)	TKA; pregabalin, control	I, II, III	1 h before surgery: 75 mg pregabalin orally; 48 h after surgery: 75 mg dose per night	No effect on postoperative opioid dose, pain scores, or functional outcomes

3.2. *Pain Intensity at Rest (0–10 Scale)*

The pain intensity score at rest on the Numerical Rating Scale (NRS) and Visual Analog Scale (VAS) is presented in a forest plot in Figure 2. As can be seen from the forest plots, the experimental group tended to have lower pain scores at almost all the time periods, although the difference in pain scores was not statistically significant. However, on POD 3, the experimental group had higher pain scores than the controls (MD = 0.21 [0.08, 0.35], p = 0.002). All of the time periods pooled together show an overall effect favoring the gabapentinoid group (MD = −0.30 [−0.55,−0.05], p-value = 0.02). This difference is not clinically meaningful. The result is sensitive to the exclusion of some studies (e.g., Carmichael et al., 2019 [21]). The model shows moderate heterogeneity (I^2 = 74%).

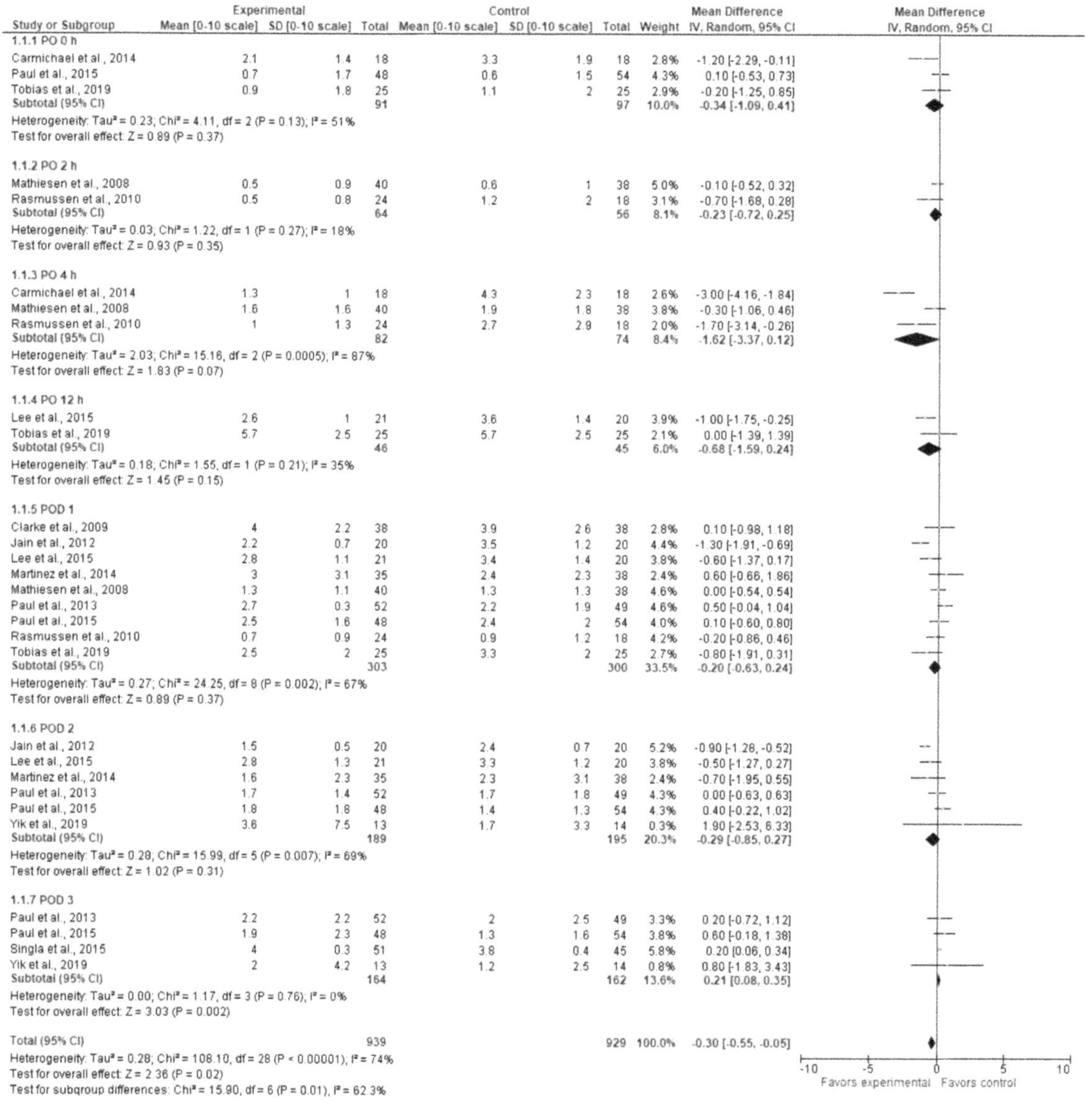

Figure 2. Pain intensity at rest [5,9,20–29].

3.3. Pain Intensity Score on Movement (0–10 Scale)

Similar to pain at rest, pain on movement tended to be lower in the experimental group up to day three (Figure 3). Immediately post-surgery, the gabapentinoid group had significantly lower pain scores (MD = −0.86 [−1.61, −0.10], p = 0.03). After that, the difference in pain scores was not statistically significant between the two groups. When pooled together, the cumulative pain at all the time periods was lower in the experimental group (MD = −0.41 [−0.68, −0.13], p-value = 0.004). The result is not sensitive to the exclusion of any study. The model shows moderate heterogeneity (I^2 = 53%).

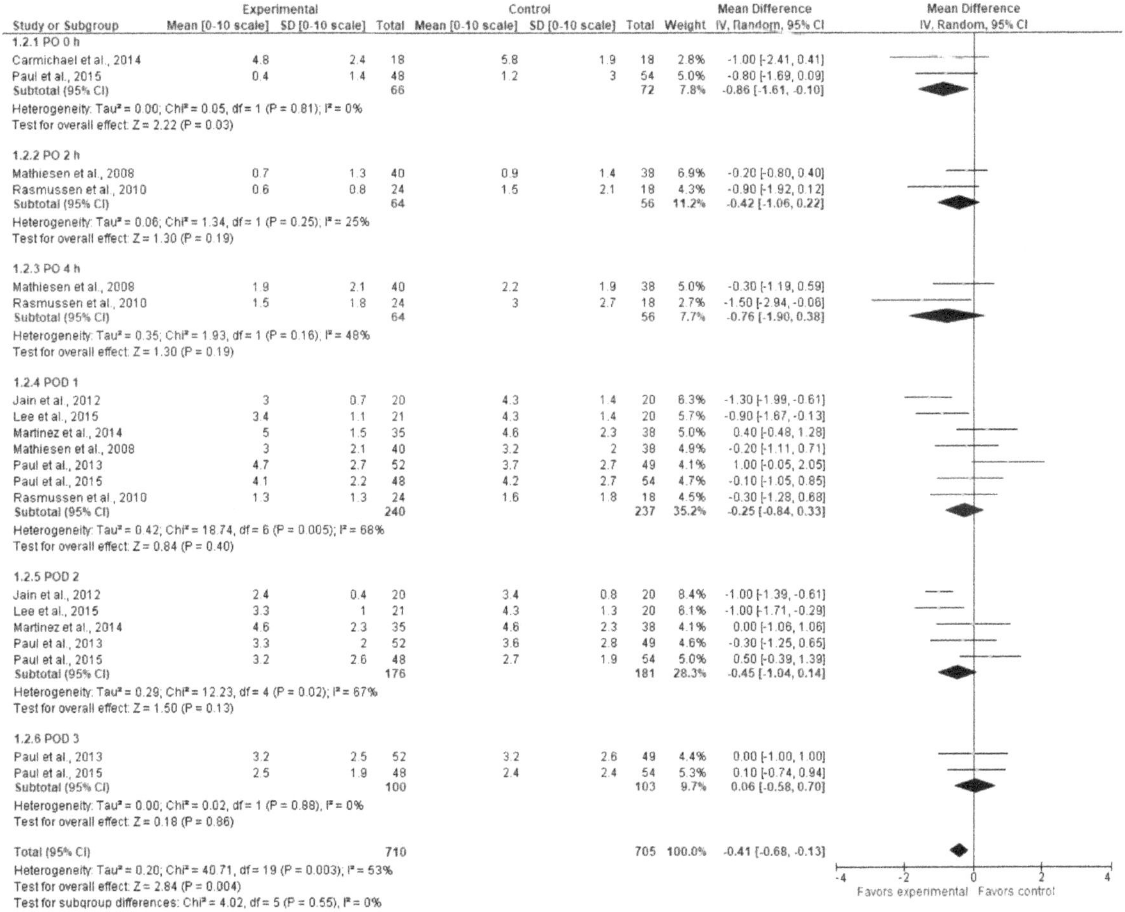

Figure 3. Pain intensity score on movement [9,20–27].

3.4. Postoperative Opioid Consumption in Morphine Equivalents (mg)

Many studies reported opioid consumption in morphine equivalents in mg (Figure 4). Since fentanyl is almost 100 times more potent than morphine, we converted the fentanyl consumption reported in Lee et al. 2015 [9] in μg into morphine equivalents by dividing the fentanyl values (μg) by 1000 to have in mg and then multiplying by 100. We should also note that Lee et al. 2015 [9] reported tramadol consumption as a rescue medication, so we have not counted it as an opioid in morphine equivalents. Tramadol consumption in two groups "showed no significant difference" [9]. Tobias et al. 2019 [23] reported the consumption of morphine, tramadol, and ketoprofen. However, the latter two were not counted in our report because ultimately "intravenous morphine was administered until pain control" [23].

Opioid consumption was lower in the gabapentinoid group on POD 1 (MD = −7.28 [−11.61, −2.96], $p = 0.001$), POD 2 (MD = −9.29 [−15.26, −3.32], $p = 0.002$), and week 1 (MD = −1.00 [−1.57, −0.43], $p < 0.001$). The overall result of the model favors the gabapentinoid group (MD = −6.42 [−9.07, −3.78], $p < 0.001$). The result is insensitive to the exclusion of any study. The model shows considerable heterogeneity ($I^2 = 96\%$).

Study or Subgroup	Experimental Mean [mg]	Experimental SD [mg]	Experimental Total	Control Mean [mg]	Control SD [mg]	Control Total	Weight	Mean Difference IV, Random, 95% CI
1.3.1 POD 1								
Clarke et al., 2015	40	4.8	92	53.9	5.1	92	7.1%	-13.90 [-15.33, -12.47]
Jain et al., 2012	3.6	1.2	20	7.2	3	20	7.1%	-3.60 [-5.02, -2.18]
Lee et al., 2015	43.6	7.5	21	57.8	22.5	20	3.4%	-14.20 [-24.57, -3.83]
Mathiesen et al., 2008	24	14	40	47	28	38	3.6%	-23.00 [-32.90, -13.10]
Paul et al., 2013	27.9	22.9	52	27	19	49	4.3%	0.90 [-7.29, 9.09]
Paul et al., 2015	19.7	16.3	48	25.1	14.4	54	5.3%	-5.40 [-11.40, 0.60]
Rasmussen et al., 2010	13	12	24	22	18	18	3.7%	-9.00 [-18.60, 0.60]
Singla et al., 2015	50.6	4.7	85	56	4.9	84	7.1%	-5.40 [-6.85, -3.95]
Tobias et al., 2019	0.7	1.3	25	0.7	1.3	25	7.3%	0.00 [-0.72, 0.72]
YaDeau et al., 2015	45.4	24.3	26	50.3	28.5	28	2.4%	-4.90 [-19.00, 9.20]
Subtotal (95% CI)			**433**			**428**	**51.4%**	**-7.28 [-11.61, -2.96]**
Heterogeneity: Tau² = 37.14; Chi² = 321.75, df = 9 (P < 0.00001); I² = 97%								
Test for overall effect: Z = 3.30 (P = 0.0010)								
1.3.2 POD 2								
Carmichael et al., 2014	144.2	85	18	177.6	101	18	0.2%	-33.40 [-94.38, 27.58]
Jain et al., 2012	3.3	1.1	20	6	2.4	20	7.2%	-2.70 [-3.86, -1.54]
Lee et al., 2015	70.2	12.6	21	85.7	23.2	20	3.1%	-15.50 [-27.01, -3.99]
Martinez et al., 2014	44	20	35	77	36	38	2.6%	-33.00 [-46.23, -19.77]
Paul et al., 2013	30.2	30.3	52	30.1	22.9	49	3.4%	0.10 [-10.34, 10.54]
Paul et al., 2015	22.7	18.1	48	23.4	19.4	54	4.7%	-0.70 [-7.98, 6.58]
Singla et al., 2015	28.8	4	82	40.9	4.1	83	7.2%	-12.10 [-13.34, -10.86]
YaDeau et al., 2015	59.2	25.3	26	70.7	35.3	28	1.9%	-11.50 [-27.80, 4.80]
Yik et al., 2019	56.3	119.6	13	29.1	56	14	0.1%	27.20 [-44.13, 98.53]
Subtotal (95% CI)			**315**			**324**	**30.4%**	**-9.29 [-15.26, -3.32]**
Heterogeneity: Tau² = 45.55; Chi² = 141.88, df = 8 (P < 0.00001); I² = 94%								
Test for overall effect: Z = 3.05 (P = 0.002)								
1.3.3 POD 3								
Paul et al., 2013	17.5	22.3	52	15.5	16.2	49	4.6%	2.00 [-5.57, 9.57]
Paul et al., 2015	15.5	25.6	48	10.3	13.2	54	4.4%	5.20 [-2.85, 13.25]
YaDeau et al., 2015	33.3	23.4	26	53	36.9	28	1.9%	-19.70 [-36.06, -3.34]
Yik et al., 2019	56.3	119.6	13	33.7	65.9	14	0.1%	22.60 [-51.01, 96.21]
Subtotal (95% CI)			**139**			**145**	**11.0%**	**-1.13 [-11.33, 9.08]**
Heterogeneity: Tau² = 55.06; Chi² = 7.58, df = 3 (P = 0.06); I² = 60%								
Test for overall effect: Z = 0.22 (P = 0.83)								
1.3.4 PO 1 w								
Singla et al., 2015	12.1	1.8	84	13.1	1.9	81	7.3%	-1.00 [-1.57, -0.43]
Tobias et al., 2019	0.7	1.3	25	0	0	25		Not estimable
Subtotal (95% CI)			**109**			**106**	**7.3%**	**-1.00 [-1.57, -0.43]**
Heterogeneity: Not applicable								
Test for overall effect: Z = 3.47 (P = 0.0005)								
Total (95% CI)			**996**			**1003**	**100.0%**	**-6.42 [-9.07, -3.78]**
Heterogeneity: Tau² = 24.98; Chi² = 617.91, df = 23 (P < 0.00001); I² = 96%								
Test for overall effect: Z = 4.76 (P < 0.00001)								
Test for subgroup differences: Chi² = 15.13, df = 3 (P = 0.002), I² = 80.2%								

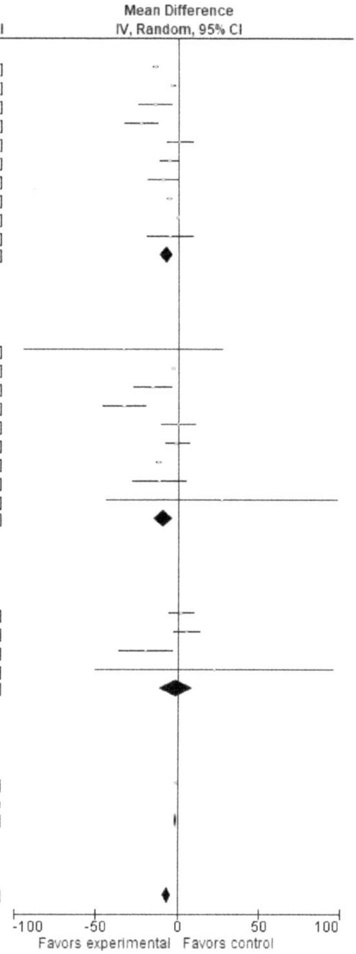

Figure 4. Postoperative opioid consumption in morphine equivalents (mg) [9,20–30,32].

3.5. Postoperative Nausea (n)

The incidence of nausea was comparable between the two groups at two and four hours after surgery and on postoperative days 1 and 2 (Figure 5). The incidence of nausea was lower in the experimental group in the "all PO periods" subgroup. In this subgroup, Tobias et al., 2020 [23] reported data values measured two months after surgery, while Jain et al., 2012 [26] and Singla et al., 2015 [29] reported data values for all study periods (i.e., total numbers). Combining all these periods shows a lower overall incidence of nausea in the gabapentinoid group (RR = 0.69 [0.55, 0.86], p-value = 0.0009, I^2 = 5%).

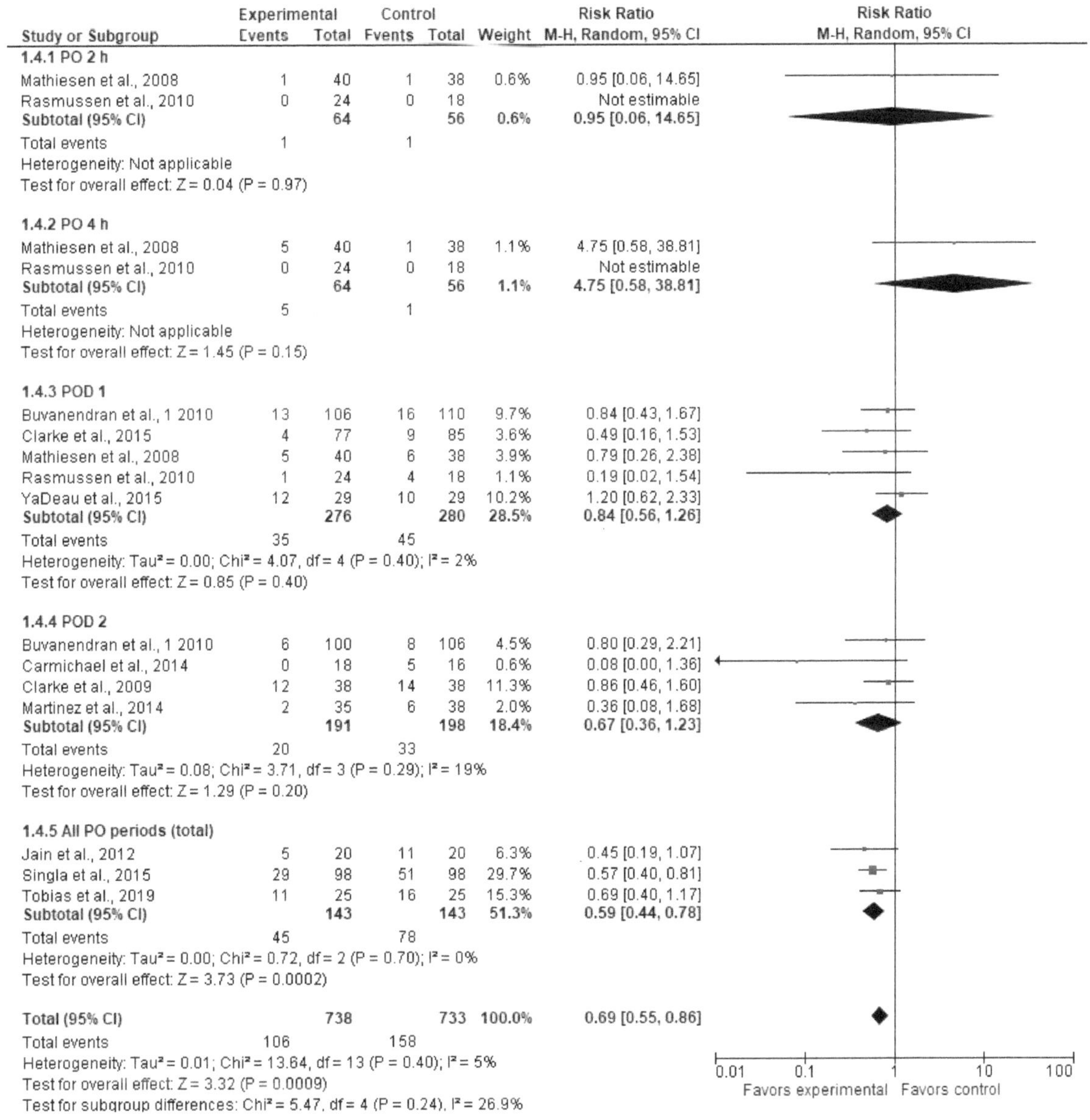

Figure 5. Postoperative nausea (n) [5,23–27,29–32].

3.6. Postoperative Vomiting (n)

The incidence of postoperative vomiting on POD 1 and 2 was comparable between the two groups (Figure 6). In the "all PO periods" subgroup, Tobias et al., 2020 [23] reported data values measured two months after surgery, while Jain et al., 2012 [26], Rasmussen et al., 2010 [25], and Singla et al., 2015 [29] reported data values for all study periods (i.e., total numbers). In this subgroup, the gabapentinoid arm had a lower incidence of vomiting (RR = 0.49 [0.31, 0.79, $p = 0.004$, $I^2 = 5\%$). Overall, the model does not favor the experimental group over the control group (RR = 0.72 [0.46, 1.14], p-value = 0.16, $I^2 = 32\%$).

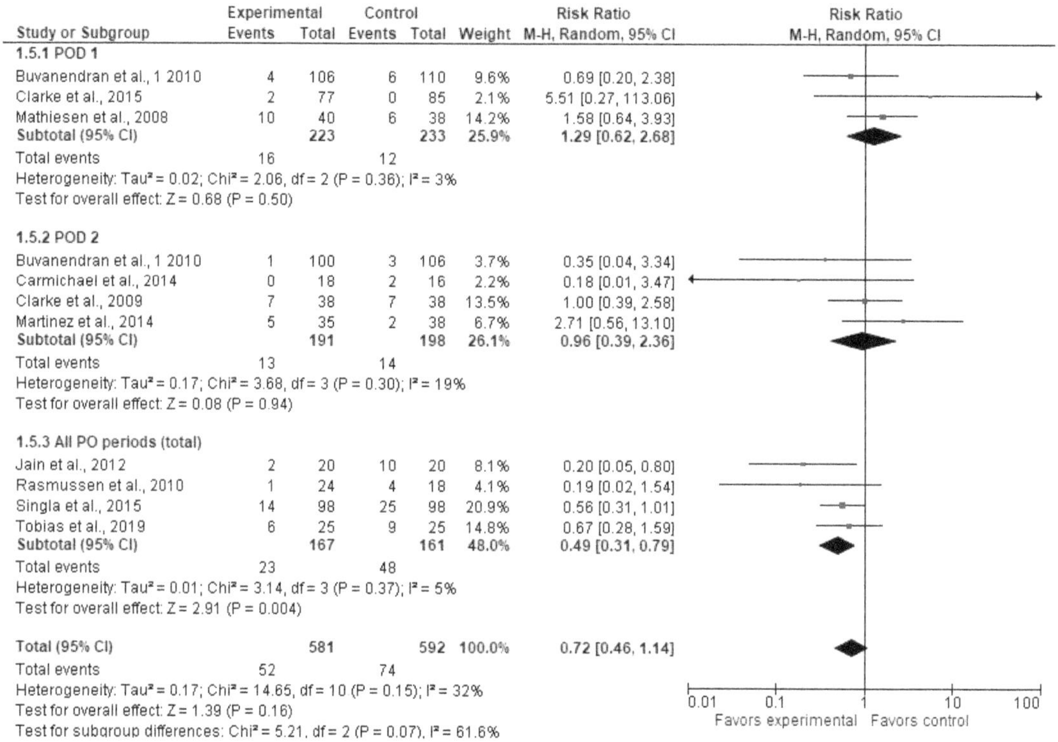

Figure 6. Postoperative vomiting (n) [5,21,23–27,29,31,32].

3.7. Subgroup Analysis for TKA and THA: Pain at Rest

As evident from Figure 7A (upper part), there is no significant difference between TKA and THA versus the control in pain intensity at rest on POD 1. The result of TKA vs. the control is sensitive to the exclusion of a study by Paul et al. (2013) [20], in which case the model would favor TKA over the control. If we had used the fixed effect model, it would have favored TKA over the control. Similar results were observed on POD 2 (Figure 7B).

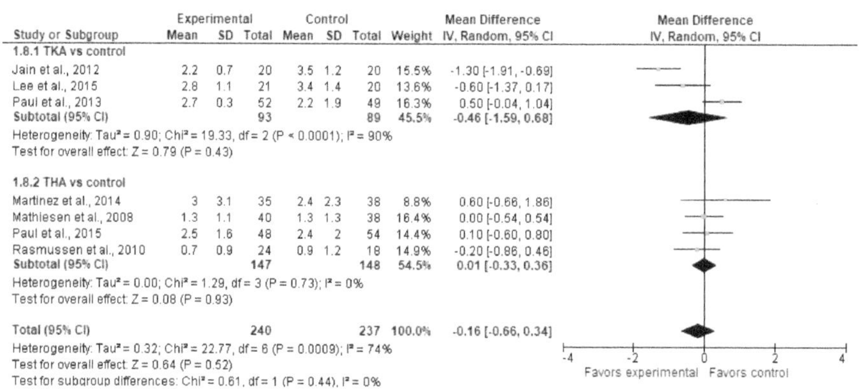

(A)

Figure 7. *Cont.*

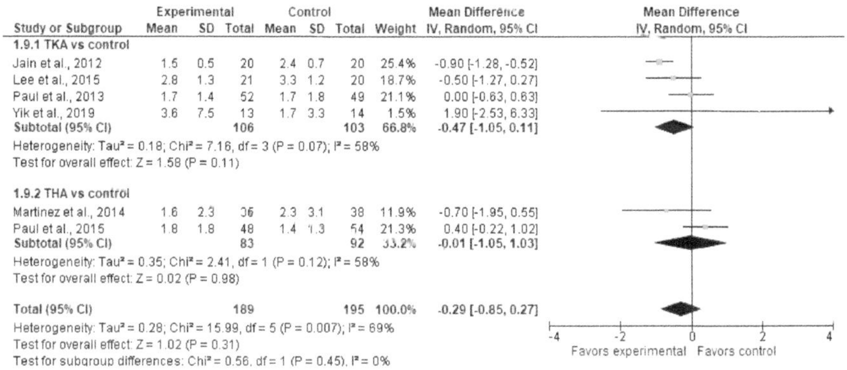

(B)

Figure 7. Postoperative pain at rest for THA and TKA on (**A**) POD 1 (upper) and (**B**) POD 2 (lower) [9,20,22,26–28].

3.8. Subgroup Analysis for TKA and THA: Pain on Movement

As shown in Figure 8A (upper part), there is no significant difference in pain on movement between TKA and THA versus the control. The result of TKA vs. the control is sensitive to the exclusion of a study by Paul et al. (2013) [20], in which case the model would favor TKA over the control. If we had used the fixed effect model, it would have favored TKA over the control.

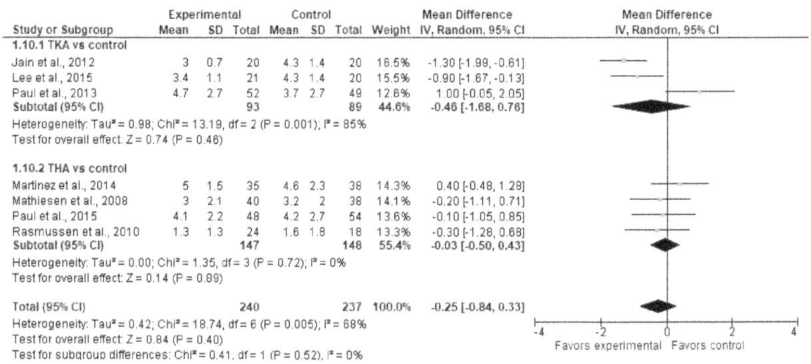

(A)

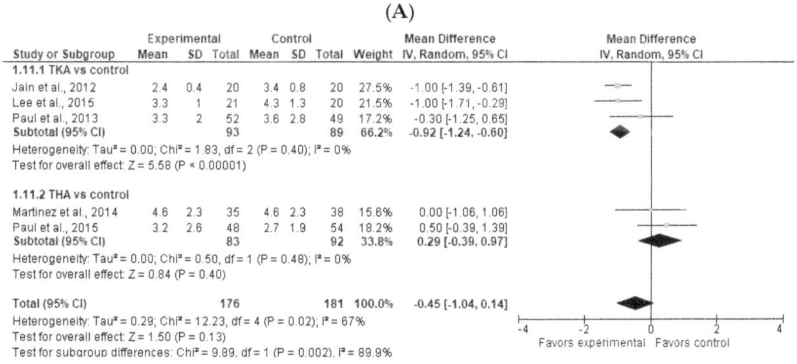

(B)

Figure 8. Postoperative pain on movement for THA and TKA on (**A**) POD 1 (upper) and (**B**) POD 2 (lower) [9,20,22,24–27].

3.9. Quality Assessment

The results of the Cochrane risk of bias tool 2 assessment are presented in Table 2. Seven studies had a "low risk" of bias, and eight studies had "some concerns" with regard to the risk of bias.

Table 2. Cochrane risk of bias.

Study Reference	D1	D2	D3	D4	D5	Overall
YaDeau et al., 2015 [30]	+	+	+	+	+	+
Buvanendran et al., 2010 [31]	+	+	?	?	+	?
Clarke et al., 2009 [5]	+	+	+	+	?	?
Paul et al., 2015 [22]	+	+	+	+	+	+
Clarke et al., 2015 [32]	+	+	?	?	+	?
Tobias et al., 2019 [23]	+	+	?	+	+	?
Yik et al., 2019 [28]	+	+	+	+	+	+
Lee et al., 2015 [9]	+	?	?	+	+	?
Paul et al., 2013 [20]	+	+	+	+	+	+
Jain et al., 2012 [26]	+	+	+	+	+	+
Martinez et al., 2014 [27]	+	+	+	+	+	+
Singla et al., 2014 [29]	+	+	+	+	+	+
Carmichael et al., 2014 [21]	+	?	?	+	+	?
Mathiesen et al., 2008 [24]	+	?	+	+	+	?
Rasmussen et al., 2010 [25]	+	?	+	+	+	?

+	Low risk
?	Some concerns
-	High risk
D1	Randomization process
D2	Deviations from the intended interventions
D3	Missing outcome data
D4	Measurement of the outcome
D5	Selection of the reported result

The results of the GRADE assessment of the main outcomes are presented in Table 3. Two outcomes had "high" and three outcomes had a "moderate" level of certainty of evidence.

Table 3. Summary of findings. Abbreviations: CI, confidence interval; GRADE, Grading of Recommendations Assessment, Development, and Evaluation; N, number; and RCT, randomized controlled trial. ⊕⊕⊕○, moderate certainty of evidence; ⊕⊕⊕⊕, high certainty of evidence.

Outcome	Study Design	N of Patients (Studies)	Mean Difference/Relative Risk [95% CI]	Certainty of Evidence (GRADE)
Overall pain scores at rest (0–10)	RCT	1868 (11)	−0.30 [−0.55, −0.05]	⊕⊕⊕○ Moderate
Overall pain scores on movement (0–10)	RCT	1415 (8)	−0.41 [−0.68, −0.13]	⊕⊕⊕○ Moderate

Table 3. *Cont.*

Outcome	Study Design	N of Patients (Studies)	Mean Difference/Relative Risk [95% CI]	Certainty of Evidence (GRADE)
Overall postoperative opioid use in morphine equivalent (mg)	RCT	2081 (12)	−6.42 [−9.07, −3.78]	⊕⊕⊕○ Moderate
Overall postoperative nausea	RCT	1471 (11)	0.69 [0.55, 0.86]	⊕⊕⊕⊕ High
Overall postoperative vomiting	RCT	1173 (11)	0.72 [0.46, 1.14]	⊕⊕⊕⊕ High

4. Discussion

4.1. Interpretations of Results

4.1.1. Pain

In this meta-analysis, pain scores at rest and on movement were lower for the gabapentinoid group from the first postoperative hours up to day three. Although this difference was not statistically significant across most time periods, the analysis may have lacked the power to reach significance due to the small number of participants. Gabapentinoids may provide effective pain management in the first hours post-surgery, and this effect declines by day three. In fact, in our analysis, pain scores at rest on day three were statistically significantly higher for the experimental group, even though the effect size was negligible. Potential contributing factors to such a trend may be the pharmacokinetics and temporal profiles of gabapentinoids, the role of central sensitization, the combination of gabapentinoids with other analgesic agents, or the "rebound pain" effect.

The previous literature has demonstrated varying findings. Similar to our results, pain at rest on days one and two, but not three was found to be lower in the pregabalin group following THA and TKA [33]. Likewise, a meta-analysis of 322 clinical trials comprising all types of surgeries also found the preoperative administration of gabapentinoids effective in alleviating postoperative pain at six, twelve, twenty-four, and forty-eight but not at seventy-two hours post-surgery [34]. It is worth noting that in their subgroup analysis, this remained true for gabapentin, while for pregabalin, the difference in pain intensity lost statistical significance between the two groups at 48 h. This may be associated with pregabalin's faster absorption: its maximum concentration in the serum is one hour, as opposed to two to four hours for gabapentin [35]. On the other hand, in a meta-analysis of gabapentin use in TKA patients, Han et al. did not find any difference in pain scores at 12, 24, or 48 h [11]. Similarly, Mao et al. did not find differences in pain scores at rest and on movement at 24 and 48 h following THA [36].

In our study, the reduction in pain scores was not clinically meaningful as defined by previous research [37]. Verret et. al. mention that in their study, the pain-sparing effect was more evident in the first hours following the surgery [34]. This again suggests that gabapentinoids are more active in the first postoperative hours. Interestingly, their subgroup analysis showed that the mean difference between the gabapentinoid and control groups for almost all the periods was higher for the gabapentin group rather than pregabalin [34], although the latter is considered to be more potent [35].

4.1.2. Opioid Consumption

Similar to pain intensity, our results showed that there was a significant difference in opioid use on the first two postoperative days, while on day three, the use of opioids was already comparable between the two groups. Lower opioid consumption in the first two days following TKA was observed between the gabapentin and control groups [11] and between the gabapentinoids and control groups following lower limb arthroplasty [13]. Both gabapentin and pregabalin have been found to be effective in reducing opioid use on the first and second postoperative days after THA [36]. Pregabalin substantially decreased morphine consumption following both THA and TKA for 48 h post-surgery [33]. The large meta-analysis comprising various surgeries by Verret et al. found lower cumulative opioid consumption in the gabapentinoid group on postoperative days one (117 trials), two (24 trials), and, unlike our study, three (four trials), compared to controls [34]. One explanation for this opioid-sparing observation may be attributed to gabapentinoids' ability to strengthen opioids' effect when taken concurrently [35]. In other words, it might be that fewer opioids were consumed in the experimental group because their effect became more substantial in the presence of gabapentinoids. Another meta-analysis observed a lowered use of opioids for three days following both the knee and hip arthroplasty between the pregabalin and placebo groups but no difference in opioid use between the gabapentin and placebo arms [14]. This, again, may be attributed to pregabalin's higher potency and, potentially, a higher synergistic effect on opioids.

4.1.3. Postoperative Nausea and Vomiting

We found the cumulative all-period incidence of nausea, but not vomiting, to be lower in the gabapentinoid group. This is consistent with the observed lower consumption of opioids, a factor often associated with postoperative nausea. However, the reduction in opioid consumption was more significant than that of the incidence of nausea, which poses the question of whether the latter was a result of the former. Indeed, Verret et al. found no association between a lower incidence of postoperative nausea and vomiting in the gabapentinoid group with morphine consumption [34]. A lower incidence of nausea, but not vomiting, was observed in the gabapentin group following THA [12]. Han et al. observed a comparable incidence of nausea between the gabapentin and placebo groups following lower limb arthroplasty [11]. Hannon et al. also observed no difference in the incidence of nausea between the gabapentin and placebo groups following TKA; however, their analysis did show a lower incidence of nausea in the pregabalin group compared to the placebo [14]. Likewise, pregabalin was shown effective in lowering the incidence of nausea in TKA but not THA [33].

4.1.4. Chronic Pain

We initially aimed to examine the impact of gabapentinoids on chronic postoperative pain. However, we lacked sufficient data to investigate this relationship in our meta-analysis. This aspect is crucial because while acute pain can be managed with various medications and nerve blocks, there are limited options proven to prevent or reduce chronic pain after surgery. Previously, in a meta-analysis of almost 3200 patients undergoing various types of surgeries, no association was found between preoperative administration of gabapentinoids with chronic pain within three to twelve months [34]. This result held across different gabapentin/pregabalin doses and administration methods. Exploring gabapentinoids' specific effects on chronic pain following knee surgery might require a longer usage period for their anti-inflammatory effects to become evident. Moreover, the relationship between neuropathic pain in acute settings and the development of chronic postsurgical or neuropathic pain is still not fully understood. Sensitization in central or peripheral nerves is complex and involves changes in how nerves function. Therefore, while gabapentinoids might offer pain relief to some extent, it is important to manage acute postoperative pain using multimodal analgesia.

4.2. Study Limitations

Our study has several limitations. First, relatively small RCTs were included in the meta-analysis, and since these reported the outcomes of interest at various times, our study had a small sample size for the majority of the time periods. Second, including studies using either pregabalin or gabapentin and in varying dosages introduced variability in the results, potentially impacting the overall findings. Third, the absence of standardization in surgical procedures across the studies may have contributed to varying pain experiences, making it challenging to draw universal conclusions. Moreover, the demographic variations among patients, including age, gender, and underlying health conditions, might have influenced individual responses to gabapentinoids, further complicating the interpretation of the results. Finally, the lack of long-term follow-up limited our understanding of the sustained effects and potential long-term side effects of gabapentinoids in postoperative pain management.

4.3. Implications for Research and Practice

Given what is mentioned above, large and high-quality randomized controlled trials on the topic should be conducted to be able to draw more definitive conclusions. Furthermore, exploring the neurobiological mechanisms, including central sensitization modulation and neuroinflammatory processes, can deepen our understanding of gabapentinoids' analgesic actions and the temporal effects, potentially leading to the development of more targeted interventions. The synergistic effects of gabapentinoids in combination with other analgesic agents, both opioid and non-opioid, should be studied in-depth to optimize multimodal pain management strategies. Future studies should also focus on examining the effect of gabapentinoid use, especially in conjunction with opioids, on postoperative nausea and vomiting. Further research should also explore the long-term effects of gabapentinoids on postoperative pain management, especially focusing on chronic pain development following knee surgeries. Longitudinal studies with extended follow-up periods are essential to assess the persistence of gabapentinoids' effects and their role in preventing chronic postoperative pain. As for practical implications, while our results have little clinical importance on their own, they might be useful for developing effective multimodal analgesic interventions for knee and hip surgical procedures.

5. Conclusions

This meta-analysis demonstrated that gabapentinoids were associated with reductions in postoperative pain at rest and with movement (however, the reduction was not clinically relevant), morphine consumption, and incidence of postoperative nausea over two postoperative days when knee and hip surgery were combined in the same model. The subgroup analysis showed that gabapentinoids reduced pain on movement on postoperative day two after total knee arthroplasty but not after total hip arthroplasty. Pain reduction was not clinically relevant. Sedation has not been evaluated in this work and, if performed, this may have influenced the conclusions. There was no significant difference between the groups in terms of vomiting during the early postoperative period. There was an insufficient amount of data to support the efficacy of gabapentinoids in the prevention or reduction of chronic postoperative pain in knee and hip surgery. An important limitation of this study is that different gabapentinoids, their administration times and dosages, as well as varying intraoperative management protocols, were pooled together. Having standardized protocols would facilitate further investigation of this issue. Future large, high-quality RCTs are warranted to study the role of gabapentoids in orthopedic surgery, with a focus on the incidence of chronic postoperative pain.

Author Contributions: Conceptualization, D.V.; methodology, D.V.; data extraction, M.A. and N.S.; software, A.S., D.K. and Y.G.A.; formal analysis, A.S., D.K. and Y.G.A.; quality assessment, M.A. and N.S.; funding acquisition, D.V., R.T. and Y.G.A.; writing—original draft preparation, D.V.; writing—review and editing, D.V., M.A., A.S., D.K., N.S., R.T. and Y.G.A. All authors have read and agreed to the published version of the manuscript.

Funding: This work was supported in part by Nazarbayev University Faculty Development Competitive Research Grants No. SOM2024005 and 11022021FD2906. The authors have no other relevant affiliations or financial involvement with any organization or entity with a financial interest in or financial conflict with the subject matter or materials discussed in this manuscript apart from those disclosed.

Institutional Review Board Statement: Not applicable.

Informed Consent Statement: Not applicable.

Data Availability Statement: The datasets are available upon request from the corresponding author.

Conflicts of Interest: The authors declare no conflicts of interest.

References

1. Fingar, K.R.; Stocks, C.; Weiss, A.J.; Steiner, C.A. Most Frequent Operating Room Procedures Performed in U.S. Hospitals, 2003–2012. In *Healthcare Cost and Utilization Project (HCUP) Statistical Briefs*; Agency for Healthcare Research and Quality: Rockville, MD, USA, 2006.
2. Trousdale, R.T.; McGrory, B.J.; Berry, D.J.; Becker, M.W.; Harmsen, W.S. Patients' Concerns Prior to Undergoing Total Hip and Total Knee Arthroplasty. *Mayo Clin. Proc.* **1999**, *74*, 978–982. [CrossRef] [PubMed]
3. Gaffney, C.J.; Pelt, C.E.; Gililland, J.M.; Peters, C.L. Perioperative Pain Management in Hip and Knee Arthroplasty. *Orthop. Clin. N. Am.* **2017**, *48*, 407–419. [CrossRef] [PubMed]
4. Joshi, G.P.; Ogunnaike, B.O. Consequences of Inadequate Postoperative Pain Relief and Chronic Persistent Postoperative Pain. *Anesthesiol. Clin. N. Am.* **2005**, *23*, 21–36. [CrossRef] [PubMed]
5. Clarke, H.; Pereira, S.; Kennedy, D.; Andrion, J.; Mitsakakis, N.; Gollish, J.; Katz, J.; Kay, J. Adding Gabapentin to a Multimodal Regimen Does Not Reduce Acute Pain, Opioid Consumption or Chronic Pain after Total Hip Arthroplasty. *Acta Anaesthesiol. Scand.* **2009**, *53*, 1073–1083. [CrossRef] [PubMed]
6. Halawi, M.J.; Vovos, T.J.; Green, C.L.; Wellman, S.S.; Attarian, D.E.; Bolognesi, M.P. Opioid-Based Analgesia: Impact on Total Joint Arthroplasty. *J. Arthroplast.* **2015**, *30*, 2360–2363. [CrossRef] [PubMed]
7. Wheeler, M.; Oderda, G.M.; Ashburn, M.A.; Lipman, A.G. Adverse Events Associated with Postoperative Opioid Analgesia: A Systematic Review. *J. Pain* **2002**, *3*, 159–180. [CrossRef] [PubMed]
8. Sharma, S.; Iorio, R.; Specht, L.M.; Davies-Lepie, S.; Healy, W.L. Complications of Femoral Nerve Block for Total Knee Arthroplasty. *Clin. Orthop. Relat. Res.* **2010**, *468*, 135–140. [CrossRef] [PubMed]
9. Lee, J.K.; Chung, K.-S.; Choi, C.H. The Effect of a Single Dose of Preemptive Pregabalin Administered with COX-2 Inhibitor: A Trial in Total Knee Arthroplasty. *J. Arthroplast.* **2015**, *30*, 38–42. [CrossRef] [PubMed]
10. Kremer, M.; Salvat, E.; Muller, A.; Yalcin, I.; Barrot, M. Antidepressants and Gabapentinoids in Neuropathic Pain: Mechanistic Insights. *Neuroscience* **2016**, *338*, 183–206. [CrossRef]
11. Turan, A.; White, P.F.; Karamanlioglu, B.; Pamukçu, Z. Premedication with Gabapentin: The Effect on Tourniquet Pain and Quality of Intravenous Regional Anesthesia. *Anesth. Analg.* **2007**, *104*, 97–101. [CrossRef]
12. Han, C.; Li, X.; Jiang, H.; Ma, J.; Ma, X. The Use of Gabapentin in the Management of Postoperative Pain after Total Knee Arthroplasty. *Medicine* **2016**, *95*, e3883. [CrossRef] [PubMed]
13. Campbell, R.; Khuong, J.N.; Liu, Z.; Borg, C.; Jackson, S.; Ramson, D.M.; Kok, J.; Douglas, N.; Penny-Dimri, J.C.; Perry, L.A. Perioperative Gabapentinoid Use Lowers Short-Term Opioid Consumption Following Lower Limb Arthroplasty: Systematic Review and Meta-Analysis. *J. Opioid Manag.* **2021**, *17*, 251–272. [CrossRef] [PubMed]
14. Hannon, C.P.; Fillingham, Y.A.; Browne, J.A.; Schemitsch, E.H.; Mullen, K.; Casambre, F.; Visvabharathy, V.; Hamilton, W.G.; Della Valle, C.J. The Efficacy and Safety of Gabapentinoids in Total Joint Arthroplasty: Systematic Review and Direct Meta-Analysis. *J. Arthroplast.* **2020**, *35*, 2730–2738.e6. [CrossRef] [PubMed]
15. Page, M.J.; McKenzie, J.E.; Bossuyt, P.M.; Boutron, I.; Hoffmann, T.C.; Mulrow, C.D.; Shamseer, L.; Tetzlaff, J.M.; Akl, E.A.; Brennan, S.E.; et al. The PRISMA 2020 Statement: An Updated Guideline for Reporting Systematic Reviews. *BMJ* **2021**, *372*, n71. [CrossRef] [PubMed]
16. Sterne, J.A.C.; Savović, J.; Page, M.J.; Elbers, R.G.; Blencowe, N.S.; Boutron, I.; Cates, C.J.; Cheng, H.-Y.; Corbett, M.S.; Eldridge, S.M.; et al. RoB 2: A Revised Tool for Assessing Risk of Bias in Randomised Trials. *BMJ* **2019**, *366*, l4898. [CrossRef]
17. Guyatt, G.H.; Oxman, A.D.; Schünemann, H.J.; Tugwell, P.; Knottnerus, A. GRADE Guidelines: A New Series of Articles in the Journal of Clinical Epidemiology. *J. Clin. Epidemiol.* **2011**, *64*, 380–382. [CrossRef]
18. Luo, D.; Wan, X.; Liu, J.; Tong, T. Optimally Estimating the Sample Mean from the Sample Size, Median, Mid-Range, and/or Mid-Quartile Range. *Stat. Methods Med. Res.* **2018**, *27*, 1785–1805. [CrossRef]
19. Wan, X.; Wang, W.; Liu, J.; Tong, T. Estimating the Sample Mean and Standard Deviation from the Sample Size, Median, Range and/or Interquartile Range. *BMC Med. Res. Methodol.* **2014**, *14*, 135. [CrossRef]
20. Paul, J.E.; Nantha-Aree, M.; Buckley, N.; Cheng, J.; Thabane, L.; Tidy, A.; DeBeer, J.; Winemaker, M.; Wismer, D.; Punthakee, D.; et al. Gabapentin Does Not Improve Multimodal Analgesia Outcomes for Total Knee Arthroplasty: A Randomized Controlled Trial. *Can. J. Anaesth.* **2013**, *60*, 423–431. [CrossRef]
21. Carmichael, N.M.E.; Katz, J.; Clarke, H.; Kennedy, D.; Kreder, H.J.; Gollish, J.; McCartney, C.J.L. An Intensive Perioperative Regimen of Pregabalin and Celecoxib Reduces Pain and Improves Physical Function Scores Six Weeks after Total Hip Arthroplasty: A Prospective Randomized Controlled Trial. *Pain Res. Manag.* **2013**, *18*, 127–132. [CrossRef]
22. Paul, J.E.; Nantha-Aree, M.; Buckley, N.; Shahzad, U.; Cheng, J.; Thabane, L.; Tidy, A.; DeBeer, J.; Winemaker, M.; Wismer, D.; et al. Randomized Controlled Trial of Gabapentin as an Adjunct to Perioperative Analgesia in Total Hip Arthroplasty Patients. *Can. J. Anaesth.* **2015**, *62*, 476–484. [CrossRef] [PubMed]
23. Tobias, A.F.; Moura, E.C.R.; Honda, C.A.D.O.; Pereira, E.C.; de Oliveira, C.M.B.; Leal, P.D.C.; Sakata, R.K. Evaluation of the Efficacy of Prolonged Pregabalin Administration Before and After Surgery in Patients Undergoing Arthroscopic Anterior Cruciate Ligament Repair: A Prospective, Randomized, Double-Blind Study. *Clin. J. Pain* **2020**, *36*, 584–588. [CrossRef] [PubMed]
24. Mathiesen, O.; Jacobsen, L.S.; Holm, H.E.; Randall, S.; Adamiec-Malmstroem, L.; Graungaard, B.K.; Holst, P.E.; Hilsted, K.L.; Dahl, J.B. Pregabalin and Dexamethasone for Postoperative Pain Control: A Randomized Controlled Study in Hip Arthroplasty. *Br. J. Anaesth.* **2008**, *101*, 535–541. [CrossRef] [PubMed]

25. Rasmussen, M.L.; Mathiesen, O.; Dierking, G.; Christensen, B.V.; Hilsted, K.L.; Larsen, T.K.; Dahl, J.B. Multimodal Analgesia with Gabapentin, Ketamine and Dexamethasone in Combination with Paracetamol and Ketorolac after Hip Arthroplasty: A Preliminary Study. *Eur. J. Anaesthesiol.* **2010**, *27*, 324–330. [CrossRef] [PubMed]
26. Jain, P.; Jolly, A.; Bholla, V.; Adatia, S.; Sood, J. Evaluation of Efficacy of Oral Pregabalin in Reducing Postoperative Pain in Patients Undergoing Total Knee Arthroplasty. *Indian J. Orthop.* **2012**, *46*, 646–652. [CrossRef] [PubMed]
27. Martinez, V.; Cymerman, A.; Ben Ammar, S.; Fiaud, J.F.; Rapon, C.; Poindessous, F.; Judet, T.; Chauvin, M.; Bouhassira, D.; Sessler, D.; et al. The Analgesic Efficiency of Combined Pregabalin and Ketamine for Total Hip Arthroplasty: A Randomised, Double-Blind, Controlled Study. *Anaesthesia* **2014**, *69*, 46–52. [CrossRef] [PubMed]
28. Yik, J.H.; Tham, W.Y.W.; Tay, K.H.; Shen, L.; Krishna, L. Perioperative Pregabalin Does Not Reduce Opioid Requirements in Total Knee Arthroplasty. *Knee Surg. Sports Traumatol. Arthrosc.* **2019**, *27*, 2104–2110. [CrossRef] [PubMed]
29. Singla, N.K.; Chelly, J.E.; Lionberger, D.R.; Gimbel, J.; Sanin, L.; Sporn, J.; Yang, R.; Cheung, R.; Knapp, L.; Parsons, B. Pregabalin for the Treatment of Postoperative Pain: Results from Three Controlled Trials Using Different Surgical Models. *J. Pain Res.* **2015**, *8*, 9–20. [CrossRef] [PubMed]
30. YaDeau, J.T.; Lin, Y.; Mayman, D.J.; Goytizolo, E.A.; Alexiades, M.M.; Padgett, D.E.; Kahn, R.L.; Jules-Elysee, K.M.; Ranawat, A.S.; Bhagat, D.D.; et al. Pregabalin and Pain after Total Knee Arthroplasty: A Double-Blind, Randomized, Placebo-Controlled, Multidose Trial. *Br. J. Anaesth.* **2015**, *115*, 285–293. [CrossRef]
31. Buvanendran, A.; Kroin, J.S.; Della Valle, C.J.; Kari, M.; Moric, M.; Tuman, K.J. Perioperative Oral Pregabalin Reduces Chronic Pain after Total Knee Arthroplasty: A Prospective, Randomized, Controlled Trial. *Anesth. Analg.* **2010**, *110*, 199–207. [CrossRef]
32. Clarke, H.; Pagé, G.M.; McCartney, C.J.L.; Huang, A.; Stratford, P.; Andrion, J.; Kennedy, D.; Awad, I.T.; Gollish, J.; Kay, J.; et al. Pregabalin Reduces Postoperative Opioid Consumption and Pain for 1 Week after Hospital Discharge, but Does Not Affect Function at 6 Weeks or 3 Months after Total Hip Arthroplasty. *Br. J. Anaesth.* **2015**, *115*, 903–911. [CrossRef] [PubMed]
33. Li, F.; Ma, J.; Kuang, M.; Jiang, X.; Wang, Y.; Lu, B.; Zhao, X.; Sun, L.; Ma, X. The Efficacy of Pregabalin for the Management of Postoperative Pain in Primary Total Knee and Hip Arthroplasty: A Meta-Analysis. *J. Orthop. Surg. Res.* **2017**, *12*, 49. [CrossRef] [PubMed]
34. Verret, M.; Lauzier, F.; Zarychanski, R.; Perron, C.; Savard, X.; Pinard, A.-M.; Leblanc, G.; Cossi, M.-J.; Neveu, X.; Turgeon, A.F.; et al. Perioperative Use of Gabapentinoids for the Management of Postoperative Acute Pain: A Systematic Review and Meta-Analysis. *Anesthesiology* **2020**, *133*, 265–279. [CrossRef] [PubMed]
35. Evoy, K.E.; Peckham, A.M.; Covvey, J.R.; Tidgewell, K.J. Gabapentinoid Pharmacology in the Context of Emerging Misuse Liability. *J. Clin. Pharma* **2021**, *61*, S89–S99. [CrossRef]
36. Mao, Y.; Wu, L.; Ding, W. The Efficacy of Preoperative Administration of Gabapentin/Pregabalin in Improving Pain after Total Hip Arthroplasty: A Meta-Analysis. *BMC Musculoskelet. Disord.* **2016**, *17*, 373. [CrossRef]
37. Laigaard, J.; Pedersen, C.; Rønsbo, T.N.; Mathiesen, O.; Karlsen, A.P.H. Minimal Clinically Important Differences in Randomised Clinical Trials on Pain Management after Total Hip and Knee Arthroplasty: A Systematic Review. *Br. J. Anaesth.* **2021**, *126*, 1029–1037. [CrossRef]

Journal of
Clinical Medicine

MDPI

Article

Transversus Abdominis Plane Block Following Cesarean Section: A Prospective Randomized Controlled Study Comparing the Effects on Pain Levels of Bupivacaine, Bupivacaine + Dexmedetomidine, and Bupivacaine + Dexamethasone

Senem Urfalı *, Sedat Hakimoğlu, Selim Turhanoğlu and Onur Koyuncu

Department of Anesthesiology and Reanimation, Tayfur Ata Sokmen Medical Faculty, Hatay Mustafa Kemal University, 31040 Hatay, Turkey; sedathakimoglu@gmail.com (S.H.); adat63@gmail.com (S.T.); dronurkoyuncu@gmail.com (O.K.)

* Correspondence: senemurfali@gmail.com; Tel.: +90-5326331797

Abstract: Background: The transversus abdominis plane (TAP) block is providing effective postoperative analgesia in patients undergoing cesarean section (CS). This study aims to evaluate and compare the effects on pain levels of bupivacaine alone versus bupivacaine combined with dexmedetomidine and bupivacaine combined with dexamethasone in ultrasound-guided TAP block for postoperative pain after CS. **Material and Method**: In this randomized controlled trial, 120 patients with American Society of Anesthesiologists (ASA) physical status I and II scheduled for elective cesarean section under spinal anesthesia were randomly divided into three groups. At the end of the surgery, an ultrasound-guided TAP block was performed on all patients: bupivacaine 0.5% (Group B), bupivacaine 0.5% + dexmedetomidine (1 μg/kg) (Group BD), and bupivacaine 0.5% + dexamethasone (4 mg) (Group BDx). Postoperatively, all patients were evaluated at 0, 1, 4, 8, 16, and 24 h for visual analog scores VASs, tramadol consumption, complications, and patient satisfaction. A p value of < 0.05 is statistically significant. **Results**: At 0 h, VASs in the sitting and supine positions were significantly higher in the BDx group (0.85 ± 1.61 and 0.85 ± 1.36, respectively) compared to the B group (0.05 ± 0.32 in both positions) and the BD group (0.15 ± 0.48 in both positions) ($p = 0.005$ and $p = 0.001$, respectively). At the 24th hour, VASs in the sitting and supine positions were significantly lower in the BDx group (1.7 ± 1.2 and 1.43 ± 1.05) compared to the B group (2.3 ± 0.68 and 2.2 ± 0.72) and the BD group (2.57 ± 1.01 and 2.28 ± 0.78) ($p = 0.005$ and $p = 0.001$, respectively). At 0 h, the tramadol requirement was highest in the BDx group at 12.5%, while it was not required in the B and BD groups ($p = 0.005$). At 0 h, the rate of nausea and vomiting was highest in the BDx group at 17.5%, compared to 2.5% in the BD group and 0% in the B group ($p = 0.003$). Patient satisfaction scores were higher in the dexamethasone group compared to the other groups. This was significant between Group B and Group BDx ($p = 0.009 < 0.05$). **Conclusions**: Adding dexmedetomidine or dexamethasone to bupivacaine in ultrasound-guided TAP blocks reduces postoperative pain and increases patient satisfaction after cesarean sections. Dexamethasone, due to its delayed onset but extended duration, achieves lower pain scores and higher satisfaction. Further research is necessary to confirm these findings.

Keywords: bupivacaine; dexmedetomidine; dexamethasone; postoperative analgesia; cesarean section

1. Introduction

Cesarean section (CS) is one of the most common surgeries and usually causes moderate to severe pain for up to 48 h [1]. The rate of CS, which is a life-saving surgical procedure in cases of certain complications that occur during pregnancy and birth, has exceeded 20% worldwide [2,3]. Pain control after CS has crucial importance, especially in the first 24 h, to facilitate early ambulation and the establishment of breastfeeding [4]. Insufficient analgesia in the postoperative period may cause a number of undesirable effects, such as patient discomfort, thromboembolism due to extended immobilization, and decreased pulmonary clearance resulting in complications [5].

Postoperative CS pain arises mainly from somatic and visceral components. Surgical incision of the tissue leads to somatic pain, while visceral pain is mainly associated with inflammation [6]. The transversus abdominis plane (TAP) block has gained increasing importance as a very effective pain relief in abdominal surgery since Rafi's application in 2001 [7]. The transversus abdominis plane (TAP) block comprises the administration of a local anesthetic agent between the transverse and internal oblique muscles of the abdominal wall, targeting spinal T7-L1 levels, which attenuates somatic pain by inhibiting neural afferents within the transversus abdominis plane [4,8]. This reduces postoperative pain from lower abdominal surgeries, including cesarean sections [9]. Although commonly used nonsteroidal anti-inflammatory drugs and paracetamol can only supplement other modes of analgesia, they are not sufficient for their own population. In this context, many studies are being conducted to increase the TAP blockage duration [10].

A variety of anesthetic agents such as bupivacaine, levobupivacaine, and ropivacaine are commonly used in TAP blocks [9]. These drugs provide short-term analgesia and primarily alleviate somatic pain [11,12]. To extend the duration of analgesic efficacy, various adjuvants such as opioids, ketamine, clonidine, and alpha-2 agonists like dexmedetomidine have been added [9]. Studies have consistently shown that optimizing analgesia reduces opioid consumption and alleviates postoperative symptoms such as nausea and sedation [1].

Bupivacaine is one of the widely used local analgesics [13]. Dexmedetomidine is a highly selective central alpha-2 adrenergic agonist. It strengthens local anesthetic effects and prolongs analgesic duration by blocking the transmission of nerve signals through C and A delta fibers [4,14]. For these reasons, dexmedetomidine is commonly used as an adjuvant to local anesthetics in many studies [4,5,15]. Dexamethasone, a corticosteroid, provides analgesia owing to its anti-inflammatory properties. It also potentiates the effect of local anesthetics [16]. In light of this knowledge, dexamethasone has been used as an adjuvant in various studies to improve the anesthetic effects of TAP block postoperative CS operations [1,4].

Recent studies have highlighted the potential of non-opioid analgesic techniques in managing various pain conditions. For example, laser therapy has proven effective in alleviating chronic headache symptoms by targeting mucosal contact points in the nasal cavity [17]. Similarly, fractional CO_2 laser technology has provided significant relief for patients with Lichen Sclerosus, offering a non-invasive alternative that improves histological outcomes and reduces discomfort without requiring general anesthesia [18]. These advancements underscore the importance of exploring non-opioid treatments, such as TAP blocks and laser therapy, alongside adjuvants, particularly in mitigating postoperative pain following cesarean sections.

This study aimed to assess and compare the effects on pain levels of bupivacaine alone versus bupivacaine combined with dexmedetomidine and bupivacaine combined with dexamethasone in an ultrasound-guided TAP block for managing postoperative pain after cesarean section. Our primary outcome was pain score, while the secondary outcomes were analgesic requirements, complications, and patient satisfaction.

2. Materials and Methods

2.1. Study Design

The study was conducted between February 2020 and September 2021 at Hatay Mustafa Kemal University, following the approval from the Clinical Research Ethics Committee (meeting date: 20 February 2020, decision no: 05). Written informed consent was obtained from all participants in accordance with the principles of the Declaration of Helsinki [19].

Pregnant women with an American Society of Anesthesiologists (ASA) score of I or II who were scheduled for cesarean section under spinal anesthesia were included in the study. The exclusion criteria were as follows:

- Refusal to participate in the study;
- Known allergies to local anesthetics/opioids/nonsteroidal anti-inflammatory drugs;
- Presence of infection at the needle entry site for the block;
- Recent use of glucocorticoids;
- Diabetes mellitus;
- Pregnancy-induced hypertension;
- Use of chronic pain medications;
- Body mass index (BMI) > 35.

In the operating room, electrocardiography, pulse oximetry, and noninvasive blood pressure were monitored for all patients from the beginning of the procedure until they left the operating room. After monitoring the patients, spinal anesthesia was administered in a seated position with 2 to 2.2 mL of 0.5% heavy bupivacaine (Marcaine®, Astra-Zeneca, Istanbul, Turkey) between the L3 and L4 vertebrae after confirming the proper flow of cerebrospinal fluid.

Subjects included in the study were randomly assigned to three groups using a computer-generated sequence of random numbers, regardless of their demographic characteristics.

Patients were equally (40 per group) allocated to three TAP block groups as follows:

1. Group B: Bupivacaine 0.5% 10 mL + physiological saline 10 mL;
2. Group BD: Bupivacaine 0.5% 10 mL + physiological saline 9 mL + dexmedetomidine 1 mL (1 μg/kg);
3. Group BDx: Bupivacaine 0.5% 10mL + physiological saline 9 mL + dexamethasone 1mL (4 mg).

At the end of the surgery, in all patients, a single-injection, ultrasound-guided (SonoSite M-Turbo) Transversus Abdominis Plane (TAP) block was administered utilizing a linear ultrasound probe (12 MHz). With the patient positioned supine, the ultrasound probe was placed transversely on the lateral abdominal wall, in the midaxillary line, between the lower edge of the ribcage and the iliac crest. The needle was inserted in-plane directly beneath the ultrasound probe and advanced until it reached the layer between the internal oblique and transversus abdominis muscles. Once this layer was reached, the local anesthetic (LA) solution was injected, causing the TAP to expand and appear as a hypoechoic area. To prevent vascular puncture, careful aspiration was performed before the injection. The procedure was then repeated on the contralateral side using the same technique. Post-surgery, patients were transferred to the post-anesthesia care unit.

Patients transferred to the post-anesthesia care unit were routinely given paracetamol (1 mg) intravenously for 24 h, every 6 h. Visual analog scores (VASs) were evaluated at 0, 1, 4, 8, 16 and 24 h. VASs were evaluated in both sitting and supine positions. Pain levels were assessed using visual analog scores (VASs), with scores of 2–4 considered mild pain, 5–7 considered moderate pain, and 8–10 considered severe pain [20]. Those with a VAS $\geq$ 4 were given 0.5 mg/kg tramadol intravenously.

Bradycardia was defined as HR < 50 bpm and was treated with an intravenous injection of 0.5 mg of atropine. Hypotension was defined by a mean arterial pressure decrease of more than 30% from baseline and was treated with a 200 mL fluid bolus and a 5 mg intravenous injection of ephedrine. Nausea and vomiting were assessed using a 4-point scale (0 = none, 1 = nausea, 2 = retching, 3 = vomiting). Patients who scored $\geq$1 were treated with 4 mg of IV ondansetron.

Instant and total analgesic consumption and complications were intermittently recorded during the first 24 h postoperatively. Patient satisfaction was evaluated after 24 h.

Statistical Method

In this study, which was designed as an active Randomized Controlled Trial, patients who underwent cesarean section were randomized into three treatment groups: Bupivacaine (Group B), Bupivacaine + Dexmedetomidine (Group BD), and Bupivacaine + Dexamethasone (Group BDx). The primary outcome variable, VAS scale scores, was compared between treatment groups. Based on a minimum clinically significant mean difference of 0.2 on the VAS scale (Cohen's d effect size) and allowing for a maximum type I error of 5% and a minimum power of 80%, the sample size for each group has been determined to be 40 patients.

Statistical analysis of the data was performed using IBM SPSS Version 21 and the MedCalc statistical package program. Due to the suitability of the Central Limit Theorem, parametric tests were used for continuous measurements without normality testing [21]. However, since VAS and Satisfaction Scores were ordinal variables, non-parametric testing was used. When making statistical analysis of continuous data on scales, mean ± standard deviation, median, and 25%-75% values are used. Frequency and percentage values were used to describe categorical variables.

The One-Way ANOVA test and Kruskal–Wallis H statistics were used to compare continuous measurement averages in three groups. If a difference was detected, pairwise comparisons were evaluated with Tukey statistics as a post hoc test. The chi-square test was used to evaluate the relationship between categorical variables. If a relationship was detected, z-test statistics were used to evaluate the difference in pairwise ratio.

For statistical significance, $p < 0.05$ was accepted.

3. Results

A total of 120 pregnant women, aged between 18 and 42 years (with a mean age of 30.1 ± 5.6), scheduled to undergo cesarean section under spinal anesthesia were included in the study. The relationship between socio-demographic and operational characteristics is presented in Table 1. There was no significant difference between the groups in terms of mean age (p * = 0.23 > 0.05). The ASA score was 1 in 48.3% of the patients and 2 in 51.7%, with no significant differences between the groups in terms of ASA status (p * = 0.85 > 0.05). BMI values were 29.41 ± 2.89 for Group B, 29.03 ± 2.98 for Group BD, and 27.62 ± 2.34 for Group BDx, with significant differences observed between the groups (p * = 0.01 < 0.05). This significance was particularly notable between Group B and Group BDx (p ** = 0.01 < 0.05). While the operating time (minute) was 77.1 ± 17.7 in Group B and 68 ± 11.6 in Group BD, it was lower in Group BDx, at 66.8 ± 14.8. There was a significant difference between the mean operation times according to the groups (p * = 0.004 < 0.05). This difference was between Group B and Group BD, and Group B and Group BDx (p ** = 0.02, 0.007 < 0.05).

The mean block time (in minutes) was also a significant difference between the groups (p * = 0.001 <0.05). This difference was between Group B and Group BD, and Group B and Group BDx (p ** = 0.001, 0.002 < 0.05). The mean block times were 10.9 ± 2.4 in Group B, 9.1 ± 1.5 in Group BD, and 9.2 ± 2.4 in Group BDx.

As explained in Table 2, the 0-h instant analgesic tramadol requirement was 12.5% in the BDx group, it was not required in the B and BD groups (p * = 0.005 < 0.05). The difference was also significant at the 1st hour [between Group B and Group BDx (p ** = 0.01 < 0.05), and Group BD and Group BDx (p ** = 0.003 < 0.05)] and at the 8th hour [between Group B and Group BD (p ** = 0.008 < 0.05), and Group BD and Group BDx (p ** = 0.03 < 0.05)], however no significant differences were observed at the 4th, 16th, and 24th hours. The 0-h total analgesic tramadol requirement was 12.5% in the BDx group, it was not required in the B and BD groups. This difference between the groups was significant (p * = 0.005 < 0.05). While this difference was significant at the 1st hour between Group B and Group BDx (p ** = 0.001 < 0.05), and Group BD and Group BDx (p ** = 0.001 < 0.05) and 4th hour between Group B and Group BDx (p ** = 0.004 < 0.05), and Group BD and

Group BDx (p ** = 0.01 < 0.05), there was no significant difference at the 8th, 16th and 24th hours.

Table 1. Socio-demographic characteristics, operation, and block times of the groups (n = 120).

	Bupivacaine (n = 40)	**Bupivacaine +Dexmedetomidin (n = 40)**	**Bupivacaine + Dexametazon (n = 40)**		
	Mean ± SD	**Mean ± SD**	**Mean ± SD**	***p* Value ***	***p* Value ** 1 vs. 2, 1 vs. 3, 2 vs. 3**
Age	30.1 ± 5.4	31.5 ± 5.9	28.9 ± 5.2	0.23	–
BMI	29.41 ± 2.89	29.03 ± 2.98	27.62 ± 2.34	**0.01**	0.82, **0.01**, 0.06
ASA score	**n (%)**	**n (%)**	**n (%)**		
I	19 (47.5)	18 (45)	21 (52.5)	0.85	–
II	21 (52.5)	22 (55)	19 (17.5)		
Operation time	77.1 ± 17.7	68 ± 11.6	66.8 ± 14.8	**0.004**	**0.02**, **0.007**, 0.93
Block time	10.9 ± 2.4	9.1 ± 1.5	9.2 ± 2.4	**0.001**	**0.001**, **0.002**, 0.91

* One-Way ANOVA test | Chi-square test, ** Post Hoc test-Tukey; $p < 0.05$ is significant. BMI: body mass index above, ASA: American Society of Anesthesiologists, SD: Standard deviation.

Table 2. Assessment of clinical relationship between groups (n = 120).

	Bupivacaine (n = 40)	**Bupivacaine +Dexmedeto-midin (n = 40)**	**Bupivacaine + Dexametazon (n = 40)**		
Hour	**n (%)**	**n (%)**	**n (%)**	***p* Value ***	***p* Value ** 1 vs. 2, 1 vs. 3, 2 vs. 3**
Instant analgesictramadol requirement					
0	0 (0)	0 (0)	5 (12.5)	**0.005**	–**0.02**, **0.02**
1	2 (5)	1 (2.5)	10 (25)	**0.002**	0.56, **0.01**, **0.003**
4	9 (22.5)	9 (22.5)	12 (30)	0.67	–
8	18 (45)	7 (17.5)	16 (40)	**0.02**	**0.008**, 0.65, **0.03**
16	12 (30)	13 (32.5)	10 (25)	0.75	–
24	1 (2.5)	6 (15)	2 (5)	0.08	–
Total analgesic tramadol requirement					
0	0 (0)	0 (0)	5 (12.5)	**0.005**	–**0.02**, **0.02**
1	2 (5)	1 (2.5)	14 (35)	**0.001**	0.56 **0.001**, **0.001**
4	11 (27.5)	9 (22.5)	20 (50)	**0.02**	0.61 **0.04**, **0.01**
8	20 (50)	16 (40)	24 (60)	0.2	–
16	21 (52.5)	21 (52.5)	27 (67.5)	0.29	–
24	19 (47.5)	23 (57.5)	27 (67.5)	0.20	–
Nausea and/or vomiting					
0	0 (0)	1 (2.5)	7 (17.5)	**0.003**	0.31, **0.006**, **0.03**
1	5 (12.5)	5 (12.5)	9 (22.5)	0.37	–
4	6 (15)	9 (22.5)	10 (25)	0.52	–
8	8 (20)	12 (30)	10 (25)	0.59	–
16	7 (17.5)	12 (30)	11 (27.5)	0.39	–
24	7 (17.5)	13 (32.5)	11 (27.5)	0.3	–
Complication					
0	0 (0)	1 (2.5)	6 (15)	**0.009**	0.31 **0.01**, **0.04**
1	5 (12.5)	3 (7.5)	3 (7.5)	0.67	–
4	2 (5)	4 (10)	1 (2.5)	0.35	–
8	3 (7.5)	3 (7.5)	1 (2.5)	0.55	–
16	0 (0)	0 (0)	1 (2.5)	0.36	–
24	0 (0)	1 (2.5)	0 (0)	0.377	–

Table 2. *Cont.*

	Bupivacaine (n = 40)	Bupivacaine +Dexmedeto-midin (n = 40)	Bupivacaine + Dexametazon (n = 40)		
Hour	**n (%)**	**n (%)**	**n (%)**	**p Value ***	**p Value ** 1 vs. 2, 1 vs. 3, 2 vs. 3**
Total analgesic tramadol requirement	21 (52.5)	23 (57.5)	27 (67.5)	0.38	–
Total antiemetic requirement	10 (25)	12 (30)	13 (32.5)	0.75	–
Nausea and/or vomiting	10 (25)	12 (30)	12 (30)	0.85	–

* Chi-square test, ** z test; $p < 0.05$ is significant.

At hour 0, there was a significant relationship between the groups regarding the incidence of nausea and vomiting (p * = 0.003 < 0.05). The rates of nausea and vomiting in group 3 were significantly different compared to groups 1 and 2 (p ** = 0.006, 0.03 < 0.05). Additionally, at hour 0, there was a significant relationship between the groups concerning the occurrence of complications (p * = 0.009 < 0.05). The complication rates in group 3 were significantly different compared to groups 1 and 2 (p ** = 0.01, 0.04 < 0.05). However, at hours 1, 4, 8, 16, and 24, there was no significant relationship between the three groups regarding nausea, vomiting, and complications (p * > 0.05). At hours 1, 4, 8, 16, and 24, there was no significant relationship between the three groups regarding antiemetic usage (p * > 0.05).

Headache, hypotension, bradycardia, arrhythmia, tinnitus, and numbness around the mouth were not observed in all three groups.

In Table 3, there was a significance at hour 1 in terms of instant analgesic amount (p * = 0.04 < 0.05). The average amounts of tramadol used were 45 ± 0, 40 (only one patient), and 37.2 ± 3.67 mg in Group B, Group BD and Group BDx, respectively. In the comparison between groups for hour 1, the difference between Group B and Group BDx was significant (p ** = 0.04 < 0.05). No significant relationship was observed at other follow-up hours for instant analgesic tramadol usage amount (p * = 0.6, 0.06, 0.22, and 0.27 > 0.05 for the 4th, 8th, 16th, and 24th hours, respectively).

Significant differences in total tramadol consumption were observed at the 8th hour (p * = 0.003 < 0.05); 55.47 ± 19.81 mg for Group B, 41.13 ± 11.16 mg for Group BD, and 65.33 ± 26.04 mg for Group BDx and at the 16th hour (p * = 0.04 < 0.05); 77.97 ± 31.31 mg for Group B, 55.57 ± 19.38 mg for Group BD, and 71.78 ± 34.96 mg for Group BDx. At the 8th hour, a significant difference was observed between Group BD and Group BDx (p ** = 0.002 < 0.05). At the 16th hour, the significant difference was between Group B and Group BD (p ** = 0.04 < 0.05). No significant differences in total tramadol consumption were found at other follow-up times (p * = 0.86, 0.39, and 0.18 for the 1st, 4th, and 24th hours, respectively).

Evaluation according to the visual analog score (VAS) was presented in Table 4. In the sitting position, the difference in mean VASs between the groups was significant at hour 0 (p * = 0.005 < 0.05). These scores were significant between Group B and Group BDx as well as in Group BD and Group BDx (p ** = 0.001, 0.005 <0.05, respectively). In Group B, the mean VAS was 0.05 ± 0.32, with a median and quartiles of 0 (0–0). In Group BD, the mean VAS was 0.15 ± 0.48, with a median and quartiles of 0 (0–0). In Group BDx, the mean VAS was 0.85 ± 1.61, with a median and quartiles of 0 (0-2). The mean VASs between the groups were also significant at the 24th hour (p * = 0.005 < 0.05). These scores were significant between Group B and Group BDx as well as between Group BD and Group BDx (p ** = 0.03, 0.001 < 0.05 respectively). In Group B, the mean VAS was 2.3 ± 0.68 with a median and quartiles of 2 (2–3). In Group BD, the mean VAS was 2.57 ± 1.01, with a median and quartiles of 2 (2–3); and in Group BDx, the mean VAS was 1.7 ± 1.2, with a median and quartiles of 1 (1–3). There were no significant differences at other follow-up hours.

Table 3. Evaluation of instantaneous analgesic amounts between groups (n = 120).

	Bupivacaine (n = 40)	**Bupivacaine +Dexmedetomidin (n = 40)**	**Bupivacaine + Dexametazon (n = 40)**		
Hour	**Mean ± SD**	**Mean ± SD**	**Mean ± SD**	***p* Value ***	***p* Value ** 1 vs. 2, 1 vs. 3, 2 vs. 3**
Instant analgesic tramadol amount (mg)					
0	–	–	–	–	–
1	45 ± 0	40 ± –	37.2 ± 3.67	**0.04**	–**0.04**–
4	38.61 ± 3.33	38.06 ± 3.14	35.83 ± 3.68	0.16	–
8	39.56 ± 3.62	39.36 ± 5.37	36.37 ± 3.71	0.06	–
16	40.67 ± 4.22	38.5 ± 6	37 ± 3.77	0.22	–
24	37.5 ± -	42.67 ± 7.52	32.5 ± 3.53	0.27	–
Total analgesic tramadol amount (mg)					
0	–	–	–	-	–
1	45 ± 0	40 ± –	39.71 ± 13.21	0.86	–
4	39.77 ± 3.94	42.5 ± 14.39	47.65 ± 19.54	0.39	–
8	55.47 ± 19.81	41.13 ± 11.16	65.33 ± 26.04	**0.003**	0.11, 0.27, **0.002**
16	77.97 ± 31.31	55.57 ± 19.38	71.78 ± 34.96	**0.04**	**0.04**, 0.76, 0.14
24	80 ± 36.14	61.5 ± 27.38	74.19 ± 35.93	0.18	–

* One-Way ANOVA test, ** Post Hoc test-Tukey; $p < 0.05$ is significant. SD: Standard deviation.

Table 4. Assessment of visual analog score and satisfaction scale between groups (n = 120).

	Bupivacaine (n = 40)	**Bupivacaine +Dexmedetomidin (n = 40)**	**Bupivacaine + Dexametazon (n = 40)**		
Hour	**Mean ± SD**	**Mean ± SD**	**Mean ± SD**	***p* Value ***	***p* Value ** 1 vs. 2, 1 vs. 3, 2 vs. 3**
VAS sitting position					
0	0 (0–0) 0.05 ± 0.32	0 (0–0) 0.15 ± 0.48	0 (0–2) 0.85 ± 1.61	**0.005**	0.89, **0.001**, **0.005**
1	0.5 (0–2) 1.03 ± 1.21	0 (0–1) 0.7 ± 1.04	0 (0–2) 1.38 ± 1.76	0.33	–
4	2 (1–3) 2.28 ± 1.37	2 (1–2) 2.32 ± 1.47	2 (1–3) 2.42 ± 1.75	0.95	–
8	2.5 (2–3) 3.02 ± 1.38	2 (2–3) 2.57 ± 1.01	2 (1–3) 2.85 ± 1.65	0.19	–
16	2 (2–3) 2.88 ± 1.24	2 (2–3) 2.83 ± 1.1	2 (0.25–3) 2.25 ± 1.48	0.14	–
24	2 (2–3) 2.3 ± 0.68	2 (2–3) 2.57 ± 1.01	1 (1–3) 1.7 ± 1.2	**0.005**	0.45, **0.03**, **0.001**
VAS supine position					
0	0 (0–0) 0.05 ± 0.32	0 (0–0) 0.15 ± 0.48	0 (0–0) 0.85 ± 1.36	**0.001**	0.86, **0.001**, **0.001**
1	1 (0–2) 0.85 ± 0.97	0 (0–1) 0.63 ± 0.89	0 (0–3.75) 1.13 ± 1.32	0.29	–
4	2 (1–3) 2.07 ± 1.22	2 (1–3) 1.78 ± 1.12	2 (1–4) 1.98 ± 1.32	0.47	–

Table 4. *Cont.*

Hour	Bupivacaine (n = 40) Mean ± SD	Bupivacaine +Dexmedetomidin (n = 40) Mean ± SD	Bupivacaine + Dexametazon (n = 40) Mean ± SD	*p* Value *	*p* Value ** 1 vs. 2, 1 vs. 3, 2 vs. 3
8	3 (2–4) 2.38 ± 1.03	3 (2–3) 2.18 ± 0.87	3 (2–4) 2.1 ± 1.23	0.43	–
16	3 (2–4) 2.25 ± 0.83	3 (2–4) 2.25 ± 0.92	2 (1–3.75) 1.73 ± 1.03	0.1	–
24	2 (2–3) 2.2 ± 0.72	3 (2–3) 2.28 ± 0.78	2 (1–3.5) 1.43 ± 1.05	**0.001**	0.92, **0.001**, **0.001**
Satisfaction Scale	3 (2–3) 2.73 ± 0.98	3 (3–4) 3.05 ± 0.78	3 (3–4) 3.3 ± 0.79	**0.02**	0.21, **0.009**, 0.39

* Kruskal–Wallis H test, ** Post Hoc test-Tukey; $p < 0.05$ is significant. Q1–Q3: 25%-75%. SD: Standard deviation, VAS: visual analog score.

At the supine position, the difference in mean VASs between the groups was significant at 0 h (p * = 0.001 < 0.05). These scores were significant between Group B and Group BDx as well as between Group BD and Group BDx (p ** = 0.001, 0.001 < 0.05, respectively). In Group B, the mean VAS was 0.05 ± 0.32, with a median and quartiles of 0 (0–0); in Group BD, the mean VAS was 0.15 ± 0.48, with a median and quartiles of 0 (0–0); and in Group BDx, the mean VAS was 0.85 ± 1.36, with a median and quartiles of 0 (0–0). Similarly, the VASs between the groups were also significant at the 24th hour (p * = 0.001 < 0.05) (p ** = 0.001 and 0.001 < 0.05 for Group B and in Group BD as well as in Group B and Group BDx, respectively). In Group B, the mean VAS was 2.2 ± 0.72 with a median and quartiles of 2 (2–3); in Group BD, the mean VAS was 2.28 ± 0.78 with a median and quartiles of 3 (2–3); and in Group BDx, the mean VAS was 1.43 ± 1.05 with a median and quartiles of 2 (1–3.5). There were no significant differences at other follow-up hours.

The difference between the mean satisfaction scale was significant (p* = 0.02 < 0.05) These scores were significant between Group B and Group BDx (p** = 0.009 < 0.05). In Group B, the mean satisfaction scale was 2.73 ± 0.98 with a median and quartiles of 3 (2–3); in Group BD, the mean satisfaction scale was 3.05 ± 0.78 with a median and quartiles of 3 (3–4); and in Group BDx, the mean the satisfaction scale was 3 ± 0.79 with a median and quartiles of 3 (3–4) (Table 4).

4. Discussion

Cesarean section is one of the major surgical procedures and, as expected, there is significant postoperative discomfort and pain [22]. Post-cesarean analgesia aims to balance maternal comfort and newborn safety, but opioids, despite their effectiveness, can cause side effects like nausea, vomiting, and dizziness, reducing patient satisfaction [11,22,23]. Hence, various drugs or techniques such as non-opioids, adjuvants, and TAP block have been used to reduce perioperative opioid consumption and thus its adverse effects [24]. The TAP block, beneficial for pain management during cesarean delivery, shares similarities with minimally invasive laparoscopic techniques that aim to reduce surgical pain and enhance recovery [25]. An ideal local anesthetic should provide complete sensory blockade and have an optimal duration of action. Among commonly used local anesthetics, bupivacaine has a significantly longer duration of action compared to lidocaine and ropivacaine [13,26]. Adding adjuvants to local anesthetics prolongs postoperative analgesia and decreases the necessity for rescue analgesics [27,28]. Recent studies indicate that adding adjuvants such as dexmedetomidine and dexamethasone into TAP block effectively lowers pain scores and reduces the need for additional analgesics while keeping side effects minimal [11,29,30]. A study found that the time to first rescue analgesia was significantly longer with ropivacaine plus dexamethasone compared to ropivacaine alone (19.04 ± 4.13 h vs. 11.62 ± 3.80 h; p <

0.001) [27]. Another study showed lower tramadol consumption in the bupivacaine plus dexamethasone group compared to bupivacaine alone (50.0 ± 35 mg vs. 92.9 ± 36 mg; $p < 0.001$) [28]. McDonnell et al. reported that pregnant women receiving a TAP block with ropivacaine had over a 70% reduction in morphine requirements and a delayed time to the first PCA morphine request compared to the placebo group. Additionally, postoperative VAS pain scores, both at rest and during movement, were lower in the TAP block group [22].

Ramya et al. reported in their study that the block duration was 14 h in the bupivacaine + dexmedetomidine TAP block and 8 h in the bupivacaine TAP block alone [15].

While Sachdeva et al. found that the combination of dexamethasone and ropivacaine significantly extended the time to the first analgesic requirement (5.92 vs. 3.11 h) and reduced postoperative tramadol use (100 mg vs. 140 mg) compared to ropivacaine alone, these findings do not align with our study. However, the improvement in patient satisfaction (57.14% vs. 25.71%) is consistent with our results [1].

In the study by Thakur et al., where dexmedetomidine and dexamethasone were added to bupivacaine in TAP block during cesarean sections, similar to our findings, higher pain levels and analgesic requirements were observed in the dexamethasone group during the initial hours [31]. In another study by Sinha et al., where dexamethasone and bupivacaine were added to levobupivacaine in the TAP block during hysterectomies, similar to our study, higher VASs and shorter time to the first rescue analgesia were observed in the dexamethasone group within the first hour. However, unlike our study, the patient satisfaction scale was higher in the dexmedetomidine group [32]. We hypothesize that the higher VASs and analgesic requirements observed in the dexamethasone group within the first hour are due to the delayed onset of action of dexamethasone. Additionally, Sinha et al. observed higher rates of nausea and vomiting in the dexmedetomidine group at the end of 24 h. In contrast, we found higher rates of nausea and vomiting in the dexamethasone group within the first hour [32].

The differences in results could also be due to variations in study designs, patient demographics, and dosages administered. For instance, a higher body mass index (BMI) in certain patient groups, as observed in our study, may influence the distribution and effectiveness of the local anesthetics and adjuvants.

5. Study's Limitations

This study is limited by its single-center design, which may affect the results. A larger, multi-center study is recommended to validate these findings across different populations. Additionally, the study only evaluated analgesia and associated outcomes within the first 24 h postoperatively. Longer follow-up periods are necessary to assess the sustained efficacy and potential long-term impacts of the interventions.

6. Conclusions

The addition of dexmedetomidine or dexamethasone to bupivacaine for ultrasound-guided TAP blocks improves postoperative analgesia and patient satisfaction in cesarean section patients. Dexamethasone as an adjuvant appears to be beneficial, providing lower pain scores and higher satisfaction levels with a late onset but long-lasting effect. Further research with follow-up periods is suggested to confirm these findings and optimize postoperative pain management strategies.

Author Contributions: S.U. and O.K. conceptualized and designed the study; S.U., O.K. and S.H. collected the original data; S.U. and O.K. analyzed the data; S.U., O.K. and S.T. interpreted the analysis; S.U. and O.K. prepared the original draft; S.U., O.K., S.H. and S.T. reviewed and edited the draft, and revised the manuscript. All authors have read and agreed to the published version of the manuscript.

Funding: This research received no external funding.

Institutional Review Board Statement: This study was conducted in accordance with the Declaration of Helsinki and approved by the Clinical Research Ethics Committee of Hatay Mustafa Kemal University (meeting date: 20 February 2020, decision no: 05).

Informed Consent Statement: Informed consent was obtained from all subjects involved in this study.

Data Availability Statement: The datasets generated during and/or analyzed during the current study are available from the corresponding author upon reasonable request.

Conflicts of Interest: The authors declare no conflicts of interest.

References

1. Sachdeva, J.; Sinha, A. Randomized Controlled Trial to Study the Effect of Dexamethasone as Additive to Ropivacaine on Duration of Ultrasound-guided Transversus Abdominis Plane Block in Cesarean Section. *Indian. J. Pain.* **2016**, *30*, 181–185. [CrossRef]
2. Betran, A.P.; Ye, J.; Moller, A.B.; Zhang, J.; Gulmezoglu, A.M.; Torloni, M.R. The Increasing Trend in Caesarean Section Rates: Global, Regional and National Estimates: 1990–2014. *PLoS ONE* **2016**, *11*, e0148343. [CrossRef]
3. Betran, A.P.; Ye, J.; Moller, A.B.; Souza, J.P.; Zhang, J. Trends and projections of caesarean section rates: Global and regional estimates. *BMJ Glob. Health* **2021**, *6*, e005671. [CrossRef]
4. Singla, N.; Garg, K.; Jain, R.; Malhotra, A.; Singh, M.R.; Grewal, A. Analgesic efficacy of dexamethasone versus dexmedetomidine as an adjuvant to ropivacaine in ultrasound-guided transversus abdominis plane block for post-operative pain relief in caesarean section: A prospective randomised controlled study. *Indian. J. Anaesth.* **2021**, *65*, S121–S126. [CrossRef]
5. Neethirajan, S.G.R.; Kurada, S.; Parameswari, A. Efficacy of dexmedetomidine as an adjuvant to bupivacaine in ultrasound-guided transverse abdominis plane block for laparoscopic appendicectomy: A randomised controlled study. *Turk. J. Anaesthesiol. Reanim.* **2020**, *48*, 364.
6. Storti, E.; Vaccari, S.; Bruno, R.; Ricchi, A.; Buffagni, J.; Neri, I. Guidelines for management of analgesics after caesarean section: Cognitive survey. *Int. J. Womens Health Wellness* **2018**, *4*, 075.
7. Rafi, A.N. Abdominal field block: A new approach via the lumbar triangle. *Anaesthesia* **2001**, *56*, 1024–1026. [CrossRef]
8. Vincent, M.; Mathieu, O.; Nolain, P.; Menace, C.; Khier, S. Population Pharmacokinetics of Levobupivacaine During Transversus Abdominis Plane Block in Children. *Ther. Drug Monit.* **2020**, *42*, 497–502. [CrossRef]
9. Thakur, S.; Sharma, A.; Kaushal, S.; Sharma, A.; Sharma, N.; Thakur, P.S. Comparison of Clonidine with Bupivaicaine vs Plain Bupivaicaine in Transversus Abdominis Plane (TAP) Block in Women Undergoing Cesarean Delivery Under Spinal Anesthesia: Randomized Clinical Trial. *J. Pharm. Bioallied Sci.* **2023**, *15*, S299–S302. [CrossRef]
10. Sujata, N.; Hanjoora, V. Pain control after cesarean birth–What are the options. *J. Gen. Pract.* **2014**, *2*, 1000164. [CrossRef]
11. Jadon, A.; Jain, P.; Chakraborty, S.; Motaka, M.; Parida, S.S.; Sinha, N.; Agrawal, A.; Pati, A.K. Role of ultrasound guided transversus abdominis plane block as a component of multimodal analgesic regimen for lower segment caesarean section: A randomized double blind clinical study. *BMC Anesthesiol.* **2018**, *18*, 53. [CrossRef]
12. Abdallah, F.W.; Laffey, J.G.; Halpern, S.H.; Brull, R. Duration of analgesic effectiveness after the posterior and lateral transversus abdominis plane block techniques for transverse lower abdominal incisions: A meta-analysis. *Br. J. Anaesth.* **2013**, *111*, 721–735. [CrossRef]
13. Collins, J.B.; Song, J.; Mahabir, R.C. Onset and duration of intradermal mixtures of bupivacaine and lidocaine with epinephrine. *Can. J. Plast. Surg.* **2013**, *21*, 51–53. [CrossRef]
14. Sivakumar, R.K.; Panneerselvam, S.; Cherian, A.; Rudingwa, P.; Menon, J. Perineural vs. intravenous dexmedetomidine as an adjunct to bupivacaine in ultrasound guided fascia iliaca compartment block for femur surgeries: A randomised control trial. *Indian. J. Anaesth.* **2018**, *62*, 851–857.
15. Ramya Parameswari, A.; Udayakumar, P. Comparison of efficacy of bupivacaine with dexmedetomidine versus bupivacaine alone for transversus abdominis plane block for post-operative analgesia in patients undergoing elective caesarean section. *J. Obstet. Gynecol. India* **2018**, *68*, 98–103. [CrossRef]
16. Zhang, P.; Liu, S.; Zhu, J.; Rao, Z.; Liu, C. Dexamethasone and dexmedetomidine as adjuvants to local anesthetic mixture in intercostal nerve block for thoracoscopic pneumonectomy: A prospective randomized study. *Reg. Anesth. Pain Med.* **2019**, *44*, 917–922. [CrossRef]
17. Maniaci, A.; Lechien, J.R.; Calvo-Henriquez, C.; Iannella, G.; Leigh, S.; Ingrassia, A.; Merlino, F.; Bannò, V.; Cocuzza, S.; La Mantia, I. Long-term stability of outcomes of endoscopic surgery for rhinogenic contact point headache (Sluder"s neuralgia). *Am. J. Otolaryngol.* **2022**, *43*, 103368. [CrossRef]
18. Teodoro, M.; Scibilia, G.; Lomeo, E.; Pecorino, B.; Galia, A.; Scollo, P. Carbon dioxide laser as a new valid treatment of lichen sclerosus. *Clin. Exp. Obstet. Gynecol.* **2019**, *46*, 206–210. [CrossRef]
19. Association, W.M. World Medical Association Declaration of Helsinki: Ethical principles for medical research involving human subjects. *JAMA* **2013**, *310*, 2191–2194.
20. Huskisson, E.C. Measurement of pain. *Lancet* **1974**, *304*, 1127–1131. [CrossRef]
21. Norman, G. Likert scales, levels of measurement and the "laws" of statistics. *Adv. Health Sci. Educ. Theory Pract.* **2010**, *15*, 625–632. [CrossRef]
22. McDonnell, J.G.; Curley, G.; Carney, J.; Benton, A.; Costello, J.; Maharaj, C.H.; Laffey, J.G. The analgesic efficacy of transversus abdominis plane block after cesarean delivery: A randomized controlled trial. *Anesth. Analg.* **2008**, *106*, 186–191. [CrossRef]

23. Benyamin, R.; Trescot, A.M.; Datta, S.; Buenaventura, R.M.; Adlaka, R.; Sehgal, N.; Glaser, S.E.; Vallejo, R. Opioid complications and side effects. *Pain Physician* **2008**, *11*, S105.
24. Imani, F.; Rahimzadeh, P.; Faiz, H.-R.; Abdullahzadeh-Baghaei, A. An evaluation of the adding magnesium sulfate to ropivacaine on ultrasound-guided transverse abdominis plane block after abdominal hysterectomy. *Anesthesiol. Pain Med.* **2018**, *8*, e74124. [CrossRef]
25. Scibilia, G.; Pecorino, B.; Pagano, I.; Scollo, P. Case report: Laparoscopic uterovaginal anastomosis for congenital isolated cervical agenesis. *J. Minim. Invasive Gynecol.* **2017**, *24*, 677–682. [CrossRef]
26. Cummings, K.C., III; Napierkowski, D.; Parra-Sanchez, I.; Kurz, A.; Dalton, J.; Brems, J.; Sessler, D. Effect of dexamethasone on the duration of interscalene nerve blocks with ropivacaine or bupivacaine. *Br. J. Anaesth.* **2011**, *107*, 446–453. [CrossRef]
27. Gupta, A.; Gupta, A.; Yadav, N. Effect of dexamethasone as an adjuvant to ropivacaine on duration and quality of analgesia in ultrasound-guided transversus abdominis plane block in patients undergoing lower segment cesarean section-A prospective, randomised, single-blinded study. *Indian J. Anaesth.* **2019**, *63*, 469–474. [CrossRef]
28. Akkaya, A.; Yildiz, I.; Tekelioglu, U.; Demirhan, A.; Bayir, H.; Ozlu, T.; Bilgi, M.; Kocoglu, H. Dexamethasone added to levobupivacaine in ultrasound-guided tranversus abdominis plain block increased the duration of postoperative analgesia after caesarean section: A randomized, double blind, controlled trial. *Eur. Rev. Med. Pharmacol. Sci.* **2014**, *18*, 717–722.
29. Talebi, G.; Moayeri, H.; Rahmani, K.; Nasseri, K. Comparison of three different doses of dexmedetomidine added to bupivacaine in ultrasound-guided transversus abdominis plane block; a randomized clinical trial. *Anesthesiol. Pain Med.* **2021**, *11*, e113778. [CrossRef]
30. Ammar, A.S.; Mahmoud, K.M. Effect of adding dexamethasone to bupivacaine on transversus abdominis plane block for abdominal hysterectomy: A prospective randomized controlled trial. *Saudi J. Anaesth.* **2012**, *6*, 229–233.
31. Thakur, J.; Gupta, B.; Gupta, A.; Verma, R.K.; Verma, A.; Shah, P. A prospective randomized study to compare dexmedetomidine and dexamethasone as an adjunct to bupivacaine in transversus abdominis plane block for post-operative analgesia in caesarean delivery. *Int. J. Reprod. Contracept. Obstet. Gynecol.* **2019**, *8*, 4903–4908. [CrossRef]
32. Sinha, J.; Pokhriyal, A.S.; Asthana, V.; Nautiyal, R. Dexmedetomidine vs Dexamethasone as an Adjuvant to Levobupivacaine in Ultrasound-Guided Transversus Abdominis Plane Block for Postoperative Analgesia in Patients Undergoing Total Abdominal Hysterectomies. *Anesthesiol. Pain Med.* **2023**, *13*, e142059. [CrossRef]

Journal of
Clinical Medicine

MDPI

Article

A Comparison of the Effectiveness of the Serratus Anterior Plane Block and Erector Spinae Plane Block to that of the Paravertebral Block in the Surgical Treatment of Breast Cancer—A Randomized, Prospective, Single-Blinded Study

Michał But [1,*], Krzysztof Wernicki [2], Jacek Zieliński [3] and Weronika Szczecińska [4]

1 Pain Treatment Clinic, Polyclinic in Koszalin, 75-720 Koszalin, Poland
2 The Department of Anesthesiology and Intensive Care, Provincial Hospital in Koszalin, 75-581 Koszalin, Poland; contact@krzysztofwernicki.pl
3 The Department of Surgical Oncology, Provincial Hospital in Słupsk, 76-200 Słupsk, Poland; jaziel@gumed.edu.pl
4 The Department of General Surgery, Hospital Copernicus in Gdańsk, 80-803 Gdańsk, Poland; ik5men@wp.pl
* Correspondence: contact@mikebut.com

Abstract: Background/Objectives: The paravertebral block (PVB) is a well-studied, effective method of analgesia for breast surgery. Alternative techniques involving the blockage of intercostal nerve branches are the serratus anterior plane block (SAPB) and the erector spinae plane block (ESPB). However, no studies comparing both fascial blocks to PVB in breast surgery have been published to date. We evaluated the effectiveness of ESPB and SAPB vs. PVB, expressed as the requirement for intraoperative fentanyl, pain intensity at rest and during coughing, and morphine consumption on the first postoperative day. Additional aims were to perform an evaluation of the safety of the block types used. **Materials and Methods**: A total of 77 women and 1 man with stage I and II clinical breast cancer, aged 18–85 years, were randomized into one of three study groups: SAPB, PVB, and ESPB. **Results:** There were no statistically significant differences in fentanyl consumption during surgery with respect to the type of block used ($p = 0.4246$). Morphine consumption in the postoperative period was highest in the ESPB group, averaging 9.4 mg. There was a statistically significant difference in pain intensity from 4 pm on the day of surgery to 8 am the following morning. No complications related to the blocks were observed on the first postoperative day. **Conclusions:** Both the serratus anterior plane block and the erector spinae plane block were as effective as the paravertebral block in achieving intraoperative analgesia. The serratus anterior plane block was equally as effective as the paravertebral block in achieving postoperative analgesia. The erector spinae plane block was significantly less effective in achieving postoperative analgesia than both the paravertebral block and serratus anterior plane block.

Keywords: regional anesthesia; breast surgery; paravertebral block; erector spinae plane block; serratus anterior plane block

1. Introduction

Breast cancer is one of the most frequently diagnosed cancers in the adult population worldwide (over 2.2 million new cases in 2022) [1], as well as in Poland (over 21,000 new cases in 2021) [2]. The standard procedure is surgery, the extent of which is defined by the stage of the disease. Surgical procedures include breast-conserving treatment (BCT), mastectomy, and axillary lymphadenectomy—removal of the sentinel node or all nodes in the axillary region. The specific and complex innervation of the surgical area originating from both the brachial plexus and intercostal nerves causes these procedures to be associated with significant nociceptive stimulation, resulting in severe postoperative pain and a high risk of persistent postoperative pain in 25 to 60% of cases [3] (Figure 1).

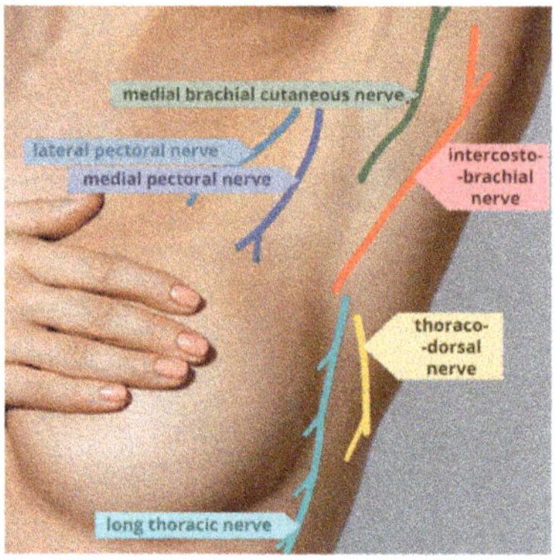

Figure 1. Innervation of the skin and subcutaneous tissue of the axillary line originating from the brachial plexus along with the intercostobrachial nerve originating from intercostal nerves Th2-3.

A well-documented and effective technique for disrupting intercostal nociception is the paravertebral block (PVB) [4]. Unfortunately, due to the anatomy of the paravertebral space, it carries a risk of pleural puncture and pneumothorax [5], as well as other potentially serious complications [6]. With the dynamic development of regional anesthesia, many new promising fascial blocks have emerged recently which can positively affect postoperative pain intensity and opioid consumption during and after surgery. Alternative blocks involving the anesthesia of intercostal nerve branches include the serratus anterior plane block (SAPB) and the erector spinae plane block (ESPB) [7–10]. There are many studies in the literature comparing the effectiveness of PVB to that of ESPB or SAPB. So far, there are no studies comparing the effectiveness of both fascial blocks to the paravertebral block. In accordance with PROSPECT recommendations, the researchers of this study decided not to create a control group in which no method of regional anesthesia was used. The control group included patients who underwent a PVB.

2. Materials and Methods

The main objective of this study was to compare the efficacy of the fascial blocks ESPB (erector spinae plane block) and SAPB (serratus anterior plane block) to that of PVB (paravertebral block) in breast surgery.

The specific objectives of this study were as follows:

1. To assess the impact of SAPB, ESPB, and PVBs on fentanyl consumption during surgery.
2. To assess the impact of SAPB, ESPB, and PVBs on the amount of morphine administered to patients postoperatively.
3. To assess the impact of SAPB, ESPB, and PVBs on pain intensity during coughing and at rest on the first day post-surgery six times daily from the first hour post-operation until the end of the second postoperative day.
4. To evaluate the safety of the paravertebral block and the applied fascial blocks SAPB and ESPB.

After obtaining written consent for the study, patient numbers were assigned, and the block was performed according to a randomization table. For all blocks, patients were positioned on the side opposite to the operative side. All regional blocks were performed under ultrasound guidance (Mindray TE7) using a linear probe by a single experienced anesthesiologist. For the blocks, 20 mL of local anesthetic (10 mL of 2% lidocaine with 10 mL of 0.5% bupivacaine) was used.

This study included patients diagnosed with breast cancer at clinical stages I and II, aged between 18 and 85 years. Patients excluded from the study were those who were unable to provide informed consent, had undergone previous breast surgery on the same side, reported chronic pain with an intensity of NRS > 3, had been taking opioids chronically up to 2 weeks before the surgery, had contraindications to regional anesthesia (such as allergies to local anesthetics, with dermatological conditions preventing regional block), had a BMI > 40, or had consciousness disorders or difficulty with verbal communication (Figure 2). Patients were prospectively and randomly assigned to groups with a single-blind design. A computer-generated table in Microsoft Excel assigned patients to the appropriate groups.

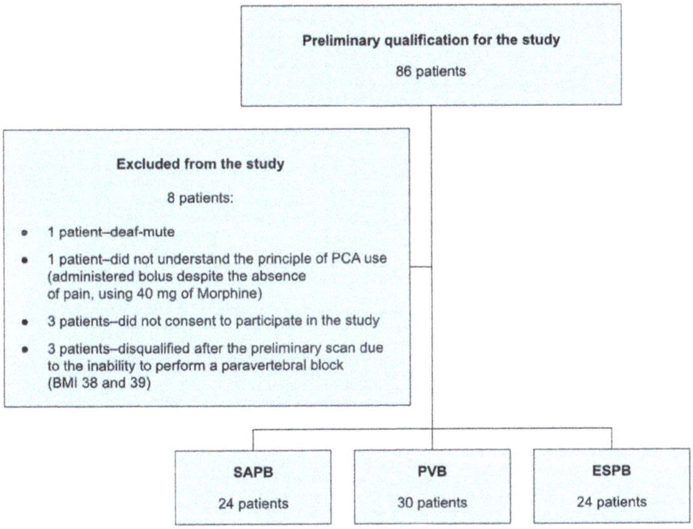

Figure 2. Qualification for the study.

2.1. Serratus Anterior Plane Block (SAPB)

The probe was placed on the mid-axillary line at the level of the fourth rib to visualize the serratus anterior and latissimus dorsi muscles (Figure 3). After establishing the correct level, the skin was anesthetized with 1 mL of 1% lidocaine, and a SonoPlex Pajunk 50 mm needle was introduced in-plane. After puncturing the serratus muscle and contacting the rib, 20 mL of local anesthetic was deposited between the serratus muscle fascia and the rib periosteum, termed a deep serratus anterior plane block.

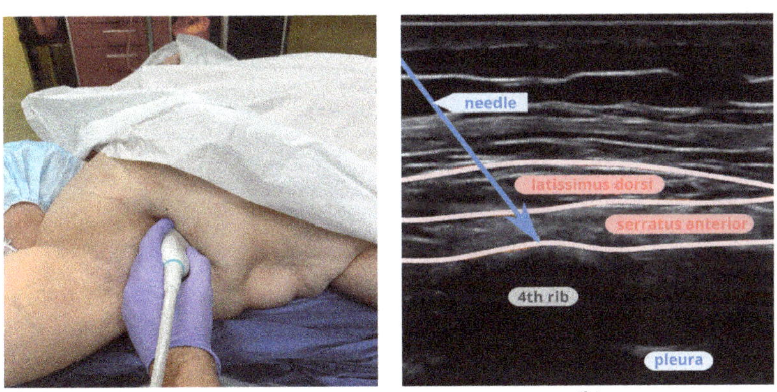

(a) (b)

Figure 3. Serratus anterior plane block: (**a**) placement of the probe at the fourth-rib level for SAPB; (**b**) an ultrasound image of the serratus anterior and latissimus dorsi muscles.

2.2. Paravertebral Block (PVB)

The probe was placed between the fourth and fifth ribs. After establishing the correct plane, the skin was locally anesthetized with 1 mL of 1% lidocaine. The needle was introduced in-plane under the internal intercostal membrane (Figure 4). Following negative aspiration, 20 mL of local anesthetic was deposited, showing the retraction of the pleura.

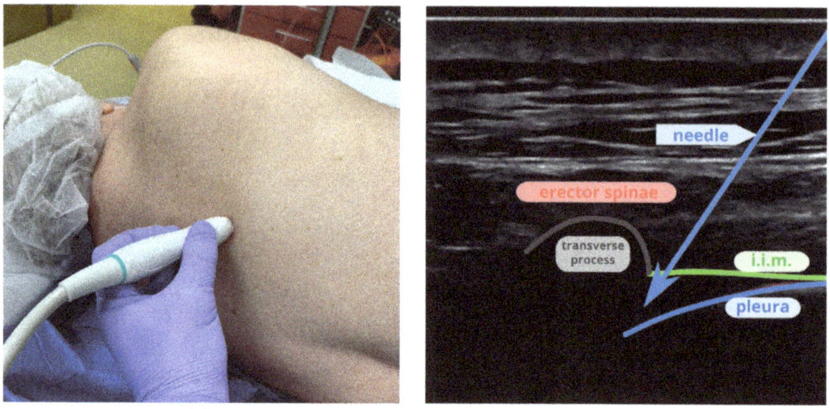

(**a**) (**b**)

Figure 4. Paravertebral block: (**a**) placement of the probe between the fourth and fifth ribs for PVB; (**b**) an ultrasound image of the costotransverse joint and internal intercostal membrane (i.i.m.).

2.3. Erector Spinae Plane Block (ESPB)

The probe was placed in the paravertebral area to visualize the transverse process and the fifth rib. After establishing the correct plane, the skin was anesthetized with 1 mL of 1% lidocaine. A SonoPlex Pajunk needle was introduced out-of-plane until contact with the periosteum. The probe was then rotated 90 degrees to visualize the needle throughout its course (Figure 5). Following negative aspiration, 20 mL of local anesthetic was deposited between the fascia of the erector spinae muscle and the periosteum of the transverse process.

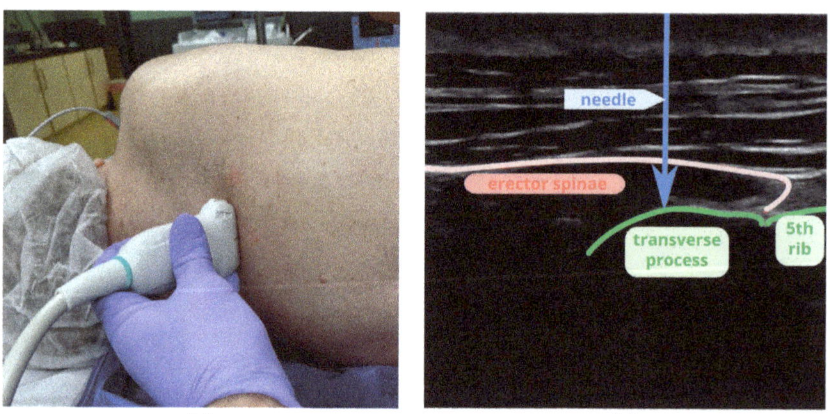

(**a**) (**b**)

Figure 5. *Cont.*

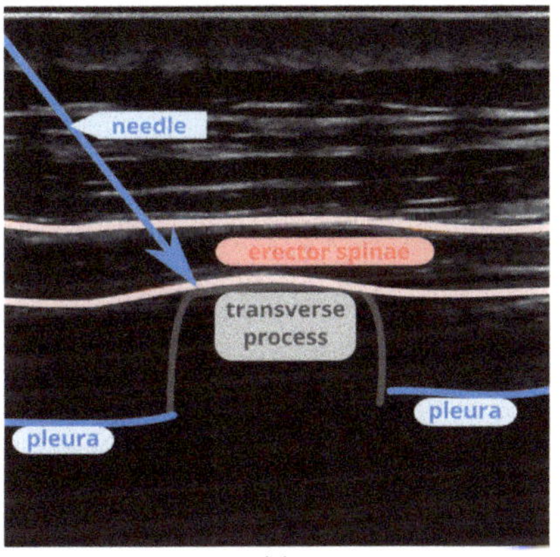

(c)

Figure 5. Erector spinae plane block: (**a**) placement of the probe at the fifth-rib level for ESPB; (**b**) a scan at the level of the costotransverse joint, where the probe is placed in a transverse projection; (**c**) a scan showing the transverse process, where the probe is placed in a longitudinal projection.

2.4. Perioperative Management

After performing the block in the operating room, general balanced anesthesia was conducted following a standardized protocol. Co-induction included 2 mg of midazolam and 0.1 mg of intravenous fentanyl. Pre-oxygenation with 100% oxygen was followed by intravenous induction with propofol at a dose of 2 mg/kg of body weight. Muscle relaxation was achieved with rocuronium 0.6 mg/kg, dosed based on ideal body weight, and maintenance was carried out with inhaled desflurane. Additional doses of 0.1 mg fentanyl were administered if blood pressure exceeded 120% of the baseline values. Post-surgery, patients were monitored in the recovery room until fully conscious, and then connected to a PCA pump with morphine.

2.5. Postoperative Pain Intensity Measurement

During the one-hour observation period in the recovery room, vital signs and pain intensity were monitored using an 11-point Numerical Rating Scale (NRS). Patients were asked to rate their pain at rest and then to cough and rate their pain during coughing on a scale from 0 to 10, with 0 indicating no pain and 10 indicating the worst pain imaginable. The highest reported pain score during the first hour post-operation was recorded. Subsequent measurements were conducted by a nurse in the ward at scheduled intervals, assessing pain both at rest and during coughing in the same manner using the same NRS.

2.6. Complication Evaluation

Before transferring patients to the ward, the regional anesthesia site of the block was scanned using ultrasound by a skilled radiologist for adverse events such as hematoma or pneumothorax.

2.7. Statistical Analysis

All statistical calculations were performed using TIBCO Software Inc. (Palo Alto, CA, USA) (2017), Statistica (data analysis software system), version 13 and Microsoft Excel. Quantitative variables were characterized by the arithmetic mean, standard deviation, median, minimum and maximum values (range), and 95% confidence interval (CI). Qualitative variables are presented as frequencies and percentages.

2.8. Sample Size and Power of the Study

An ANOVA was conducted. An analysis of PCA morphine requirements on the first postoperative day was performed for three independent groups. Under the conditions of $\alpha = 0.05$ and power = 80–90%, the minimum sample size obtained was 3–24. Assuming equal numbers in all the studied groups and a population standard deviation value at even a high level of 4–5, the minimum sample size for each group should be approximately 20–24 patients.

As a second variable, pain intensity was analyzed, measured one hour after the procedure, and then every 6 h. Under the conditions of $\alpha = 0.05$ and power = 80–90%, the minimum sample size obtained was 4–16. Assuming equal numbers in all studied groups and the number of pain/rest intensity measurements at the level of 8, the sample size for each group should be approximately 20 patients.

Additionally, a power analysis was conducted for the following calculations. The power obtained was 97% for both variables.

3. Results

The average ages of patients in the SAPB, PVB, and ESPB groups were 66.5, 66.5, and 62.5 years, respectively. No statistically significant differences in age were found between the block types ($p = 0.4577$). The average body weights of patients in the SPB, PVB, and ESPB groups were 74.1, 69.3, and 73.9 kg, respectively. No statistically significant differences in body weight were found between the block types ($p = 0.2898$). The average heights of patients in the SAPB, PVB, and ESPB groups were 159.5, 158.7, and 163.9 cm, respectively. Patients in group 2 were significantly shorter than those in group 3 ($p = 0.0291$). The average BMIs of patients in the SPB, PVB, and ESPB groups were 28.9, 27.4, and 27.8, respectively. No statistically significant differences in BMI were found between the block types ($p = 0.7089$).

A total of 78 procedures were performed. The majority were breast-conserving surgeries with sentinel lymph node excision, totaling 47. Twelve mastectomies with sentinel lymph node excision were performed, along with ten Maddens' mastectomies, three tumorectomies, two BCTs (breast-conserving treatments), and one quadrantectomy. Detailed numbers and percentages of the procedures are presented in Table 1. There were no statistically significant differences in the types of procedures with respect to the type of block used ($p = 0.8031$).

Table 1. Comparative characteristics of the studied groups (SAPB—serratus anterior plane block; PVB—paravertebral block; ESPB—erector spinae plane block) regarding the type of procedure.

	SAPB (n = 24)	PVB (n = 30)	ESPB (n = 24)	Total (n = 78)	p-Value
Procedure					0.8031 [1]
Mastectomy + SNLD	4 (16.7%)	5 (17.9%)	3 (12.5%)	12 (15.8%)	
BCT + SNLD	16 (66.7%)	16 (57.1%)	15 (62.5%)	47 (61.8%)	
Madens' mastectomy	2 (8.3%)	4 (14.3%)	4 (16.7%)	10 (13.2%)	
Quadrantectomy + SNLD	0 (0.0%)	1 (3.6%)	0 (0.0%)	1 (1.3%)	
Tumorectomy	2 (8.3%)	0 (0.0%)	1 (4.2%)	3 (3.9%)	
Quadrantectomy	0 (0.0%)	1 (3.6%)	0 (0.0%)	1 (1.3%)	
BCT	0 (0.0%)	1 (3.6%)	1 (4.2%)	2 (2.6%)	

[1] Chi-square.

The percentages of patients with ASA scale 1 in the SAPB, PVB, and ESPB groups were 4.2%, 3.4%, and 8.3%, respectively, and those of patients with ASA scale 2 were 95.8%, 96.6%, and 91.7%. No statistically significant differences in ASA scale were found between the block types ($p = 0.7008$). The average NRS pain scale scores of patients in the SAPB, PVB, and ESPB groups were 0.48, 0.41, and 0.29, respectively. No statistically significant differences in preoperative NRS pain scale scores were found between the block types ($p = 0.7710$).

3.1. Intraoperative Fentanyl Consumption and Postoperative Morphine Consumption

The average fentanyl consumption values during surgery for patients in the SAPB, PVB, and ESPB groups were 0.12 mg, 0.12 mg, and 0.11 mg, respectively. There were no statistically significant differences in fentanyl consumption during surgery with respect to the type of block used ($p = 0.4246$). The average postoperative morphine consumption values for patients in the SAPB, PVB, and ESPB groups were 5.4 mg, 4.4 mg, and 9.4 mg, respectively. In the ESPB group (erector spinae plane block), consumption was significantly higher compared to the SAPB group ($p = 0.0074$) and the PVB group ($p = 0.0005$) (Table 2).

Table 2. Comparative characteristics of the studied groups (SAPB—serratus anterior plane block; PVB—paravertebral block; ESPB—erector spinae plane block) regarding intraoperative fentanyl consumption and postoperative morphine consumption.

	SAPB (n = 24)	PVB (n = 30)	ESPB (n = 24)	Total (n = 78)	p-Value
Fentanyl (mg)					0.4246 [1]
Mean (SD)	0.12 (0.04)	0.12 (0.05)	0.11 (0.03)	0.12 (0.04)	
Range	0.10–0.20	0.10–0.30	0.10–0.20	0.10–0.30	
Median	0.10	0.10	0.10	0.10	
95% CI	[0.10;0.14]	[0.10;0.14]	[0.10;0.12]	[0.11;0.13]	
Morphine (mg)					0.0004 [1]
Mean (SD)	5.4 (3.7)	4.4 (2.1)	9.4 (5.5)	6.3 (4.4)	[a] 0.0074 [2]
Range	1.0–15.0	1.0–18.0	3.0–23.0	1.0–23.0	[b] 0.0005 [2]
Median	4.0	4.0	8.0	5.0	
95% CI	[3.8;6.9]	[3.6;5.2]	[7.1;11.7]	[5.3;7.3]	

[1] ANOVA Kruskal–Wallis; [2] post hoc tests; [a] SAPB vs ESPB; [b] PVB vs ESPB.

3.2. Pain Intensity at Rest

The first measurement of pain intensity at rest was conducted in the recovery room. Subsequent measurements were carried out by a nurse in the patient's room.

The average pain intensity at rest 1 h after the procedure for patients in the SAPB, PVB, and ESPB groups was 4.1, 4.0, and 3.9, respectively, according to the NRS. There were no statistically significant differences in pain intensity at rest 1 h after the procedure with respect to the type of block used ($p = 0.8651$).

The average pain intensities at 4:00 PM for patients in the SAPB, PVB, and ESPB groups were 2.6, 2.6, and 3.6, respectively, according to the NRS. At 4:00 PM, there were significant differences in pain levels at rest depending on the type of anesthesia block used ($p = 0.0017$). Detailed post hoc tests showed that in the ESPB group (erector spinae plane block), pain intensity was significantly higher compared to the SAPB group ($p = 0.0129$) and the PVB group ($p = 0.0071$). No significant differences were found for the other comparisons.

The average pain intensities at 8:00 PM for patients in the SAPB, PVB, and ESPB groups were 2.6, 2.6, and 3.6, respectively, according to the NRS. There were statistically significant differences in pain intensity at rest at 8:00 PM with respect to the type of block used ($p = 0.0017$). Detailed post hoc tests showed that in the ESPB group, pain intensity was significantly higher compared to the SAPB group ($p = 0.0129$) and the PVB group ($p = 0.0071$). No significant differences were found for the other comparisons.

For the times 12:00 AM and 4:00 AM, statistical tests could not be calculated due to small or absent sample sizes.

The average pain intensities at 8:00 AM the next day for patients in the SAPB, PVB, and ESPB groups were 2.1, 2.0, and 2.7, respectively, according to the NRS. There were statistically significant differences in pain intensity at rest at 8:00 AM with respect to the type of block used ($p = 0.0176$). Detailed post hoc tests showed that in the ESPB group, pain intensity was significantly higher compared to the PVB group ($p = 0.0388$). No significant differences were found for the other comparisons.

The average pain intensities at 12:00 PM the next day for patients in the SAPB, PVB, and ESPB groups were 1.8, 1.9, and 2.4, respectively, according to the NRS. There were no statistically significant differences in pain intensity at 12:00 PM with respect to the type of block used ($p > 0.05$).

The average pain intensities at 4:00 PM the next day for patients in the SAPB, PVB, and ESPB groups were 1.8, 1.8, and 2.2, respectively, according to the NRS. There were no statistically significant differences in pain intensity at 4:00 PM with respect to the type of block used ($p = 0.2182$) (Table 3).

Table 3. Comparative characteristics of the studied groups (SAPB—serratus anterior plane block; PVB—paravertebral block; ESPB—erector spinae plane block) regarding pain intensity at rest.

		SAPB ($n = 24$)	PVB ($n = 30$)	ESPB ($n = 24$)	Total ($n = 78$)	p-Value
1 h after the procedure		$n = 20$	$n = 28$	$n = 23$	$n = 71$	0.8651 [1]
	mean (SD) median (range) 95%CI	4.1 (1.8) 4.0 (2.0–9.0) [3.3;4.9]	4.0 (1.7) 4.0 (1.0–7.0) [3.3;4.7]	3.9 (1.6) 3.0 (2.0–8.0) [3.2;4.6]	4.0 (1.6) 4.0 (1.0–9.0) [3.6;4.4]	
4:00 PM		$n = 24$	$n = 27$	$n = 24$	$n = 75$	0.0017 [1]
	mean (SD) median (range) 95%CI	2.6 (0.8) 2.0 (2.0–5.0) [2.3;3.0]	2.6 (0.9) 2.0 (1.0–5.0) [2.2;2.9]	3.6 (1.2) 4.0 (1.0–5.0) [3.1;4.1]	2.9 (1.1) 3.0 (1.0–5.0) [2.7;3.2]	[a] 0.0129 [2] [b] 0.0071 [2]
8:00 PM		$n = 24$	$n = 27$	$n = 24$	$n = 75$	0.0017 [1]
	mean (SD) median (range) 95%CI	2.6 (0.8) 2.0 (2.0–5.0) [2.3;3.0]	2.6 (0.9) 2.0 (1.0–5.0) [2.2;2.9]	3.6 (1.2) 4.0 (1.0–5.0) [3.1;4.1]	2.9 (1.1) 3.0 (1.0–5.0) [2.7;3.2]	[a] 0.0129 [2] [b] 0.0071 [2]
12:00 AM		$n = 2$	$n = 7$	$n = 6$	$n = 15$	--
	mean (SD) median (range) 95%CI	2.5 (0.7) 2.5 (2.0–3.0) [-3.9;8.9]	2.4 (0.5) 2.0 (2.0–3.0) [1.9;2.9]	2.8 (1.2) 2.5 (2.0–5.0) [1.6;4.1]	2.6 (0.8) 2.0 (2.0–5.0) [2.1;3.1]	
4:00 AM		$n = 0$	$n = 1$	$n = 1$	$n = 2$	--
	mean (SD) median (range) 95%CI		2.0 (0.0) 2.0 (2.0–2.0) [0.0;0.0]	1.0 (0.0) 1.0 (1.0–1.0) [0.0;0.0]	1.5 (0.7) 1.5 (1.0–2.0) [0.0;0.0]	
8:00 AM		n =24	$n = 28$	$n = 24$	$n = 76$	0.0176 [1]
	mean (SD) median (range) 95%CI	2.1 (0.7) 2.0 (1.0–4.0) [1.8;2.4]	2.0 (0.7) 2.0 (1.0–4.0) [1.7;2.3]	2.7 (1.0) 3.0 (1.0–4.0) [2.3;3.1]	2.3 (0.9) 2.0 (1.0–4.0) [2.1;2.5]	[a] 0.0388 [2]
12:00 PM		$n = 24$	$n = 29$	$n = 24$	$n = 77$	>0.05 [1]
	mean (SD) median (range) 95%CI	1.8 (0.5) 2.0 (1.0–3.0) [1.6;2.0]	1.9 (0.8) 2.0 (1.0–4.0) [1.6;2.2]	2.4 (1.0) 2.5 (1.0–4.0) [2.0;2.8]	2.0 (0.8) 2.0 (1.0–4.0) [1.8;2.2]	
4:00 PM		$n = 24$	$n = 29$	$n = 24$	$n = 77$	0.2182 [1]
	mean (SD) median (range) 95%CI	1.8 (0.6) 2.0 (1.0–3.0) [1.5;2.0]	1.8 (0.8) 2.0 (1.0–4.0) [1.5;2.1]	2.2 (0.9) 2.0 (1.0–4.0) [1.8;2.5]	1.9 (0.8) 2.0 (1.0–4.0) [1.8;2.1]	

[1] ANOVA Kruskal–Wallis; [2] post hoc tests; [a] SAPB vs ESPB; [b] PVB vs ESPB.

3.3. Pain Intensity during Coughing

Similarly to the pain measurement at rest, the first pain intensity measurement was conducted in the recovery room. Subsequent measurements were carried out by nurses on the ward. During the measurement, patients were asked to cough.

The average pain intensities during coughing 1 h post-operation for patients in the SAPB, PVB, and ESPB groups were 4.8, 4.8, and 4.8, respectively, according to the NRS. No statistically significant differences in pain intensity during coughing were found 1 h post-operation among the types of block ($p = 0.8809$).

The average pain intensities at 4:00 PM for patients in the SAPB, PVB, and ESPB groups were 3.5, 3.5, and 4.5, respectively, according to the NRS. Statistically significant differences in pain intensity during coughing were found at 4:00 PM among the types of block ($p = 0.0010$). Detailed post hoc tests showed that in the ESPB group (erector spinae plane block), pain intensity was significantly higher compared to the SAPB group ($p = 0.0080$) and PVB group ($p = 0.0045$). No other statistically significant differences were observed.

The average pain intensities at 8:00 PM for patients in the SAPB, PVB, and ESPB groups were 3.5, 3.5, and 4.5, respectively, according to the NRS. Statistically significant differences in pain intensity during coughing were found at 8:00 PM among the types of block ($p = 0.0010$).

Detailed post hoc tests showed that in the ESPB group (erector spinae plane block), pain intensity was significantly higher compared to the SAPB group ($p = 0.0080$) and PVB group ($p = 0.0045$). No other statistically significant differences were observed.

For 12:00 AM and 4:00 AM, statistical tests could not be performed due to small sample sizes.

The average pain intensities at 8:00 AM the next day for patients in the SAPB, PVB, and ESPB groups were 3.1, 3.1, and 3.7, respectively, according to the NRS. Statistically significant differences in pain intensity during coughing were found at 8:00 AM among the types of block ($p = 0.0128$). Detailed post hoc tests showed that in the ESPB group (erector spinae plane block), pain intensity was significantly higher compared to the PVB group ($p = 0.0478$). No other statistically significant differences were observed.

The average pain intensities at 12:00 PM the next day for patients in the SAPB, PVB, and ESPB groups were 2.8, 2.8, and 3.4, respectively, according to the NRS. Statistically significant differences in pain intensity during coughing were found at 12:00 PM among the types of block ($p = 0.0097$). Detailed post hoc tests showed that in the ESPB group (erector spinae plane block), pain intensity was significantly higher compared to the PVB group ($p = 0.0253$). No other statistically significant differences were observed.

The average pain intensities during coughing at 4:00 PM the next day for patients in the SAPB, PVB, and ESPB groups were 2.8, 2.6, and 3.2, respectively, according to the NRS. No statistically significant differences in pain intensity during coughing were found at 4:00 PM among the types of block ($p > 0.05$) (Table 4).

Table 4. Comparative characteristics of the studied groups (SAPB—serratus plane block; PVB—paravertebral block; ESPB—erector spinae plane block) regarding pain intensity during coughing.

		SAPB ($n = 24$)	PVB ($n = 30$)	ESPB ($n = 24$)	Total ($n = 78$)	p-Value
1 h after the procedure		$n = 20$	$n = 28$	$n = 23$	$n = 71$	0.8809 [1]
	mean (SD)	4.8 (1.6)	4.8 (1.7)	4.8 (1.4)	4.8 (1.6)	
	median (range)	5.0 (2.0–8.0)	5.0 (1.0–8.0)	4.0 (3.0–8.0)	5.0 (1.0–8.0)	
	95%CI	[4.1;5.5]	[4.2;5.5]	[4.2;5.4]	[4.4;5.2]	

Table 4. *Cont.*

		SAPB (*n* = 24)	PVB (*n* = 30)	ESPB (*n* = 24)	Total (*n* = 78)	*p*-Value
4:00 PM		*n* = 24	*n* = 28	*n* = 24	*n* = 76	0.0010 [1]
	mean (SD) median (range) 95%CI	3.5 (0.9) 3.0 (1.0–5.0) [3.1;3.9]	3.5 (0.9) 3.0 (2.0–5.0) [3.2;3.8]	4.5 (1.1) 4.5 (2.0–6.0) [4.0;4.9]	3.8 (1.0) 4.0 (1.0–6.0) [3.5;4.0]	[a] 0.0080 [2] [b] 0.0045 [2]
8:00 PM		*n* = 24	*n* = 28	*n* = 24	*n* = 76	0.0010 [1]
	mean (SD) median (range) 95%CI	3.5 (0.9) 3.0 (1.0–5.0) [3.1;3.9]	3.5 (0.9) 3.0 (2.0–5.0) [3.2;3.8]	4.5 (1.1) 4.5 (2.0–6.0) [4.0;4.9]	3.8 (1.0) 4.0 (1.0–6.0) [3.5;4.0]	[a] 0.0080 [2] [b] 0.0045 [2]
12:00 AM		*n* = 2	*n* = 7	*n* = 6	*n* = 15	--
	mean (SD) median (range) 95%CI	3.5 (0.7) 3.5 (3.0–4.0) [−2.9;9.9]	3.6 (0.8) 3.0 (3.0–5.0) [2.8;4.3]	3.7 (0.8) 3.5 (3.0–5.0) [2.8;4.5]	3.6 (0.7) 3.0 (3.0–5.0) [3.2;4.0]	
4:00 AM		*n* = 0	*n* = 1	*n* = 1	*n* = 2	--
	mean (SD) median (range) 95%CI		3.0 (0.0) 3.0 (3.0–3.0) [0.0;0.0]	1.0 (0.0) 1.0 (1.0–1.0) [0.0;0.0]	2.0 (1.4) 2.0 (1.0–3.0) [0.0;0.0]	
8:00 AM		*n* =24	*n* = 28	*n* = 24	*n* = 76	0.0128 [1]
	mean (SD) median (range) 95%CI	3.1 (0.7) 3.0 (2.0–5.0) [2.8;3.4]	3.1 (0.8) 3.0 (2.0–5.0) [2.8;3.4]	3.7 (0.9) 4.0 (2.0–5.0) [3.3;4.1]	3.3 (0.8) 3.0 (2.0–5.0) [3.1;3.5]	[a] 0.0478 [2]
12:00 PM		*n* = 24	*n* = 29	*n* = 24	*n* = 77	0.0097 [1]
	mean (SD) median (range) 95%CI	2.8 (0.5) 3.0 (2.0–4.0) [2.6;3.0]	2.8 (0.8) 3.0 (2.0–5.0) [2.5;3.1]	3.4 (0.9) 3.0 (2.0–5.0) [3.0;3.7]	3.0 (0.8) 3.0 (2.0–5.0) [2.8;3.1]	[a] 0.0253 [2]
4:00 PM		*n* = 24	*n* = 29	*n* = 24	*n* = 77	>0.05 [1]
	mean (SD) median (range) 95%CI	2.8 (0.6) 3.0 (2.0–4.0) [2.5;3.0]	2.6 (0.7) 3.0 (2.0–5.0) [2.3;2.9]	3.2 (0.9) 3.0 (2.0–5.0) [2.8;3.5]	2.8 (0.8) 3.0 (2.0–5.0) [2.7;3.0]	

[1] ANOVA Kruskal–Wallis; [2] post hoc tests; [a] SAPB vs ESPB; [b] PVB vs ESPB.

4. Discussion

4.1. Intraoperative Analgesia

In this study, both the serratus anterior plane block and the erector spinae plane block were as effective as the paravertebral block in achieving intraoperative analgesia. Intraoperative fentanyl use was similar in all groups, which is in line with the study by Gabriel [11].

4.2. SAPB vs. PVB in Postoperative Analgesia

In our study, SAPB was equally as effective as PVB in achieving postoperative analgesia. The reported pain levels and opioid use were similar in both groups.

In the study by Gabriel et al., the serratus anterior plane block was reported to be less effective than the paravertebral block. The reported pain levels and postoperative opioid use were higher in the serratus plane block group compared to the paravertebral block group [11]. The discrepancies between their results and ours may be attributable to several factors. Gabriel et al. describe non-mastectomy procedures primarily performed on outpatients. Additionally, some blocks, particularly serratus anterior plane blocks, were performed by less experienced practitioners in training, which may have affected their effectiveness. Our study also includes radical procedures, exclusively in inpatients, with all blocks performed by a single experienced anesthesiologist.

In the study by Gupta et al., it was reported that the duration of analgesia from SAPB was significantly shorter compared to PVB. The reported pain levels and postoperative opioid use were higher in the SAPB group than in the PVB group. The authors speculated that the greater effectiveness of PVB is associated with a larger extent of the block [12].

Although the study by Gupta seems to lack the disadvantages of the study by Gabriel, both studies used the superficial serratus plane block, whereas in our study, we employed the deep serratus plane block. The more efficient option for mastectomy remains unclear [13–15].

4.3. *ESPB vs. PVB in Postoperative Analgesia*

In our study, ESPB was significantly less effective than PVB in achieving postoperative analgesia, which is consistent with findings from other similar studies [16–18] where opioid use and/or reported pain intensity were higher in the ESPB group compared to the PVB group. The greater effectiveness of PVB is likely associated with a larger extent of the block [19].

4.4. *ESPB vs. SAPB in Postoperative Analgesia*

In our study, ESPB was significantly less effective than SAPB in achieving postoperative analgesia. The patients from the erector spinae plane block group reported higher pain intensity despite using, on average, twice the amount of opioid compared to both other groups.

Elsabeeny et al. found no difference between ESPB and SPB in breast cancer surgeries. The reported pain intensity was comparable in both groups. The main limitation of their study was the control group, where morphine was used instead of PVB; therefore, only the need for rescue ketorolac analgesia was measured instead of opioid requirements [20].

In the study by Mekhaeil et al., SAPB provided more effective postoperative analgesia in patients undergoing modified radical mastectomy, with lower pain scores, less peri operative analgesic consumption, and longer duration of analgesia than ESPB [21].

The study by Ahuja et al. failed to show statistically significant differences in postoperative analgesia between ESPB and SAPB, and only the percentage of patients requiring rescue analgesia was recorded instead of those requiring a PCA pump like in our study, which could have affected the accuracy of the comparison [22].

4.5. *Limitations*

Only the first pain assessment was conducted exactly one hour after the surgery, while the subsequent assessments were carried out at fixed times, which may affect the accuracy of our results. Furthermore, variations in surgeons and the durations of procedures were not considered during randomization.

5. Conclusions

1. Both the serratus anterior plane block and the erector spinae plane block were as effective as the paravertebral block in achieving intraoperative analgesia.
2. The serratus anterior plane block was equally as effective as the paravertebral block in achieving postoperative analgesia.
3. The erector spinae plane block was significantly less effective in achieving postoperative analgesia than both the paravertebral block and serratus anterior plane block.

Author Contributions: Methodology, M.B.; software, W.S.; formal analysis, J.Z.; investigation, M.B.; writing—original draft, K.W.; project administration, M.B. All authors have read and agreed to the published version of the manuscript.

Funding: This research received no external funding.

Institutional Review Board Statement: This study was conducted in accordance with the Declaration of Helsinki, and approved by the Bioethical Committee of the Regional Medical Chamber in Koszalin (16 OCT 2020 r).

Informed Consent Statement: Informed consent was obtained from all subjects involved in this study.

Data Availability Statement: The data presented in this study are available on request from the corresponding author.

Conflicts of Interest: The authors declare no conflicts of interest.

References

1. Bray, F.; Laversanne, M.; Sung, H.; Ferlay, J.; Siegel, R.L.; Soerjomataram, I.; Jemal, A. Global cancer statistics 2022: GLOBOCAN estimates of incidence and mortality worldwide for 36 cancers in 185 countries. *CA Cancer J. Clin.* **2024**, *74*, 229–263. [CrossRef] [PubMed]
2. Didkowska, J.; Barańska, K.; Miklewska, M.J.; Wojciechowska, U. Cancer incidence and mortality in Poland in 2023. *Nowotw. J. Oncol.* **2024**, *74*, 75–93. [CrossRef]
3. Calapai, M.; Esposito, E.; Puzzo, L.; Vecchio, D.A.; Blandino, R.; Bova, G.; Quattrone, D.; Mannucci, C.; Ammendolia, I.; Mondello, C.; et al. Post-Mastectomy Pain: An updated overview on risk factors, predictors, and markers. *Life* **2021**, *11*, 1026. [CrossRef] [PubMed]
4. Rao, F.; Wang, Z.; Chen, X.; Liu, L.; Qian, B.; Guo, Y. Ultrasound-guided thoracic paravertebral block enhances the quality of recovery after modified radical mastectomy: A randomized controlled trial. *J. Pain. Res.* **2021**, *14*, 2563–2570. [CrossRef] [PubMed]
5. Niesen, A.D.; Jacob, A.K.; Law, L.A.; Sviggum, H.P.; Johnson, R.L. Complication rate of ultrasound-guided paravertebral block for breast surgery. *Reg. Anesth. Pain. Med.* **2020**, *10*, 813–817. [CrossRef] [PubMed]
6. Schnabel, A.; Reichl, S.U.; Kranke, P.; Pogatzki-Zahn, E.M.; Zahn, P.K. Efficacy and safety of paravertebral blocks in breast surgery: A meta-analysis of randomized controlled trials. *Br. J. Anaesth.* **2010**, *6*, 842–852. [CrossRef] [PubMed]
7. Blanco, R. The 'pecs block': A novel technique for providing analgesia after breast surgery. *Anaesthesia* **2011**, *9*, 847–848. [CrossRef] [PubMed]
8. Blanco, R.; Fajardo, M.; Parras Maldonado, T. Ultrasound description of Pecs II (modified Pecs I): A novel approach to breast surgery. *Rev. Esp. Anestesiol. Reanim.* **2012**, *9*, 470–475. [CrossRef]
9. Blanco, R.; Parras, T.; McDonnell, J.G.; Prats-Galino, A. Serratus plane block: A novel ultrasound-guided thoracic wall nerve block. *Anaesthesia* **2013**, *11*, 1107–1113. [CrossRef]
10. Singh, S.; Chowdhary, N.K. Erector spinae plane block an effective block for post-operative analgesia in modified radical mastectomy. *Indian. J. Anaesth.* **2018**, *2*, 148–150. [CrossRef]
11. Gabriel, R.A.; Swisher, M.W.; Sztain, J.F.; Curran, B.P.; Said, E.T.; Abramson, W.B.; Khatibi, B.; Alexander, B.S.; Finneran, J.J.; Wallace, A.M.; et al. Serratus anterior plane versus paravertebral nerve blocks for postoperative analgesia after non-mastectomy breast surgery: A randomized controlled non-inferiority trial. *Reg. Anesth. Pain. Med.* **2021**, *9*, 773–778. [CrossRef] [PubMed]
12. Gupta, K.; Srikanth, K.; Girdhar, K.K.; Chan, V. Analgesic efficacy of ultrasound-guided paravertebral block versus serratus plane block for modified radical mastectomy: A randomised, controlled trial. *Indian. J. Anaesth.* **2017**, *5*, 381–386. [CrossRef] [PubMed]
13. Edwards, J.T.; Langridge, X.T.; Cheng, G.S.; McBroom, M.M.; Minhajuddin, A.; Machi, A.T. Superficial vs. deep serratus anterior plane block for analgesia in patients undergoing mastectomy: A randomized prospective trial. *J. Clin. Anesth.* **2021**, *75*, 110470. [CrossRef]
14. Tan, K.W.; Sayed Masri, S.N.N.; Musthafa, Q.A.; Mohd Azidin, A.; Nik Mohamed Kamil, A.; Izaham, A.; Md Nor, N. Analgesic efficacy of the superficial versus deep serratus plane blocks for mastectomy with axillary clearance: A randomized controlled trial. *Medicine* **2022**, *35*, e30515. [CrossRef]
15. Abdallah, F.W.; Cil, T.; MacLean, D.; Madjdpour, C.; Escallon, J.; Semple, J.; Brull, R. Too deep or not too deep?: A propensity-matched comparison of the analgesic effects of a superficial versus deep serratus fascial plane block for ambulatory breast cancer surgery. *Reg. Anesth. Pain. Med.* **2018**, *5*, 480–487. [CrossRef]
16. Aoyama, Y.; Sakura, S.; Tsuchiya, R.; Wittayapairoj, A.; Saito, Y. Erector spinae plane block and paravertebral block for breast surgery: A retrospective propensity-matched noninferiority. *Trial. J. Pain. Res.* **2020**, *13*, 2367–2376. [CrossRef]
17. Jayakrishnan, S.; Dua, A.; Kumar, A. Comparison of fascial plane blocks (ESPB vs. TPVB) for pain relief following modified radical mastectomy. *J. Anaesthesiol. Clin. Pharmacol.* **2023**. [CrossRef]
18. Elsabeeny, W.Y.; Shehab, N.N.; Wadod, M.A.; Elkady, M.A. Perioperative analgesic modalities for breast cancer surgeries: A prospective randomized controlled trial. *J. Pain. Res.* **2020**, *13*, 2885–2894. [CrossRef]
19. Cowie, B.; McGlade, D.; Ivanusic, J.; Barrington, M.J. Ultrasound-guided thoracic paravertebral blockade: A cadaveric study. *Anesth. Analg.* **2010**, *6*, 1735–1739. [CrossRef] [PubMed]
20. Mekhaeil, M.F.W.; Abdelkader, S.F.; Marof, H.M.; Yousef, A.A.E. Prospective study: The analgesic efficacy of ultrasound-guided erector spinae plane block versus serratus plane block in patients undergoing modified radical mastectomy. *J. Adv. Med. Med. Res.* **2021**, *33*, 9–18. [CrossRef]

21. Ahuja, D.; Kumar, V.; Gupta, N.; Bharati, S.J.; Garg, R.; Mishra, S.; Khan, M.A.; Bhatnagar, S. Comparison of the efficacy of ultrasound-guided serratus anterior plane block versus erector spinae plane block for postoperative analgesia after modified radical mastectomy: A randomised controlled trial. *Turk. J. Anaesthesiol. Reanim.* **2022**, *6*, 435–442. [CrossRef] [PubMed]
22. Swisher, M.W.; Wallace, A.M.; Sztain, J.F.; Said, E.T.; Khatibi, B.; Abanobi, M.; Finneran Iv, J.J.; Gabriel, R.A.; Abramson, W.; Blair, S.L.; et al. Erector spinae plane versus paravertebral nerve blocks for postoperative analgesia after breast surgery: A randomized clinical trial. *Reg. Anesth. Pain. Med.* **2020**, *4*, 260–266. [CrossRef] [PubMed]

Journal of
Clinical Medicine

MDPI

Article

Multimodal Analgesia and Outcomes in Hysterectomy Surgery—A Population-Based Analysis

Crispiana Cozowicz [1], Hannah D. Gerner [2], Haoyan Zhong [3], Alex Illescas [3], Lisa Reisinger [3], Jashvant Poeran [3], Jiabin Liu [3,4] and Stavros G. Memtsoudis [1,3,4,*]

1 Department of Anesthesiology, Perioperative Medicine and Intensive Care Medicine, Paracelsus Medical University, Muellner Hauptstrasse 48, 5020 Salzburg, Austria; c@cozowicz.at
2 Medical University of Graz, Neue Stiftingtalstrasse 6, 8010 Graz, Austria; hannah.gerner@stud.medunigraz.at
3 Department of Anesthesiology, Critical Care & Pain Management, Weill Cornell Medical College, Hospital for Special Surgery, 535 East 70th Street, New York, NY 10021, USA; zhongh@hss.edu (H.Z.); illescasa@hss.edu (A.I.); reisingerl@hss.edu (L.R.); poeranv@hss.edu (J.P.); liuji@hss.edu (J.L.)
4 Department of Anesthesiology, Weill Cornell Medicine, New York, NY 10021, USA
* Correspondence: memtsoudiss@hss.edu; Tel.: +1-(212)-606-1036

Abstract: Objective: We aimed to investigate the impact of multimodal analgesia on postoperative complications and opioid prescription on a national level. **Methods**: This retrospective cross-sectional study included n = 1,307,923 hysterectomies (01/2006–12/2022, Premier Healthcare claims data). Multimodal analgesia was defined as opioid use with the addition of non-opioid analgesic modes, grouped into four categories: opioid-only and 1, 2, or 3 or more additional non-opioid analgesics. Multivariable regression models measured associations between multimodal categories and outcomes (composite/respiratory/cardiac/gastrointestinal/genitourinary, and CNS complications, oral morphine milligram equivalents [MME], and length of hospital stay [LOS]). Odds ratios (OR) and 95% confidence intervals (CI) are reported. **Results**: Overall, 84.3% (1,102,812/1,307,923) received multimodal analgesia, of which 58.9%, 28.0%, and 13.1% received 1, 2, or 3 or more additional non-opioid analgesics, respectively. The odds of any composite complication (any $\geq$1 complication) decreased with the addition of 1, 2, 3, or more analgesic modalities (versus opioid-only): OR 0.66 (CI 0.64; 0.68), OR 0.63 (CI 0.61; 0.66), OR 0.65 (CI 0.62; 0.67), respectively. Similar patterns existed for respiratory, cardiac, and genitourinary complications. Opioid prescription decreased incrementally with 1,2, 3, or more non-opioid analgesic modalities by 9.51 mg (CI 11.16; 7.86) and 15.29 mg (CI 17.21; 13.37) and 29.35 mg (CI 31.79; 26.91) cumulative MME. LOS was reduced by 0.52 days (CI 0.54; 0.51), 0.49 days (CI 0.51; 0.47), and 0.40 days (CI 0.43; 0.38), respectively. Costs were reduced by $765 (CI 817; 714) or $479 (CI 539; 419) with 1 or 2 multimodal modes. **Conclusions**: These findings suggest substantial benefits of multimodal analgesia, including significant decreases in serious complications (especially respiratory, cardiac, and genitourinary), opioid consumption, and hospitalizations. Multimodal analgesia may facilitate safe and efficient pain management with optimized opioid consumption.

Keywords: hysterectomy; multimodal analgesia; anesthesia; pain management; perioperative; complications; opioids

1. Introduction

In the United States, hysterectomies are the most frequent non-obstetric surgical procedures performed in women, rendering an incidence of more than 600,000 per year [1]. Regardless of surgical route, postoperative pain is significant and may escalate to chronic conditions, as reported in 10–50% [2]. While insufficient pain management presents a driver of delayed recovery and complications, the prevalent opioid crisis has raised concern for excessive perioperative opioid consumption. Thus, efforts to optimize perioperative care and accelerate patient recovery have spurred the implementation of enhanced recovery after surgery (ERAS) pathways with multimodal analgesic techniques as key interventions for improved postoperative outcomes [3]. Multimodal analgesia concurrently targets different pain pathways to facilitate additive and synergistic analgesic effects [4]. The aim is to attenuate the surgical stress response, reduce opioid consumption, and improve patient recovery. While a growing body of evidence recommends the utilization of multimodal analgesia, little is known about nationwide utilization practices and added clinical benefits in hysterectomy surgery. Moreover, population-based data on the impact of multimodal analgesia in terms of postoperative complication risk, patient recovery, and opioid consumption are lacking.

We therefore utilized national data to investigate associations between the use of multimodal analgesia and the occurrence of postoperative complications, length of hospital stay (LOS), and opioid prescription in patients undergoing hysterectomy surgery. We hypothesized that multimodal analgesia would be associated with a reduction in postoperative complications, LOS, and opioid use.

2. Methods

2.1. Study Design and Sample

This retrospective cross-sectional study was approved by the Institutional Review Board (IRB# 2012-050) of the Hospital for Special Surgery, New York. The requirement for written informed consent was waived, given the de-identified nature of these data. We identified adult patients undergoing elective hysterectomy surgery (2006–2022) from the Premier Healthcare claims dataset. (Premier Healthcare Solutions, Inc., Charlotte, NC, USA). Hysterectomy procedures were identified utilizing international classification of diseases -ninth/tenth revision (ICD-9/10 codes) and The Current Procedural Terminology (CPT) codes as shown in Appendix A. Exclusion criteria encompassed unknown sex (n = 516), unknown discharge status (n = 1533), patients without documented opioid use (n = 70,635), and cases with opioid utilization above the 95th percentile (to address outliers, n = 13,355).

2.2. Study Variables

The exposure of interest was the implementation of multimodal analgesia, defined as opioid use with the addition of 1, 2, or >2 non-opioid analgesic modes, as previously operationalized. Non-opioid analgesic modes included ketamine, non-steroidal anti-inflammatory drugs (NSAIDs), cyclooxygenase-2 inhibitors, paracetamol/acetaminophen, steroids (>1 dose of use on the day of surgery or the day after surgery), gabapentin/pregabalin, or neuraxial anesthesia. The use of multimodal analgesia components was identified from billing codes, which were published by this study group previously [4,5].

The outcomes of interest were perioperative complications (see below), opioid prescription, LOS measured in days, and cost measured in 2022 United States dollars (USD). Complications included a composite (any ≥1 complication) and individual analysis of respiratory, cardiac, gastrointestinal, genitourinary, and central nervous system (CNS) complications. All complications were defined using ICD-9 and ICD-10 diagnosis codes based on the previous literature (see Appendix B for definitions). Opioid utilization during hospitalization was based on billing for opioids (opioid type and dosage were billed by day in Premier) and then was converted into oral morphine milligram equivalents (MME) [6].

Patient-level variables included age, sex, race (black, white, other), insurance type (commercial, Medicaid, Medicare, uninsured, other), Elixhauser Comorbidity index (categorized as 0, 1, 2, 3+), history of sleep apnea, substance abuse, chronic pain, psychiatric, and opioid abuse. Procedure-level variables included the year of the procedure and type of anesthesia (general, neuraxial). Healthcare-level variables included hospital location (urban, rural), hospital size (<300, 300–499, ≥500 beds), and hospital teaching status.

2.3. Statistical Analysis

A descriptive analysis of all study variables was presented and stratified by the number of multimodal analgesia modalities used. Categorical variables were presented as counts and percentages, and continuous variables were presented as median and interquartile ranges (IQR). Given our large sample size, univariable differences between groups easily reach statistical significance; therefore, we applied standardized differences instead of p-values. An absolute standardized difference of $\geq$0.1 (or 10%) generally indicates a meaningful difference in covariate distribution between groups [7].

Multivariable multilevel logistic regression models were run to compare associations between the use of multimodal analgesia categories for all binary outcomes (composite complication and individual complications). Odds ratios (OR) and 95% confidence intervals (CI) were reported. The models were adjusted for all priori-determined covariates, including age, race, gender, Elixhauser Comorbidity index group, insurance type, year of surgery, hospital location, bed size, and hospital teaching status, type of anesthesia, history of sleep apnea, substance abuse, chronic pain, psychiatric history, and opioid abuse, based in their potential association with exposure and outcome, as previously described [5,8]. A generalized linear model was applied to compare associations between the use of multimodal analgesia categories (categorized as opioid-only, 1, 2, or >2 non-opioid analgesic modes) and continuous outcomes (opioid utilization, LOS, and cost), adjusting the same covariates as in the logistic regression model. Estimates were presented as least square means differences compared with the reference group along with 95% CIs. For the opioid utilization outcome, we additionally adjusted for substance use/abuse (including smoking), chronic pain conditions, psychiatric comorbidity variables, and opioid use disorder, given their association with opioid use. The outcome of LOS was modeled using only the inpatient cohort. A p-value <0.01 was used as the cutoff for statistical significance. Analyses were performed with SAS version 9.4 (SAS Institute, Cary, NC, USA).

3. Results

Among 1,307,923 adult women undergoing hysterectomy surgery from January 2006 to December 2022, we found that 84.3% (n = 1,102,812) received multimodal analgesia, of which 58.9%, 28.0%, and 13.1% received 1, 2 or >2 additional non-opioid analgesics, respectively. The use of >2 analgesic techniques for multimodal analgesia (compared with those on opioids only) was most common in teaching hospitals. In contrast, in non-teaching hospitals, a lower number of analgesic modalities were utilized more frequently. Multimodal analgesia utilization was slightly higher among those with an increased comorbidity burden and a history of substance abuse, while lower use was seen for older patients, those on Medicare, and patients receiving general anesthesia; all standardized differences $\geq$0.1 (Table 1).

Table 1. Baseline characteristics stratified by multimodal groups; each multimodal group is compared separately with the opioid-only group.

				Multimodal			
	Opioid-Only	**1 Mode**	**Stdiff**	**2 Modes**	**Stdiff**	**3 or More Modes**	**Stdiff**
	N = 200,052	N = 649,471		N = 308,579		N = 144,762	
Age, median [IQR]	48 [41.1, 59.9]	45.1 [39, 52.4]	−0.3	45 [38, 52.9]	−0.33	44.7 [36.9, 54.6]	−0.31
Race, n (%)							
Black	30,292 (15.1)	94,903 (14.5)	−0.02	46,790 (15.1)	<0.01	26,283 (18.1)	0.08
Other	39,651 (19.7)	114,842 (17.6)	−0.06	55,087 (17.8)	−0.05	22,948 (15.8)	−0.1
White	130,961 (65.2)	443,127 (67.9)	0.06	207,457 (67.1)	0.04	95,582 (66.0)	0.02
Insurance, n (%)			0.22		0.22		0.24
Commercial	124,528 (62.0)	451,696 (69.2)		202,136 (65.3)		86,796 (59.9)	
Medicaid	22,835 (11.4)	80,029 (12.3)		49,614 (16.0)		27,805 (19.2)	
Medicare	40,617 (20.2)	77,402 (11.9)		39,092 (12.6)		21,301 (14.7)	

Table 1. *Cont.*

		Multimodal					
	Opioid-Only	**1 Mode**	**Stdiff**	**2 Modes**	**Stdiff**	**3 or More Modes**	**Stdiff**
Uninsured	5764 (2.9)	18,881 (2.9)		7999 (2.6)		4283 (3.0)	
Unknown	7160 (3.6)	24,864 (3.8)		10,493 (3.4)		4628 (3.2)	
Inpatient/outpatient, n (%)			−0.1		−0.1		0.06
Inpatient	143,079 (71.2)	433,476 (66.4)		205,441 (66.4)		107,018 (73.9)	
Outpatient	57,825 (28.8)	219,396 (33.6)		103,893 (33.6)		37,795 (26.1)	
General anesthesia, n (%)	169,508 (84.4)	549,005 (84.1)	−0.03	234,946 (76.0)	−0.33	95,309 (65.8)	−0.58
Elixhauser comorbidity group, n (%)			0.18		0.12		0.27
0	129,723 (64.6)	455,374 (69.7)		195,770 (63.3)		75,067 (51.8)	
1	32,755 (16.3)	109,647 (16.8)		60,494 (19.6)		33,106 (22.9)	
2	19,810 (9.9)	52,858 (8.1)		31,351 (10.1)		20,110 (13.9)	
3	18,616 (9.3)	34,993 (5.4)		21,719 (7.0)		16,530 (11.4)	
Sleep apnea, n (%)	4361 (2.2)	10,869 (1.7)	−0.04	6732 (2.2)	<.01	4646 (3.2)	0.06
Substance abuse, n (%)	24,323 (12.1)	86,390 (13.2)	0.04	44,193 (14.3)	0.06	26,159 (18.1)	0.17
Chronic pain	48,688 (24.2)	108,550 (16.6)	−0.19	52,110 (16.8)	−0.18	25,960 (17.9)	−0.16
Psychiatric, n (%)	24,741 (12.3)	82,118 (12.6)	0.01	39,573 (12.8)	0.01	18,658 (12.9)	0.02
Opioid abuse, n (%)	170 (0.1)	625 (0.1)	<0.01	562 (0.2)	0.03	574 (0.4)	0.06
Urban/Rural, n (%)			0.07		0.08		0.03
Rural	17,501 (8.7)	71,336 (10.9)		34,775 (11.2)		13,899 (9.6)	
Urban	183,403 (91.3)	581,536 (89.1)		274,559 (88.8)		130,914 (90.4)	
Hospital Size, n (%)							
Large	73,566 (36.6)	200,558 (30.7)	−0.13	109,264 (35.3)	−0.03	59,044 (40.8)	0.09
Medium	68,461 (34.1)	230,322 (35.3)	0.03	107,828 (34.9)	0.02	47,390 (32.7)	−0.03
Small	58,877 (29.3)	221,992 (34.0)	0.1	92,242 (29.8)	0.01	38,379 (26.5)	−0.06
Teaching hospital, n (%)			−0.05		0.1		0.32
No	114,276 (56.9)	386,814 (59.2)		159,842 (51.7)		59,751 (41.3)	
Yes	86,628 (43.1)	266,058 (40.8)		149,492 (48.3)		85,062 (58.7)	
Use of multimodal components, n (%)							
Gabapentin	-	5500 (0.8)		25,924 (8.4)		86,137 (59.5)	
Steroid	-	2835 (0.4)		8866 (2.9)		10,356 (7.2)	
Ketamine	-	3245 (0.5)		17,725 (5.7)		44,896 (31.0)	
NSAID	-	558,994 (85.6)		285,111 (92.2)		126,480 (87.3)	
Cox2	-	3456 (0.5)		9034 (2.9)		49,178 (34.0)	
Acetaminophen	-	72,041 (11.0)		233,878 (75.6)		133,243 (92.0)	
Neuraxial	-	5669 (0.9)		29,817 (9.6)		26,452 (18.3)	

Stdiff: Multimodal groups were compared with the opioid-only group. An absolute standardized difference of 0.1 (or 10%) generally indicates a meaningful difference in covariate distribution between groups.

The trend analysis showed that the practice of adding three or more non-opioid analgesic modalities to opioids has seen a steady rise from an incidence of 1.03% in 2006 to 39.57% in 2022. Concurrently, the use of just one non-opioid analgesic modality in addition to opioid analgesia decreased from 61.72% in 2006 to 18.84% in 2022. Furthermore, a drop in the use of opioid-only-based analgesia was observed from 25.31% in 2006 to 5.14% in 2022 (Figure 1). The most frequently used non-opioid analgesics were NSAIDs and acetaminophen, followed by gabapentin and neuraxial anesthesia (Table 1).

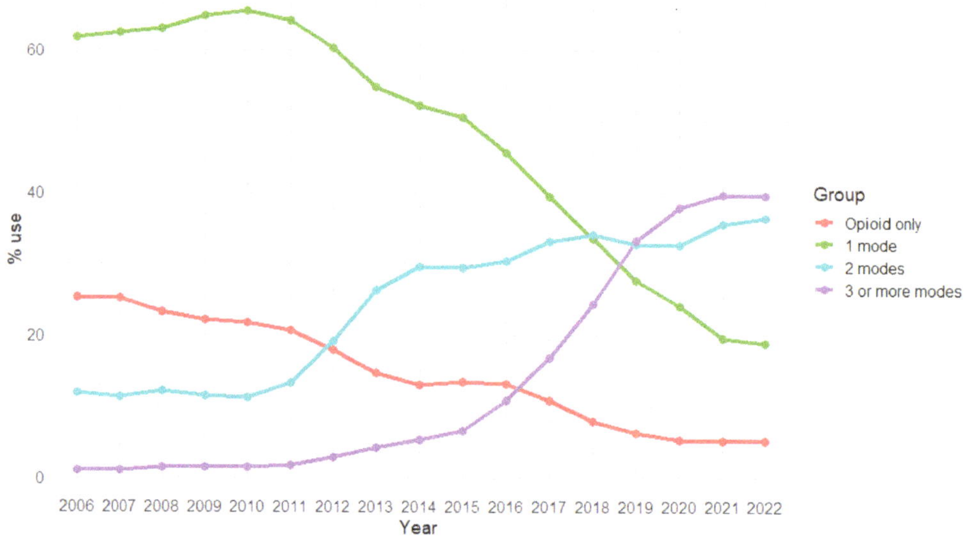

Figure 1. Trends of multimodal analgesia use among hysterotomy cases over study time.

In unadjusted outcome comparisons, patients receiving multimodal analgesia had a lower incidence of the composite of any complication and, more specifically, respiratory, cardiac, and genitourinary complications. Furthermore, opioid dispensation was lower among those receiving multimodal analgesia (Table 2).

Table 2. Outcomes stratified by multimodal groups.

	Opioid Only	1 Mode	2 Modes	3 or More Modes
	N = 200,052	**N = 649,471**	**N = 308,579**	**N = 144,762**
Composite outcome for complication, n (%)	8661 (4.3)	13,979 (2.1)	7694 (2.5)	4915 (3.4)
Respiratory	2998 (1.5)	4006 (0.6)	2330 (0.8)	1615 (1.1)
Gastrointestinal	626 (0.3)	1274 (0.2)	571 (0.2)	263 (0.2)
Genitourinary	3653 (1.8)	5446 (0.8)	2442 (0.8)	1374 (0.9)
Central nervous system	345 (0.2)	600 (0.1)	373 (0.1)	288 (0.2)
Cardiac	2489 (1.2)	4425 (0.7)	2948 (1.0)	2104 (1.5)
Total opioid use, median [IQR]	237 [124, 412]	226 [130, 385]	202 [114, 360]	173 [96, 315]
Adjusted cost, median [IQR]	9683 [6950, 13,494]	9033 [6758, 12,210]	9515 [7083, 13,041]	10,280 [7638, 14,485]
	N = 143,079	**N = 433,476**	**N = 205,441**	**N = 107,018**
Length of stay for inpatient cohort, median [IQR]	2, [2, 3]	2 [1, 3]	2 [2, 3]	2 [2, 3]

This pattern was more pronounced in adjusted models. (Table 3) Multimodal use applied as a categorical variable with four categories (1, 2, or 3 or more additional non-opioid analgesics versus opioid-only) was associated with consistent decreases in any complication (OR 0.66 CI 0.64; 0.68/OR 0.63 CI 0.61; 0.66/OR 0.65 CI 0.62; 0.67). The increased modes of analgesia did not result in more reduced odds of complications. Consistently, respiratory complications decreased by (OR 0.60 CI 0.57; 0.63/OR 0.60 CI 0.56; 0.64/OR 0.64 CI 0.60; 0.69), cardiac complications by (OR 0.71 CI 0.68, 0.75/OR 0.69 CI 0.65, 0.73/OR 0.66 CI 0.62, 0.71), and genitourinary complications decreased by (OR 0.65 CI 0.62, 0.68/OR 0.58 CI 0.55, 0.61/OR 0.61 CI 0.57, 0.66) with the addition of 1,2, or 3 or more multimodal techniques, respectively; all $p < 0.001$. A decrease in gastrointestinal complications was only observed with the addition of one non-opioid analgesic modality OR 0.81 (CI 0.74, 0.90). No effect was found for the occurrence of CNS system complications.

Table 3. Adjusted outcomes.

Binary Outcomes	Unadjusted Odds Ratio (95% CIs)	*p*-Value	Adjusted Odds Ratio (95% CIs) [a]	*p*-Value
Composite complications				
1 mode vs. opioid only	0.49 (0.47, 0.5)	<0.001	0.66 (0.64, 0.68)	<0.001
2 modes vs. opioid only	0.57 (0.55, 0.58)	<0.001	0.63 (0.61, 0.66)	<0.001
3 modes vs. opioid only	0.78 (0.75, 0.81)	<0.001	0.65 (0.62, 0.67)	<0.001
Respiratory complications				
1 mode vs. opioid only	0.41 (0.39, 0.43)	<0.001	0.6 (0.57, 0.63)	<0.001
2 modes vs. opioid only	0.5 (0.47, 0.53)	<0.001	0.6 (0.56, 0.64)	<0.001
3 modes vs. opioid only	0.74 (0.7, 0.79)	<0.001	0.64 (0.6, 0.69)	<0.001
Cardiac complications				
1 mode vs. opioid only	0.54 (0.52, 0.57)	<0.001	0.71 (0.68, 0.75)	<0.001
2 modes vs. opioid only	0.77 (0.73, 0.81)	<0.001	0.69 (0.65, 0.73)	<0.001
3 modes vs. opioid only	1.18 (1.11, 1.25)	<0.001	0.66 (0.62, 0.71)	<0.001
Gastrointestinal complications				
1 mode vs. opioid only	0.63 (0.57, 0.69)	<0.001	0.81 (0.74, 0.9)	<0.001
2 modes vs. opioid only	0.59 (0.53, 0.66)	<0.001	0.93 (0.83, 1.05)	0.242
3 modes vs. opioid only	0.58 (0.5, 0.67)	<0.001	1.08 (0.92, 1.28)	0.360
Genitourinary complications				
1 mode vs. opioid only	0.45 (0.44, 0.47)	<0.001	0.65 (0.62, 0.68)	<0.001
2 modes vs. opioid only	0.43 (0.41, 0.45)	<0.001	0.58 (0.55, 0.61)	<0.001
3 modes vs. opioid only	0.52 (0.49, 0.55)	<0.001	0.61 (0.57, 0.66)	<0.001
Central nervous system complications				
1 mode vs. opioid only	0.53 (0.47, 0.61)	<0.001	0.9 (0.79, 1.03)	0.143
2 modes vs. opioid only	0.7 (0.61, 0.81)	<0.001	0.93 (0.79, 1.09)	0.359
3 modes vs. opioid only	1.16 (0.99, 1.35)	0.066	0.99 (0.82, 1.19)	0.890
Continuous Outcomes	**Unadjusted least square means (95% CIs)**	***p*-value**	**Adjusted least square means (95% CIs) [b]**	***p*-value**
Length of stay for inpatients in days				
1 mode vs. opioid only	−0.73 (−0.74, −0.71)	<0.001	−0.52 (−0.54, −0.51)	<0.001
2 modes vs. opioid only	−0.56 (−0.58, −0.54)	<0.001	−0.49 (−0.51, −0.47)	<0.001
3 modes vs. opioid only	−0.28 (−0.31, −0.30)	<0.001	−0.40 (−0.43, −0.38)	<0.001

Table 3. *Cont.*

Continuous Outcomes	Unadjusted least square means (95% CIs)	p-value	Adjusted least square means (95% CIs) [b]	p-value
Adjusted cost in dollars				
1 mode vs. opioid only	−1506 (−1560, −1452)	<0.001	−765 (−817, −714)	<0.001
2 modes vs. opioid only	−760 (−821, −700)	<0.001	−479 (−539, −419)	<0.001
3 modes vs. opioid only	666 (594, 739)	<0.001	79 (2, 156)	0.042
Total opioid consumption				
1 mode vs. opioid only	−16.55 (−18.24, −14.85)	<0.001	−9.51 (−11.16, −7.86)	<0.001
2 modes vs. opioid only	−32.34 (−34.25, −30.43)	<0.001	−15.29 (−17.21, −13.37)	<0.001
3 modes vs. opioid only	−63.57 (−65.86, −61.27)	<0.001	−29.35 (−31.79, −26.91)	<0.001

[a]. Multiple logistic regression models were run to compare associations between the use of multimodal analgesia categories for all binary outcomes (composite complication and individual complications). Odds ratios (OR) and 95% CIs were reported. Models were adjusted using a priori-determined covariate, including age, race, gender, Elixhauser Comorbidity index group, year of surgery, hospital location, bed size, and hospital teaching status, as described previously. [b]. A generalized linear model was applied to compare associations between the use of multimodal analgesia categories (categorized as opioid-only, 1, 2, or >2 non-opioid analgesic modes) and continuous outcomes (Opioid utilization, inpatient length of stay, and cost) adjusting the same covariates in the logistic regression model. Estimates were presented as least square means differences compared with the reference group along with 95% CIs. For opioid utilization outcome, we additionally adjusted for a history of substance use/abuse (including smoking), chronic pain conditions, psychiatric comorbidity variables, and opioid use disorder, given their association with opioid use.

Notably, opioid prescription was incrementally reduced in line with additional non-opioid analgesics utilized: −9.51 mg (CI −11.16; −7.86) and −15.29 mg (CI −17.21; −13.37) and −29.35 mg (CI −31.79; −26.91). LOS decreased by 0.52 days (CI 0.54; 0.51), 0.49 days (CI 0.51; 0.47), and 0.40 days (CI 0.43; 0.38), respectively. Furthermore, cost reductions of −765 USD (CI −817; −714) and −479 USD (CI −539; −419) were observed with 1 or 2 modalities. However, a small, non-significant increase in the cost of 79 USD (CI 2; 156) emerged among those receiving >2 non-opioid analgesic modalities (Table 3).

4. Discussion

In this large national sample of more than 1.3 million women undergoing hysterectomy surgery from 2006 to 2022, we found that the use of multimodal analgesia was associated with significantly improved outcomes.

The odds of the occurrence of any postoperative complication were reduced by 35%. More specifically, respiratory complications decreased by about 40%, cardiac complications by 30%, and genitourinary complications were reduced by 40% when compared with patients without multimodal analgesia. No impact on the occurrence of CNS complications was observed. Concurrently, opioid prescription incrementally decreased with the use of increasing modes of multimodal modalities. Furthermore, we observed a reduction in LOS while costs were reduced with the addition of 1 or 2 analgesic modalities, but not when adding >2 analgesic techniques.

Trend analysis demonstrated substantial changes in the practice of perioperative pain management for hysterectomies in the last two decades. Most notably, a steep increase in the use of >2 non-opioid analgesic modalities was found, which increased from an incidence of 1.03% in 2006 to 39.57% in 2022. Concurrently, the use of just one non-opioid analgesic modality in addition to opioid analgesia decreased from 61.72% in 2006 to 18.84% in 2022.

Hysterectomy is the second most common procedure performed in women after obstetric surgery, which is in part related to gynecological malignancy affecting over 1,000,000 women per year [3,9]. Although it is known that hysterectomies often result in significant pain and slow recovery, postoperative pain is easily overlooked, and persistent opioid use is reported in 5% regardless of surgical route [9–11]. Inadequate analgesic management after gynecologic surgery is a major driver of postoperative complications, delayed recovery, and increased opioid use [12,13].

Therefore, enhanced recovery after surgery pathways have been widely implemented, including the gynecological specialties, with strong recommendations for the routine administration of multimodal analgesia. The goal is to concurrently target various pain pathways by combining different analgesic medications and techniques to achieve additive and synergistic analgesic effects while diminishing complications [12]. However, little is known about the clinical impact of multimodal analgesia in hysterectomies, and pharmacologic strategies to improve the quality of this population have yet to be examined [14]. In this context, these data demonstrate that in a large sample of hysterectomies, the use of multimodal analgesia was associated with a substantial decrease in the occurrence of serious adverse events, including respiratory, cardiac, and genitourinary complications. Pain physiologically confers several detrimental effects, such as adrenergic activation with catecholamine release, inflammatory mediator activation, hemodynamic instability, cardiac stress, and respiratory deterioration [5]. Thus, inadequate analgesia is linked to increased perioperative morbidity with a higher risk for cardiac and pulmonary complications [15–19]. It is, therefore, conceivable that multimodal analgesia, by concurrently targeting multiple pain pathways, may diminish postoperative stress and other pain-related detriments and, therefore, accelerate postoperative recovery. Consistently, these data also demonstrate a decrease in LOS among patients with multimodal analgesia. This is in line with evidence from radical laparoscopic gynecological cancer surgery, where multimodal analgesia conferred lower pain scores, earlier mobilization, and a lower incidence of severe complications [13].

While we did not have information on pain scores in these data, we found that multimodal analgesia was associated with a significant reduction in opioid prescription, which could indicate improved pain management [10]. With the opioid crisis globally expanding, the pressure to restrict or even abolish opioid use has increasingly gained popularity in clinical practice. At the same time, postoperative pain remains insufficiently managed, with reported incidences reaching 80% [20]. This is a serious concern given that pain appears to be the most prevalent, disabling, and burdensome health problem in the US, with related expenses exceeding those for cardiac disease, cancer, and diabetes. [20,21]. Therefore, perioperative clinicians are particularly challenged with facilitating adequate pain management and rapid recovery while trying to diminish drivers of persistent opioid use. In the absence of equipotent alternatives, opioids remain the mainstay for perioperative pain management based on their undisputed analgesic efficacy [20,22]. It may, therefore, be more meaningful to strive for improved postoperative pain management and fastened recovery rather than exclusive opioid reduction [20]. In fact, opioid-free strategies have not been shown to decrease the risk of persistent opioid use [23]. The complexity in hysterectomies is highlighted by evidence showing that hysterectomy surgeons appear to be among the top physician prescribers of opioids nationally, while in laparoscopic hysterectomies, it has been shown that opioid prescriptions were a four-fold of what was required for acute postoperative pain control [24,25]. Moreover, nationwide trend analysis showed a substantial increase in perioperative opioid prescriptions for hysterectomies from 2004 to 2014 despite an increase in minimally invasive surgical techniques [26]. In this national sample of hysterectomies, we observed an incremental decrease in opioid prescription with the use of increasing modes of multimodal analgesia techniques. This dose–response relationship was observed alongside a reduced risk for serious postoperative complications and a significant decrease in LOS. Consistently, opioid-sparing with multiple analgesic modalities has been shown in laparoscopic hysterectomies and cesarean deliveries [10]. Previously, however, no conclusions could have been drawn regarding patient safety and complication risk due to the lack of adequately powered data [27]. The current data supports the notion of improved postoperative outcomes with reduced opioid consumption in hysterectomy surgery. With the Society of Gynecologic Oncology encouraging limited opioid use, multimodal analgesia may prove to be crucial in the development of perioperative strategies that strike a balance between adequate pain control and the prevention of excess opioid use [9,28].

5. Limitations

This analysis is subject to several limitations, given the nature of observational data. Despite efforts to account for baseline differences, the lack of randomization bears the risk of residual confounding. Thus, causal conclusions cannot be drawn, while associations require careful interpretation in the context of plausibility based on previous scientific findings. As mentioned, patients without documentation for opioid use were excluded as reflective of either missing data or lack of opioid use. However, we would not anticipate a significant impact on our results as missing data would likely be evenly distributed, and the lack of opioid use would not comply with our predefined study question. Despite the nature of the surgery, patients with a lack of information on gender were excluded to eliminate any concerns about quality issues in these cases. Furthermore, the lack of detailed clinical information (e.g., precise timing of medication and pain scores) needs to be acknowledged, which is based on the primary purpose of the utilized billing data. Analysis specific to individual ethnicities was not possible because of changes in reporting practices over the study period. Given the skewed distribution of age, LOS, cost, and opioid use, we reported median and IQR. Nevertheless, this is a large national sample of patients undergoing hysterectomy surgery, facilitating the investigation of potential harm.

6. Conclusions

This large national sample of patients undergoing hysterectomy surgery indicates substantial benefits with the use of multimodal analgesia. A decrease in serious complications by at least 30% was accompanied by incrementally reduced opioid use and a reduction in LOS. While more evidence is needed, multimodal analgesic approaches may facilitate safe and efficient pain management with optimized opioid consumption.

Author Contributions: S.G.M., C.C., H.D.G., L.R., J.P. and J.L. have helped design the study, conduct the study and perform data analysis, write the manuscript, and approve the final manuscript. H.Z. and A.I. performed the statistical analysis, helped conduct the study, wrote the manuscript, and approved the final manuscript. All authors have read and agreed to the published version of the manuscript.

Funding: This work was supported by the Research and Education Fund, Department of Anesthesiology, Critical Care and Pain, Hospital for Special Surgery.

Institutional Review Board Statement: Institutional review board #2017-0169, provided by the institutional review board of the Hospital for Special, Surgery, Dana Center, 7 February 2020.

Informed Consent Statement: The requirement for written informed consent was waived, given the deidentified nature of the data.

Data Availability Statement: Restrictions apply to the availability of these data. Data were obtained from Premier Healthcare and are available from Stavros G. Memtsoudis with the permission of Premier Healthcare.

Conflicts of Interest: Stavros G. Memtsoudis is a one-time consultant for Sandoz Inc. and Teikoku. He is the owner of a US Patent for a Multicatheter Infusion System. US-2017-0361063. He is the owner of SGM Consulting, LLC, and co-owner of FC Monmouth, LLC. None of the above relations influenced the conduct of the present study. All authors declare no competing interest.

Appendix A

Table A1. Identifying hysterectomy procedures based on International Classification of Diseases 9th (ICD-9) and 10th Revision (ICD-10) procedure codes and The Current Procedural Terminology (CPT) codes.

ICD-9	Description
68.0x	Hysterotomy
68.3x	Subtotal abdominal hysterectomy

Table A1. *Cont.*

ICD-9	Description
68.4x	Total abdominal hysterectomy
68.5x	Vaginal hysterectomy
68.6x	Radical abdominal hysterectomy
68.7x	Radical vaginal hysterectomy
68.8x	Pelvic evisceration
68.9x	Other and unspecified hysterectomy
ICD-10	
0U54xxx	Destruction of Uterine Supporting Structure
0U55xxx	Destruction of Fallopian Tube, Right
0U56xxx	Destruction of Fallopian Tube, Left
0U57xxx	Destruction of Fallopian Tubes, Bilateral
0U59xxx	Destruction of Uterus
0U94xxx	Drainage of Uterine Supporting Structure
0U95xxx	Drainage of Fallopian Tube, Right
0U96xxx	Drainage of Fallopian Tube, Left
0U97xxx	Drainage of Fallopian Tubes, Bilateral
0U99xxx	Drainage of Uterus
0UB4xxx	Excision of Uterine Supporting Structure
0UB5xxx	Excision of Fallopian Tube, Right
0UB6xxx	Excision of Fallopian Tube, Left
0UB7xxx	Excision of Fallopian Tubes, Bilateral
0UB9xxx	Excision of Uterus
0UC4xxx	Extirpation of Uterine Supporting Structure
0UC5xxx	Extirpation of Fallopian Tube, Right
0UC6xxx	Extirpation of Fallopian Tube, Left
0UC7xxx	Extirpation of Fallopian Tubes, Bilateral
0UN4xxx	Release of Uterine Supporting Structure
0UN5xxx	Release of Fallopian Tube, Right
0UN6xxx	Release of Fallopian Tube, Left
0UN7xxx	Release of Fallopian Tubes, Bilateral
0UN9xxx	Release Uterus
0UT2xxx	Resection of Bilateral Ovaries
0UT4xxx	Resection of Uterine Supporting Structure
0UT5xxx	Resection of Fallopian Tube, Right
0UT6xxx	Resection of Fallopian Tube, Left
0UT7xxx	Resection of Fallopian Tubes, Bilateral
0UT9xxx	Resection of Uterus
0UTCxxx	Resection of Cervix
CPT	
58150	Total abdominal hysterectomy (corpus and cervix), with or without removal of tube(s), with or without removal of ovary(s)

Table A1. *Cont.*

CPT	
58152	Total abdominal hysterectomy (corpus and cervix), with or without removal of tube(s), with or without removal of ovary(s)
58180	The provider removes the uterus via an abdominal incision. The provider may also remove the fallopian tubes and ovaries.
58200	The provider removes the uterus and cervix and may also remove the fallopian tubes and ovaries, all through via an abdominal incision. The provider removes the upper one–third of the vaginal canal and some of the pelvic and para-aortic lymph nodes.
58210	The provider removes the uterus and cervix, including the parametrium, via an abdominal incision, known as a radical abdominal hysterectomy. The provider may also remove all or part of the vagina, all the pelvic lymph nodes on the right and left side, and biopsy a few of the para-aortic lymph nodes. The provider may remove part or all of the fallopian tubes and ovaries.
58240	The provider performs pelvic exenteration on patients who have had a recurrence of cancer of the cervix after they have had radiation therapy or patients who have stage IV cancer and the tumor is in the bladder and rectum. There is no standard procedure and the organs and tissues that the provider removes depend on where the cancer is located and the stage. In a total exenteration, the provider removes the uterus, tubes, ovaries, parametrial tissue, bladder, rectum, vagina, urethra, and part of the levator ani muscles. In an anterior exenteration, the provider does not remove the rectum. In a posterior exenteration, the provider does not remove the bladder and urethra. He may also resect part of the anus, urethra, and part of the vulva.
58260	In this procedure, the provider surgically removes the uterus and cervix only using a vaginal approach, known as a vaginal hysterectomy. The uterus is normal in size, which means it weighs 250 g or less.
58262	In this procedure, the provider surgically removes the uterus, cervix, fallopian tubes, and ovaries using a vaginal approach known as a vaginal hysterectomy. The uterus is normal in size, which means it weighs 250 g or less.
58263	In this procedure, the provider surgically removes the uterus, cervix, fallopian tubes, and ovaries using a vaginal approach known as a vaginal hysterectomy. Because the patient has a small bowel prolapsing into the vaginal canal, called an enterocele, he also repairs this area. The uterus is normal in size, which means it weighs 250 g or less.
58267	In this procedure, the provider surgically removes the uterus and cervix only using a vaginal approach, known as a vaginal hysterectomy. The patient also has stress urinary incontinence, which requires the suspension of the urethra. The uterus is normal in size, which means it weighs 250 g or less, and the provider may use an endoscope during the procedure.
58270	In this procedure, the provider surgically removes the uterus and cervix only using a vaginal approach, known as a vaginal hysterectomy. The provider also repairs a small bowel prolapse into the vaginal canal. The uterus is normal in size, which means it weighs 250 g or less.
58275	In this procedure, the provider surgically removes the uterus and the cervix using a vaginal approach, known as a vaginal hysterectomy. The provider also partially or completely excises the vagina.
58280	The provider surgically removes the uterus and the cervix using a vaginal approach, known as a vaginal hysterectomy. The provider also partially or completely excises the vagina and repairs a small bowel prolapse into the vaginal canal.
58285	the provider removes the uterus, fallopian tubes, and ovaries, the parametrium, which includes the uterosacral, cardinal, broad, and round ligaments, and the upper one-third of the vagina. This procedure treats cervical cancer.
58290	the physician surgically removes the uterus and cervix only using a vaginal approach. The uterus is larger than normal, usually due to the presence of fibroids, which means it weighs more than 250 g.
58291	the physician surgically removes the uterus, cervix, the fallopian tubes, and ovaries using a vaginal approach. The uterus is usually larger than normal because of the presence of fibroids, which means it weighs more than 250 g.

Table A1. *Cont.*

CPT	
58292	the physician surgically removes the uterus, cervix, fallopian tubes, and ovaries using a vaginal approach. Because the patient has small bowel prolapse into the vaginal canal, the provider also repairs this area. The uterus is usually larger than normal due to the presence of fibroids, which means it weighs more than 250 g.
58294	the physician surgically removes the uterus and cervix only using a vaginal approach. Because the patient has a small bowel prolapsing into the vaginal canal, this area is repaired. The uterus is usually larger than normal because of the presence of fibroids, which means it weighs more than 250 g.

Appendix B

Table A2. Complication identification based on the International Classification of Diseases, Ninth and Tenth Revision (ICD-9/ICD-10).

	ICD-9	ICD-10
Respiratory	518.5, 518.52, 518.51, 518.53, 518.82, 786.09, 799.02, 799.01, 518.81, 518.84	J95.2, J80, R09.02, R09.01, J95.821, J96.00, J96.01, J96.02, J96.90, J96.91, J96.92, J96.20, J96.21, J96.22, J95.822
Cardiac		
Gastrointestinal	584, N17	E879.1, V45.11, Z99.2
Genitourinary	997.4	K91.3, K91.8
CNS	997.01,780.09,780.97,799.2, 293	G97.81, G97.82, R41.82, R40.0, R40.1, F06.8, R45, F05, F6, F53

References

1. Harvey, S.V.; Pfeiffer, R.M.; Landy, R.; Wentzensen, N.; Clarke, M.A. Trends and predictors of hysterectomy prevalence among women in the United States. *Am. J. Obstet. Gynecol.* **2022**, *227*, 611.e1–611.e12. [CrossRef]
2. Brandsborg, B.; Nikolajsen, L. Chronic pain after hysterectomy. *Curr. Opin. Anaesthesiol.* **2018**, *31*, 268–273. [CrossRef] [PubMed]
3. Bisch, S.P.; Wells, T.; Gramlich, L.; Faris, P.; Wang, X.; Tran, D.T.; Thanh, N.X.; Glaze, S.; Chu, P.; Ghatage, P.; et al. Enhanced recovery after surgery (eras) in gynecologic oncology: System-wide implementation and audit leads to improved value and patient outcomes. *Gynecol. Oncol.* **2018**, *151*, 117–123. [CrossRef] [PubMed]
4. Memtsoudis, S.G.; Poeran, J.; Zubizarreta, N.; Cozowicz, C.; Morwald, E.E.; Mariano, E.R.; Mazumdar, M. Association of multimodal pain management strategies with perioperative outcomes and resource utilization: A population-based study. *Anesthesiology* **2018**, *128*, 891–902. [CrossRef] [PubMed]
5. Cozowicz, C.; Zhong, H.; Poeran, J.; Illescas, A.; Liu, J.; Poultsides, L.A.; Avgerinos, D.V.; Memtsoudis, S.G. The impact of multimodal analgesia in coronary artery bypass graft surgery-a population-based analysis. *J. Thorac. Cardiovasc. Surg.* 2023, *in press*. [CrossRef] [PubMed]
6. Dowell, D.; Ragan, K.R.; Jones, C.M.; Baldwin, G.T.; Chou, R. Cdc clinical practice guideline for prescribing opioids for pain—United States, 2022. *MMWR Recomm. Rep.* **2022**, *71*, 1–95. [CrossRef]
7. Austin, P.C. An introduction to propensity score methods for reducing the effects of confounding in observational studies. *Multivar. Behav. Res.* **2011**, *46*, 399–424. [CrossRef]
8. Liu, H.; Zhong, H.; Zubizarreta, N.; Cagle, P.; Liu, J.; Poeran, J.; Memtsoudis, S.G. Multimodal pain management and postoperative outcomes in inpatient and outpatient shoulder arthroplasties: A population-based study. *Reg. Anesth. Pain. Med.* 2024; *Online ahead of print*.
9. Hessami, K.; Welch, J.; Frost, A.; AlAshqar, A.; Arian, S.E.; Gough, E.; Borahay, M.A. Perioperative opioid dispensing and persistent use after benign hysterectomy: A systematic review and meta-analysis. *Am. J. Obstet. Gynecol.* **2023**, *229*, 23–32.e23. [CrossRef]
10. Anyaehie, K.B.; Duryea, E.; Wang, J.; Echebelem, C.; Macias, D.; Sunna, M.; Ogunkua, O.; Joshi, G.P.; Gasanova, I. Multimodal opioid-sparing pain management for emergent cesarean delivery under general anesthesia: A quality improvement project. *BMC Anesthesiol.* **2022**, *22*, 239. [CrossRef]
11. Choi, J.B.; Kang, K.; Song, M.K.; Seok, S.; Kim, Y.H.; Kim, J.E. Pain characteristics after total laparoscopic hysterectomy. *Int. J. Med. Sci.* **2016**, *13*, 562–568. [CrossRef]
12. Nelson, G.; Bakkum-Gamez, J.; Kalogera, E.; Glaser, G.; Altman, A.; Meyer, L.A.; Taylor, J.S.; Iniesta, M.; Lasala, J.; Mena, G.; et al. Guidelines for perioperative care in gynecologic/oncology: Enhanced recovery after surgery (eras) society recommendations-2019 update. *Int. J. Gynecol. Cancer* **2019**, *29*, 651–668. [CrossRef] [PubMed]

13. Dong, W.; An, B.; Wang, Y.; Cui, X.; Gan, J. Effect of multimodal analgesia on gynecological cancer patients after radical resection. *Am. J. Transl. Res.* **2021**, *13*, 2686–2693. [PubMed]
14. Castro-Alves, L.J.; Oliveira de Medeiros, A.C.; Neves, S.P.; Carneiro de Albuquerque, C.L.; Modolo, N.S.; De Azevedo, V.L.; De Oliveira, G.S., Jr. Perioperative duloxetine to improve postoperative recovery after abdominal hysterectomy: A prospective, randomized, double-blinded, placebo-controlled study. *Anesth. Analg.* **2016**, *122*, 98–104. [CrossRef]
15. Beattie, W.S.; Badner, N.H.; Choi, P. Epidural analgesia reduces postoperative myocardial infarction: A meta-analysis. *Anesth. Analg.* **2001**, *93*, 853–858. [CrossRef]
16. Beattie, W.S.; Badner, N.H.; Choi, P.T. Meta-analysis demonstrates statistically significant reduction in postoperative myocardial infarction with the use of thoracic epidural analgesia. *Anesth. Analg.* **2003**, *97*, 919–920. [CrossRef]
17. Popping, D.M.; Elia, N.; Marret, E.; Remy, C.; Tramer, M.R. Protective effects of epidural analgesia on pulmonary complications after abdominal and thoracic surgery: A meta-analysis. *Arch. Surg.* **2008**, *143*, 990–999; discussion 1000. [CrossRef]
18. Singh, N.; Sidawy, A.N.; Dezee, K.; Neville, R.F.; Weiswasser, J.; Arora, S.; Aidinian, G.; Abularrage, C.; Adams, E.; Khuri, S.; et al. The effects of the type of anesthesia on outcomes of lower extremity infrainguinal bypass. *J. Vasc. Surg.* **2006**, *44*, 964–968; discussion 968–970. [CrossRef]
19. O'Neill, A.; Lirk, P. Multimodal analgesia. *Anesthesiol. Clin.* **2022**, *40*, 455–468. [CrossRef] [PubMed]
20. Kharasch, E.D.; Avram, M.J.; Clark, J.D. Rational perioperative opioid management in the era of the opioid crisis. *Anesthesiology* **2020**, *132*, 603–605. [CrossRef]
21. Gaskin, D.J.; Richard, P. The economic costs of pain in the united states. *J. Pain.* **2012**, *13*, 715–724. [CrossRef]
22. Larach, D.B.; Hah, J.M.; Brummett, C.M. Perioperative opioids, the opioid crisis, and the anesthesiologist. *Anesthesiology* **2022**, *136*, 594–608. [CrossRef]
23. Shanthanna, H.; Ladha, K.S.; Kehlet, H.; Joshi, G.P. Perioperative opioid administration. *Anesthesiology* **2021**, *134*, 645–659. [CrossRef] [PubMed]
24. Howard, R.; Kenney, B.; Brummett, C.; Waljee, J.; Englesbe, M.; Telem, D. Prevalence and prescribers of preoperative opioid prescriptions in the us, 2008–2019. *JAMA Netw. Open* **2022**, *5*, e2147897. [CrossRef] [PubMed]
25. Wong, M.; Vogell, A.; Wright, K.; Isaacson, K.; Loring, M.; Morris, S. Opioid use after laparoscopic hysterectomy: Prescriptions, patient use, and a predictive calculator. *Am. J. Obstet. Gynecol.* **2019**, *220*, 259.e1–259.e11. [CrossRef] [PubMed]
26. Thompson, J.C.; Komesu, Y.M.; Qeadan, F.; Jeppson, P.C.; Cichowski, S.B.; Rogers, R.G.; Mazurie, A.J.; Nestsiarovich, A.; Lambert, C.G.; Dunivan, G.C. Trends in patient procurement of postoperative opioids and route of hysterectomy in the united states from 2004 through 2014. *Am. J. Obstet. Gynecol.* **2018**, *219*, 484.e1–484.e11. [CrossRef] [PubMed]
27. Lirk, P.; Thiry, J.; Bonnet, M.P.; Joshi, G.P.; Bonnet, F. Pain management after laparoscopic hysterectomy: Systematic review of literature and prospect recommendations. *Reg. Anesth. Pain. Med.* **2019**, *44*, 425–436. [CrossRef]
28. Kim, C.H.; Lefkowits, C.; Holschneider, C.; Bixel, K.; Pothuri, B. Managing opioid use in the acute surgical setting: A society of gynecologic oncology clinical practice statement. *Gynecol. Oncol.* **2020**, *157*, 563–569. [CrossRef]

Journal of
Clinical Medicine

MDPI

Article

Comparative Effects of Spinal Anesthesia and Combined Spinal with Peripheral Nerve Blocks on Postoperative Outcomes in Anterior Cruciate Ligament Repair

Sanja Berić [1,2], Tamara Murselović [1,2,*], Mark Žižak [1], Stjepan Bulat [1] and Goran Vrgoč [1,3]

1 Clinical Hospital Sveti Duh, Sveti Duh 64, 10000 Zagreb, Croatia; sanja.beric1@gmail.com (S.B.); m_zizak@hotmail.com (M.Ž.); bulatstjepan@gmail.com (S.B.); goran.vrgoc@kif.unizg.hr (G.V.)
2 Faculty of Dental Medicine and Health, Josip Juraj Strossmayer University of Osijek, Crkvena 21, 31000 Osijek, Croatia
3 Faculty of Kinesiology, University of Zagreb, Horvaćanski zavoj 15, 10110 Zagreb, Croatia
* Correspondence: murselovict@yahoo.com

Abstract: Objectives: This study aimed to compare the effectiveness of spinal anesthesia (SA) alone versus combined spinal anesthesia with adductor canal block (ACB) and sciatic nerve block (SNB) (SA + ACB + SNB) in patients undergoing arthroscopic anterior cruciate ligament (ACL) reconstruction. We hypothesized that SA + ACB + SNB would provide better analgesia, greater patient satisfaction, and shorter postanesthesia recovery times than SA alone. **Methods**: A prospective randomized controlled trial was conducted with 60 patients aged 15–49 years scheduled for elective arthroscopic ACL reconstruction. Participants were randomly assigned to receive either SA or SA + ACB + SNB. Postoperative pain was assessed using the Visual Analog Scale (VAS) at 4, 12, and 24 h post-operation. General health was evaluated using the 12-item Short Form Survey (SF-12) at 1 month postoperatively. Range of motion and analgesic consumption were also recorded. **Results**: The median VAS score at 4 h post-operation was significantly lower in the SA + ACB + SNB group compared to the SA group (0 [IQR: 0–1] vs. 2 [IQR: 1–3], $p = 0.0137$). No significant differences in VAS scores were found at 12 h ($p = 0.9282$) and 24 h ($p = 0.5809$). PCS-12 and MCS-12 scores did not differ significantly between groups. The SA group had a lower postoperative range of motion (ROM) compared to the SA + ACB + SNB group, with a mean active ROM of 40.67 degrees (±23.52) versus 72.17 degrees (±24.69), respectively ($p < 0.0001$). Analgesic consumption was similar, with 53.33% of participants in each group using postoperative analgesics ($p = 1.0$). The mean surgery duration was 74.6 min. The gender distribution was 83% male and 17% female, with an average age of 27.7 years. **Conclusions**: Adding ACB and SNB to spinal anesthesia improved immediate postoperative pain relief and preserved range of motion in patients undergoing ACL reconstruction, suggesting potential clinical benefits in pain management and functional recovery.

Keywords: arthroscopic ACL reconstruction; spinal anesthesia; adductor canal block; sciatic nerve block; postoperative pain management; orthopedic surgery

1. Introduction

Anterior cruciate ligament (ACL) reconstruction is a common orthopedic procedure aimed at restoring knee stability and function following ACL rupture. However, despite advances in surgical techniques, postoperative pain management remains a critical challenge that significantly impacts patient recovery and rehabilitation outcomes. Effective pain control not only enhances patient comfort but also facilitates earlier mobilization and reduces the risk of long-term complications such as joint stiffness and chronic pain [1,2].

Traditionally, various anesthesia techniques have been employed to manage pain after ACL reconstruction. Spinal anesthesia and femoral nerve blocks are among the most frequently used methods, each offering specific benefits and limitations. Spinal anesthesia provides excellent pain relief but lacks targeted action at the site of surgery, which femoral nerve blocks can achieve by directly blocking pain transmission from the knee [3]. Studies have shown diverging results on the efficacy of combining spinal anesthesia with peripheral nerve blocks, with some reporting enhanced pain relief and others indicating minimal additional benefits [4].

Spinal anesthesia is a regional anesthesia technique used to achieve anesthesia of the lower part of the body by injecting a local anesthetic into the subarachnoid space, where it mixes with cerebrospinal fluid. Its advantages include rapid onset of action, reliable and effective analgesia, lower risk of complications compared to general anesthesia, and reduced need for opioids in the postoperative period. Possible complications of this type of anesthesia include hypotension, bradycardia, and post-dural puncture headache [5].

The adductor canal block (ACB) is a regional anesthesia technique increasingly used in orthopedic surgeries, particularly for knee procedures. This block targets the saphenous nerve and other distal branches of the femoral nerve, providing pain relief while preserving quadriceps strength. This muscle strength preservation is a crucial advantage over the femoral nerve block (FNB), which often causes significant muscle weakness, delaying mobilization, and increasing the risk of falls after surgery [6]. Several studies have shown that ACB provides analgesia comparable to FNB but with less quadriceps weakness [7,8]. Additionally, the use of ultrasound increases the success rate of ACB by allowing precise visualization of the adductor canal, facilitating accurate delivery of the local anesthetic. This technique has become a cornerstone of multimodal analgesic regimens, promoting faster postoperative recovery and shortening hospital stays [5]. Blocking these nerves provides targeted knee analgesia, reducing the need for opioids and speeding up postoperative recovery [9].

The sciatic nerve is the largest and longest nerve in the body. It provides motor and sensory functions [10]. The sciatic nerve block (SNB) is a regional anesthesia technique used to achieve anesthesia of the lower extremities, particularly the leg, foot, and ankle. There are several approaches to performing a sciatic nerve block, including the posterior, lateral, and anterior approaches [6].

The knee joint has complex innervation, with anterior, medial, and posterior regions contributing to postoperative pain following ACL reconstruction. The combination of ACB and SNB allows for a complete sensory blockade of these regions, which can significantly reduce pain intensity and duration in the early postoperative phase compared to spinal anesthesia alone or with a single block. However, studies report mixed results regarding the added benefits of combining spinal anesthesia with peripheral nerve blocks, with some findings supporting improved pain relief and others suggesting minimal additional benefits [11].

The main aim of this work is to conduct a comprehensive comparison of spinal anesthesia alone versus its combination with adductor canal nerve block and sciatic nerve block, examining their effectiveness in controlling postoperative pain and facilitating early physical therapy and mobilization. Although spinal anesthesia and nerve blocks like ACB or SNB are individually well-documented in orthopedic pain management, there is limited research on the combined use of these techniques specifically for ACL reconstruction. Existing studies on this multimodal approach in knee surgeries offer mixed results, particularly regarding the added benefit of combining peripheral nerve blocks with spinal anesthesia for ACL procedures. This lack of consensus creates a gap in the literature on the optimal anesthesia strategy for effective postoperative recovery in ACL reconstruction. This study is significant as it contributes to the ongoing debate and development of best practices for anesthesia in ACL reconstruction, ultimately aiming to improve patient outcomes.

We performed a prospective randomized controlled study comparing preoperative spinal anesthesia (SA) to combined spinal anesthesia with adductor canal block (ACB) and sciatic nerve block (SNB) in patients undergoing arthroscopic ACL reconstruction and semitendinosus and gracilis tendon harvest for ACL graft. We hypothesized that patients who received SA + ACB + SNB would have improved analgesia measured by lower pain scores on standardized pain scales (e.g., VAS) post-treatment compared to baseline or control, longer-lasting pain relief, and reduced need for additional analgesics, as well as greater patient satisfaction.

2. Materials and Methods

This prospective randomized controlled study was conducted to compare preoperative spinal anesthesia (SA) to combined spinal anesthesia with adductor canal block (ACB) and sciatic nerve block (SNB) in patients undergoing arthroscopic ACL reconstruction. Only patients with isolated ACL injuries without any chondral damage or meniscal injuries were included in the study. All patients demonstrated positive findings on magnetic resonance imaging (MRI), as well as positive results on the anterior drawer test and Lachman test, confirming anterior cruciate ligament (ACL) rupture.

Ethical approval for the study was obtained from Institutional Review Board (IRB) approval (Approval No. 03-6544), and all participants provided written informed consent. Participants included in the study were adults aged 15–49 years undergoing elective arthroscopic ACL reconstruction with m. semitendinosus and m. gracilis tendon graft. By including patients as young as 15, we aim to capture a representative sample of the population most commonly affected by ACL injuries. Younger patients, especially those involved in sports, have specific recovery and rehabilitation needs, such as maintaining muscle strength, range of motion, and quick return to physical activity. Examining postoperative pain management techniques in this age group is therefore essential for identifying effective approaches that meet their unique demands for fast, functional recovery. Exclusion criteria were a history of chronic pain, previous knee surgery, open ACL reconstruction, contraindications to regional anesthesia, or inability to understand the study protocol.

Patients in this study were randomly assigned by an independent study coordinator to one of two groups: spinal anesthesia alone (SA) or spinal anesthesia combined with adductor canal and sciatic nerve blocks (SA + ACB + SNB). Due to the nature of the interventions, patients were aware of whether they received spinal anesthesia alone or the additional peripheral nerve blocks (ACB and SNB). Therefore, complete blinding of patients was not feasible in this study. To minimize potential bias in data collection, the doctor responsible for recording primary and secondary outcomes—postoperative pain scores (VAS), range of motion (ROM), opioid consumption, and quality of life (SF-12)—was blinded to the patients' group assignments. This approach aimed to ensure that all outcome measurements remained objective and unaffected by knowledge of the anesthesia technique used.

Patients in the SA group received spinal anesthesia with 0.5% levobupivacaine 15 mg.

Patients in the SA + ACB + SNB group received spinal anesthesia as described above, along with an adductor canal block and sciatic nerve block under ultrasound guidance. The adductor canal block was performed using 0.5% levobupivacaine 10 mL, and the sciatic nerve block was performed using 0.25% levobupivacaine 20 mL. Ultrasound was used for all peripheral nerve blocks. A total of four anesthesiologists were involved in the study. Only one anesthesiologist performed all peripheral nerve blocks (ACB and SNB) to maintain consistency in technique. The spinal anesthesia was administered by three different anesthesiologists, each trained in the procedure, ensuring standardized application across patients.

All patients underwent arthroscopic ACL reconstruction performed by a single surgeon using a standardized technique. For ACL reconstruction, the m. semitendinosus and m. gracilis tendons were harvested from the pes anserinus through a 2 cm vertical incision. The tendons were subsequently prepared on a graft preparation station. A femoral tunnel was drilled through the anteromedial portal, and a tibial tunnel was created using a tibial guide (Arthrex, Naples, FL, USA) set at an angle of 55 degrees. Proximal fixation of the ACL graft was achieved with the ACL TightRope II device (Arthrex, Naples, FL, USA), while distal fixation was secured at 20 degrees with a FastThread Biocomposite Interference Screw (Arthrex, Naples, FL, USA). Following placement and fixation of the graft, additional tightening was performed with the ACL TightRope II. At the end of the procedure, graft impingement and graft tension were assessed using a probe, and the positions of the screw and endobutton were verified via intraoperative X-ray imaging in the operating room. The duration of surgery was recorded from skin incision to skin closure. Esmarch was used in all patients to minimize bleeding. After surgery, bulky bandages were applied and left in place until the following morning, at which time they were removed and replaced with lighter bandages to facilitate range of motion (ROM) measurement. ROM was assessed before surgery and 20–24 h postoperatively, ensuring that measurements were taken without bulky bandages.

The primary outcome measure was postoperative pain, assessed using the Visual Analog Scale (VAS) at 4 h, 12 h, and 24 h post-surgery. Secondary outcomes included patient-reported general health assessed using the 12-item Short Form Survey (SF-12) version 1.0 at 1-month post-surgery, range of motion, and postoperative opioid consumption.

VAS scores were recorded at specified time points post-surgery. SF-12 scores were collected at 1 month postoperatively. The range of motion was measured using a goniometer preoperatively and postoperatively. Analgesic consumption was recorded based on patient medical records.

Data were analyzed using IBM SPSS Statistics version 29.0.2.0. The normality of continuous variables was assessed using the Shapiro–Wilk test. Independent t-tests were used for normally distributed variables, while Mann–Whitney *U* tests were applied for non-normally distributed variables. Chi-square tests were used to compare categorical variables. Statistical significance was set at $p < 0.05$.

3. Results

3.1. Participant Characteristics

A total of 60 patients were included in the study, divided into two groups based on the type of anesthesia administered: spinal anesthesia (SA) and combined spinal anesthesia with adductor canal block and sciatic nerve block (SA + ACB + SNB). The gender distribution of the study participants was 83% male and 17% female, with an average age of 27.7 years (15–49).

3.2. Visual Analog Scale (VAS) Pain Scores

The VAS pain scores were assessed at 4 h, 12 h, and 24 h post-operation. The median VAS scores for the SA group were higher compared to the SA + ACB + SNB group at 4 h post-operation. Specifically, the median VAS scores at 4 h were 2 (IQR: 1–3) for the SA group and 0 (IQR: 0–1) for the SA + ACB + SNB group, showing significantly lower pain levels in the SA + ACB + SNB group ($p = 0.0137$). However, there were no significant differences in VAS scores between the two groups at 12 h ($p = 0.9282$) and 24 h ($p = 0.5809$) post-operation. The boxplots illustrate that the combined anesthesia technique (SA + ACB + SNB) provides better pain control in the immediate postoperative period (4 h), but pain levels between the groups become similar by 12 and 24 h post-operation (Figure 1).

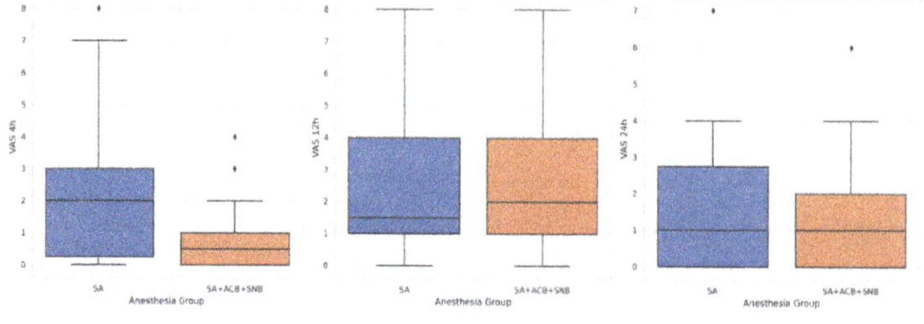

Figure 1. The boxplot displays the distribution of Visual Analog Scale (VAS) pain scores at 4 h, 12 h, and 24 h post-operation for two anesthesia groups: spinal anesthesia (SA) and combined spinal anesthesia with adductor canal block and sciatic nerve block (SA + ACB + SNB).

3.3. SF-12 Health Survey Scores

The physical component scores (PCS-12) and mental component scores (MCS-12) were evaluated using the SF-12 Health Survey. The PCS-12 scores for the SA group were lower than those for the SA + ACB + SNB group, as depicted in the boxplots (Figure 2). Despite this visual difference, the Mann–Whitney *U* test indicated no significant difference in PCS-12 scores between the two groups ($p = 0.569$). Similarly, the MCS-12 scores did not show a significant difference between the groups according to the independent *t*-test ($p = 0.787$).

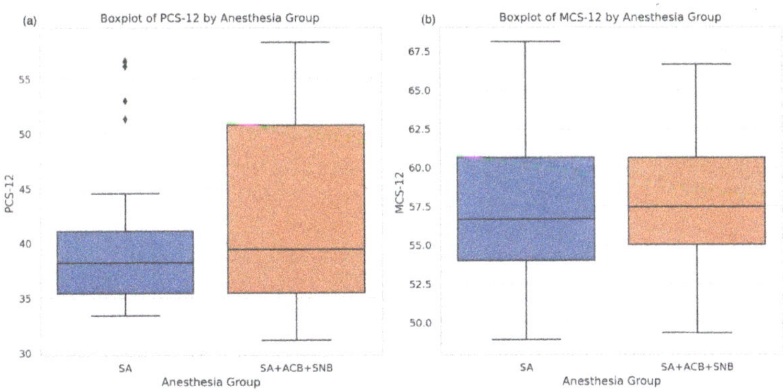

Figure 2. Boxplots for PCS-12 and MCS-12 scores by anesthesia group. (**a**) The left plot shows the distribution of PCS-12 scores for each group (SA and SA + ACB + SNB); (**b**) The right plot shows the distribution of MCS-12 scores for each group.

3.4. Range of Motion

The active range of motion (ROM) for patients before and after the procedure was analyzed and compared between the two anesthesia groups: spinal anesthesia (SA) and spinal anesthesia combined with adductor canal block and sciatic nerve block (SA + ACB + SNB) (Table 1).

Table 1. Range of motion before and after surgery for different anesthesia types.

Group	ROM Before Surgery (Mean ± std *)	ROM Before Surgery (Median)	ROM After Surgery (Mean ± std)	ROM After Surgery (Median)	Change (Mean ± std)	Change (Median)
SA	131.33 ± 3.46	130.0	40.67 ± 23.52	30.0	−90.67 ± 23.07	−100.0
SA + ACB + SNB	130.67 ± 2.54	130.0	72.17 ± 24.69	80.0	−58.50 ± 25.43	−50.0

* Standard deviation.

The mean active ROM before the procedure was similar between the two groups. The SA group had a mean ROM of 131.33 degrees (±3.46), while the SA + ACB + SNB group had a mean ROM of 130.67 degrees (±2.54). The mean active ROM after the procedure was significantly different between the two groups. The SA group had a mean active ROM of 40.67 degrees (±23.52), whereas the SA + ACB + SNB group had a higher mean active ROM of 72.17 degrees (±24.69). The change in active ROM (after minus before) also showed significant differences. The SA group experienced a larger decrease in active ROM with a mean change of −90.67 degrees (±23.07). In contrast, the SA + ACB + SNB group had a mean change of −58.50 degrees (±25.43). A Mann–Whitney *U* test was conducted to compare the change in active ROM between the two groups. The test revealed a U-statistic of 189.5 and a *p*-value of 0.000094, indicating a statistically significant difference in the change in ROM between the SA and SA + ACB + SNB groups ($p < 0.05$) (Figure 3). The analysis indicates that patients in the SA + ACB + SNB group showed improved postoperative ROM compared to the SA group.

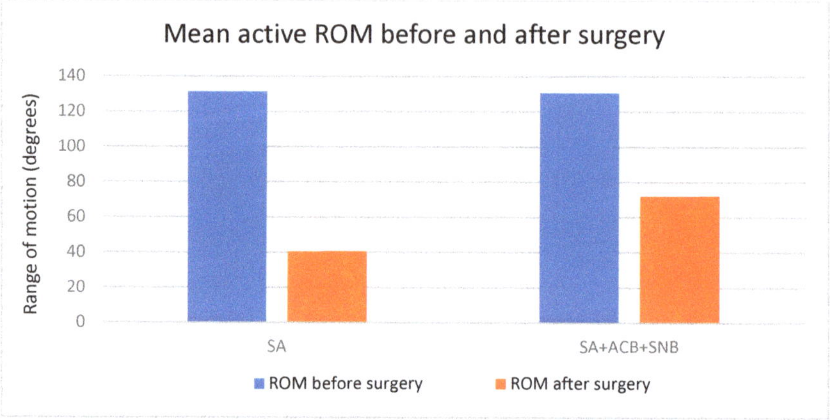

Figure 3. Mean active range of motion before and after surgery between the two groups visually demonstrates that while both groups experienced a decrease in ROM following surgery, the SA + ACB + SNB group retained a greater range of motion compared to the SA group.

3.5. Analgesic Consumption

Postoperative analgesic consumption was systematically recorded based on patient-reported use of analgesics following surgery, guided by a standardized pain management protocol. Analgesic administration was structured according to Visual Analog Scale (VAS) pain scores to ensure consistent and objective pain management across both groups:

- VAS 0–3: Patients reporting pain in this range received no analgesic intervention.
- VAS 4–6: Patients with moderate pain (VAS 4–6) were administered a combination of intravenous nonsteroidal anti-inflammatory drugs (NSAIDs) and paracetamol.
- VAS > 7: For patients experiencing severe pain (VAS > 7), intravenous tramadol at a dose of 50–100 mg was provided.

Each patient's postoperative pain scores and corresponding analgesic use were recorded by nursing staff and subsequently confirmed through patient reports during follow-up assessments. Both groups had an equal proportion of patients (53.33%) using postoperative analgesics. The chi-square test confirms that this difference is not statistically significant ($p = 1.0$), indicating that the type of anesthesia did not affect the likelihood of patients using analgesics postoperatively.

3.6. Surgery Duration

The mean surgery duration for all patients was 74.6 min, with no significant differences noted between the groups.

4. Discussion

This study aimed to compare spinal anesthesia (SA) alone versus combined spinal anesthesia with adductor canal block (ACB) and sciatic nerve block (SNB) (SA + ACB + SNB) in patients undergoing arthroscopic anterior cruciate ligament (ACL) reconstruction with m.semitendinosus and m.gracilis tendons harvesting for ACL graft. The results showed that the SA + ACB + SNB group experienced significantly lower immediate postoperative pain (4 h post-operation) compared to the SA group. Additionally, the SA + ACB + SNB group exhibited better preservation of active range of motion after knee ACL reconstruction postoperatively. There were no significant differences in pain scores at 12 and 24 h, SF-12 health survey scores, postoperative analgesic consumption, or surgery duration between the two groups.

Our findings are consistent with several previous studies demonstrating the benefits of regional anesthesia techniques in orthopedic surgeries. Naser et al. [12] reported that peripheral nerve blocks, such as the adductor canal block, provided better pain control than other methods in knee surgeries. Similarly, Sahin et al. [13] found that femoral nerve blocks significantly reduced postoperative morphine consumption and enhanced patient satisfaction following knee arthroplasty. Fowler et al. [11] also highlighted the superior analgesic efficacy of peripheral nerve blocks over epidural analgesia in major knee surgeries.

In the context of ACL reconstruction, Abdallah et al. [7] demonstrated that adductor canal block (ACB) provided noninferior analgesia and superior quadriceps strength compared to femoral nerve block (FNB). This aligns with our findings that SA + ACB + SNB improved pain control, especially in the first 4 h post-operation, without compromising functional outcomes. El Ahl [14] and Kamath and Faiaz [15] further supported the use of ACB in ACL reconstruction, noting its benefits in preserving quadriceps strength and facilitating early mobilization.

Our findings align with earlier research investigating the impact of different nerve blocks used alongside spinal anesthesia. For instance, a prospective double-blinded randomized study by Astur et al. [3] evaluated clinical outcomes using femoral nerve block with spinal anesthesia versus spinal analgesia alone in patients undergoing ACL reconstruction. They found that spinal anesthesia with a femoral nerve block provided significant pain relief shortly after surgery, but there were no additional benefits in pain control after the third postoperative day. This aligns with our findings where the SA + ACB + SNB group had superior pain relief at 4 h but showed no significant advantage at 12 and 24 h post-operation. Similarly, a randomized clinical trial by Harbell et al. [2] compared preoperative femoral nerve block alone versus combined femoral and sciatic nerve block for arthroscopic ACL reconstruction under general anesthesia. The study demonstrated improved analgesia, decreased opioid consumption perioperatively, and shorter PACU length of stay in the combined block group on the day of surgery. However, there was no significant difference in opioid consumption, pain scores, or patient satisfaction on postoperative days 1–3 between the groups. This suggests that the benefits of additional nerve blocks may be limited to the immediate postoperative period, which is in agreement with our observation that the SA + ACB + SNB group experienced better pain control at 4 h but not at later time points. The study by Frost et al. [1] evaluated the efficacy of intraoperative femoral nerve block in reducing postoperative pain following ACL hamstring reconstruction under general anesthesia. They found that femoral nerve block may reduce pain on the night of surgery, but the reduction might not be clinically significant. This further supports the notion that while nerve blocks can be effective in the immediate postoperative period, their benefits may diminish over time, as observed in our study.

The significant reduction in immediate postoperative pain observed in the SA + ACB + SNB group has important clinical implications. Effective early pain management can enhance patient comfort, reduce opioid consumption, and facilitate early mobilization and rehabilitation, ultimately improving overall recovery and patient satisfaction. The better preservation of the range of motion in the SA + ACB + SNB group is particularly crucial for functional recovery in ACL reconstruction.

For instance, Goyal et al. [16] showed that a combined femoral–obturator–sciatic nerve block provides superior postoperative pain scores and earlier mobilization compared to spinal anesthesia in patients undergoing arthroscopic ACL reconstruction. This supports our observation of better pain control and ROM in the immediate postoperative period with the combined block technique. It may be worth mentioning that a significant advantage of the ACB over the femoral block is the early activation of the quadriceps muscle, which is extremely important for the early initiation of physical therapy in patients after ACL reconstruction. This is especially important for professional athletes. The femoral block increases the risk of ACL re-injury within the first year following reconstruction [17]. Similarly, Montes et al. [18] compared sciatic–femoral nerve block with low-dose spinal anesthesia for outpatient arthroscopic knee surgery. Although knee arthroscopy is a significantly less complex surgery and causes less pain compared to arthroscopic anterior cruciate ligament reconstruction, the study found that combined nerve block offers satisfactory anesthesia with a clinical profile similar to that of low-dose spinal anesthesia and is associated with significantly lower pain scores during the first 6 postoperative hours, which parallels our findings of improved pain management at 4 h post-operation when using peripheral nerve blocks.

A systematic review by Secrist et al. [19] further corroborates these results by demonstrating that peripheral nerve blocks, when used in combination with spinal anesthesia, can reduce opioid requirements and enhance functional recovery. These studies collectively highlight the benefits of multimodal analgesia, particularly in orthopedic surgeries such as arthroscopic ACL reconstruction.

However, consistent with the findings of Astur et al. and Harbell et al. [2,3], our study did not find significant differences in pain scores at 12 and 24 h post-operation or in overall analgesic consumption. This suggests that while combined nerve blocks provide significant immediate postoperative benefits, their long-term efficacy might be limited. The variations in study designs, anesthesia protocols, and patient populations, as well as the relatively short follow-up period in our study, may contribute to these discrepancies.

A major strength of this study is the randomized controlled design, which minimizes selection bias and enhances the validity of the findings. The use of validated outcome measures (VAS and SF-12) adds robustness to the results. However, this study has limitations, including a relatively small sample size that may limit generalizability and a short follow-up period that precludes assessment of long-term outcomes.

Future research should focus on comparing different combinations of regional anesthesia techniques to optimize postoperative pain management and functional recovery in ACL reconstruction. Studies with longer follow-up periods are essential to evaluate the long-term benefits and potential complications of these techniques. Additionally, investigating the effects of these anesthesia methods in diverse patient populations, such as those with chronic pain or opioid tolerance, would provide valuable insights for personalized pain management strategies.

Overall, the combined use of spinal anesthesia with peripheral nerve blocks, specifically ACB and SNB, offers significant advantages in immediate postoperative pain control and range of motion, aligning with the broader evidence in the literature.

5. Conclusions

In conclusion, the addition of adductor canal block and sciatic nerve block to spinal anesthesia significantly improves immediate postoperative pain relief and preserves active range of motion in patients undergoing arthroscopic ACL reconstruction. Furthermore, using this combination of peripheral nerve blocks, we avoid motor inactivation of the quadriceps muscle, as seen with the use of a femoral nerve block, resulting in earlier quadriceps activation and faster recovery, which is of utmost importance in professional athletes. Further research is needed to confirm these results and investigate long-term outcomes.

Author Contributions: Conceptualization, T.M.; data curation, T.M.; formal analysis, S.B. (Stjepan Bulat); investigation, S.B. (Sanja Berić), M.Ž., S.B. (Stjepan Bulat) and G.V.; methodology, S.B. (Sanja Berić); supervision, G.V.; writing—original draft preparation, S.B. (Sanja Berić) and M.Ž.; writing—review and editing, G.V. All authors have read and agreed to the published version of the manuscript.

Funding: This research received no external funding.

Institutional Review Board Statement: This study was conducted in accordance with the Declaration of Helsinki and approved by the Ethics Committee of Clinical Hospital Sveti Duh (Approval No. 03-6544; 30 August 2023).

Informed Consent Statement: All patients who provided informed consent for anesthesia also agreed to the use of their data anonymously for scientific purposes.

Data Availability Statement: The original contributions presented in the study are included in the article; further inquiries can be directed to the corresponding author.

Conflicts of Interest: The authors declare no conflicts of interest.

References

1. Frost, S.; Grossfeld, S.; Kirkley, A.; Litchfield, B.; Fowler, P.; Amendola, A. The Efficacy of Femoral Nerve Block in Pain Reduction for Outpatient Hamstring Anterior Cruciate Ligament Reconstruction: A Double-Blind, Prospective, Randomized Trial. *Arthroscopy* **2000**, *16*, 243–248. [CrossRef] [PubMed]
2. Harbell, M.; Cohen, J.M.; Kolodzie, K.; Behrends, M.; Braehler, M.R.; Kinjo, S.; Feeley, B.; Aleshi, P. Combined Preoperative Femoral and Sciatic Nerve Blockade Improves Analgesia after Anterior Cruciate Ligament Reconstruction: A Randomized Controlled Clinical Trial. *J. Clin. Anesth.* **2016**, *33*, 68–74. [CrossRef] [PubMed]
3. Astur, D.C.; Aleluia, V.; Veronese, C.; Astur, N.; Oliveira, S.G.; Arliani, G.G.; Badra, R.; Kaleka, C.C.; Amaro, J.T.; Cohen, M. A Prospective Double Blinded Randomized Study of Anterior Cruciate Ligament Reconstruction with Hamstrings Tendon and Spinal Anesthesia with or without Femoral Nerve Block. *Knee* **2014**, *21*, 911–915. [CrossRef] [PubMed]
4. McCartney, C., McIsaac, D. Are Peripheral Nerve Blocks Indicated in Ambulatory Knee Surgery? *Anesth. Analg.* **2019**, *128*, 3–4. [CrossRef] [PubMed]
5. Gropper, M.A.; Eriksson, L.I.; Fleisher, L.A.; Wiener-Kronish, J.P.; Cohen, N.H.; Leslie, K. (Eds.) *Miller's Anesthesia*, 9th ed.; Elsevier: Amsterdam, The Netherlands, 2019.
6. Hadzic, A.; Balocco, A.L. *Hadzic's Textbook of Regional Anesthesia and Acute Pain Management. Self-Assessment and Review*; McGraw-Hill Education: New York, NY, USA, 2019.
7. Abdallah, F.; Whelan, D.; Chan, V.; Prasad, G.A.; Endersby, R.; Theodoropolous, J.; Oldfield, S.; Oh, J.; Brull, R. Adductor Canal Block Provides Noninferior Analgesia and Superior Quadriceps Strength Compared with Femoral Nerve Block in Anterior Cruciate Ligament Reconstruction. *Anesthesiology* **2016**, *124*, 1053–1064. [CrossRef] [PubMed]
8. Wang, D.; Yang, Y.; Li, Q.; Tang, S.-L.; Zeng, W.-N.; Xu, J.; Xie, T.-H.; Pei, F.-X.; Yang, L.; Li, L.-L.; et al. Adductor Canal Block versus Femoral Nerve Block for Total Knee Arthroplasty: A Meta-Analysis of Randomized Controlled Trials. *Sci. Rep.* **2017**, *7*, 40721. [CrossRef] [PubMed]
9. Barash, P.G. *Clinical Anesthesia, 8e: eBook Without Multimedia*; Wolters Kluwer Health: Philadelphia, PA, USA, 2017; ISBN 978-1-4963-3701-6.
10. Waldeyer, W. *Waldeyer Anatomie des Menschen*, 17th ed.; Walter de Gruyter: Berlin, Germany, 2003.
11. Fowler, S.J.; Symons, J.; Sabato, S.; Myles, P.S. Epidural Analgesia Compared with Peripheral Nerve Blockade after Major Knee Surgery: A Systematic Review and Meta-Analysis of Randomized Trials. *Br. J. Anaesth.* **2008**, *100*, 154–164. [CrossRef] [PubMed]
12. Naser, S.R.; Refaat, S.; Shmaa, N.S.E.; Amin, S. Comparative Study between Ultrasound-Guided Fascia Iliaca Block Versus Adductor Canal Block for Postoperative Analgesia in Patients Undergoing Knee Surgeries. *J. Adv. Med. Med. Res.* **2021**, *33*, 214–224. [CrossRef]
13. Sahin, L.; Korkmaz, H.F.; Sahin, M.; Atalan, G. Ultrasound-Guided Single-Injection Femoral Nerve Block Provides Effective Analgesia after Total Knee Arthroplasty up to 48 Hours. *Ağrı-J. Turk. Soc. Algol.* **2014**, *26*, 113–118. [CrossRef] [PubMed]
14. El Ahl, M. Femoral Nerve Block versus Adductor Canal Block for Postoperative Pain Control after Anterior Cruciate Ligament Reconstruction: A Randomized Controlled Double Blind Study. *Saudi J. Anaesth.* **2015**, *9*, 279. [CrossRef] [PubMed]
15. Faiaz, A.F.; Kamath, S.S. Randomised Controlled Trial between Ultrasound Guided Femoral Nerve Block and Adductor Canal Block for Postoperative Pain and Functional Outcome in Anterior Cruciate Ligament Reconstruction. *J. Clin. Diagn. Res.* **2019**, *13*, UC11–UC14. [CrossRef]
16. Goyal, T.; Paul, S.; Choudhury, A.K.; Das, L.; Schuh, A.; Govil, N. Combined Femoral-Obturator-Sciatic Nerve Block Has Superior Postoperative Pain Score and Earlier Ambulation as Compared to Spinal Anaesthesia for Arthroscopic Anterior Cruciate Ligament Reconstruction. *Knee Surg. Sports Traumatol. Arthrosc. Off. J. ESSKA* **2022**, *30*, 3480–3487. [CrossRef] [PubMed]
17. Everhart, J.S.; Hughes, L.; Abouljoud, M.M.; Swank, K.; Lewis, C.; Flanigan, D.C. Femoral Nerve Block at Time of ACL Reconstruction Causes Lasting Quadriceps Strength Deficits and May Increase Short-Term Risk of Re-Injury. *Knee Surg. Sports Traumatol. Arthrosc. Off. J. ESSKA* **2020**, *28*, 1894–1900. [CrossRef] [PubMed]
18. Montes, F.R.; Zarate, E.; Grueso, R.; Giraldo, J.C.; Venegas, M.P.; Gomez, A.; Rincón, J.D.; Hernadez, M.; Cabrera, M. Comparison of Spinal Anesthesia with Combined Sciatic-Femoral Nerve Block for Outpatient Knee Arthroscopy. *J. Clin. Anesth.* **2008**, *20*, 415–420. [CrossRef] [PubMed]
19. Secrist, E.S.; Freedman, K.B.; Ciccotti, M.G.; Mazur, D.W.; Hammoud, S. Pain Management After Outpatient Anterior Cruciate Ligament Reconstruction: A Systematic Review of Randomized Controlled Trials. *Am. J. Sports Med.* **2016**, *44*, 2435–2447. [CrossRef] [PubMed]

Journal of
Clinical Medicine

MDPI

Article

Learnability of Ultrasound-Guided Locoregional Anesthesia for Carotid Endarterectomy

Benjamin Seybold [1,*], Nils Gaier [2], Andreas Ofenloch [3], Dittmar Boeckler [4], Armin Kalenka [1,5] and Mascha O. Fiedler-Kalenka [1]

1 Department of Anesthesiology, Heidelberg University Hospital, Medical Faculty, University of Heidelberg, 69120 Heidelberg, Germany; armin.kalenka@med.uni-heidelberg.de (A.K.); mascha.fiedler-kalenka@med.uni-heidelberg.de (M.O.F.-K.)
2 Merck KGaA, 64293 Darmstadt, Germany
3 Department of Vascular Surgery, District Hospital Bergstrasse, 64646 Heppenheim, Germany; andreas.ofenloch@med.uni-heidelberg.de
4 Department of Vascular and Endovascular Surgery, Heidelberg University Hospital, Medical Faculty, University Heidelberg, 69120 Heidelberg, Germany; dittmar.boeckler@med.uni-heidelberg.de
5 District Hospital Bergstrasse, 64646 Heppenheim, Germany
* Correspondence: benjamin.seybold@med.uni-heidelberg.de

Abstract: Background/Objectives: There is an ongoing debate about the most advantageous anesthesia technique for carotid endarterectomy (CEA). From an anesthesiologic perspective, locoregional anesthesia (LRA) appears to offer significant benefits. However, the learning curve and complication rates for anesthesiologists newly performing ultrasound-guided LRA for CEA remain unclear and are to be examined in greater detail in this study. **Methods:** This retrospective, single-center study included all consecutive LRA administrations for CEA following the introduction of this procedure at a district hospital in Germany from November 2013 to November 2017. Nine board-certified anesthesiologists, initially inexperienced in LRA for CEA but with prior experience in other ultrasound-guided peripheral nerve blocks (PNBs), received theoretical training and supervision during their first six combined deep and superficial cervical plexus blocks under ultrasound guidance. The primary endpoint was the incidence of insufficient block quality, indicated by pain and restlessness or the additional need for analgesics. Secondary endpoints included LRA-associated complications. Patients were divided into four groups based on the number of previously performed LRA procedures by the attending anesthesiologist. **Results:** In 83 patients, LRA was performed by initially inexperienced anesthesiologists. Group A (patients managed by anesthesiologists performing their 1st to 3rd cervical plexus blockades) included 21 patients, Group B (blockades 4–6) included 12 patients, Group C (blockades 7–9) included 9 patients, and Group D ($\geq$10 blockades) included 41 patients, respectively. The overall complication rate was 22% (18/83). Insufficient block quality occurred in 18.1% of patients (15/83), resulting in three conversions to general anesthesia (3.6%). Additional complications included dysphagia (n = 2) and Horner's syndrome (n = 1). The incidence of insufficient block quality was significantly reduced ($p = 0.008$) after performing the first three blockades. **Conclusions:** Ultrasound-guided cervical plexus block for CEA appears to be a rapidly learnable anesthesia technique for anesthesiologists experienced in other ultrasound-guided PNBs, with a low risk of complications. After three supervised blockades, the failure rate of LRA decreases significantly.

Keywords: locoregional anesthesia; learning curve; cervical plexus blockade; ultrasound; carotid endarterectomy

1. Introduction

There is an ongoing debate about whether carotid endarterectomy (CEA) should be performed under locoregional anesthesia (LRA) or general anesthesia (GA). The largest randomized controlled trial (RCT), the General Anaesthesia versus Local Anaesthesia (GALA) trial, which included 3526 participants, found no significant difference in the rates of perioperative death, stroke, or myocardial infarction between GA (4.8%) and LRA (4.5%) [1]. However, a large meta-analysis found that LRA was associated with significantly shorter operation times, lower rates of perioperative stroke, fewer cardiac complications, and lower mortality in the 25 observational studies included [2]. Nevertheless, each of the six included RCTs failed to demonstrate statistically significant differences in any endpoints [2]. Some authors believe that these RCTs lacked statistical power [3]. Recent subgroup analyses from two studies suggest that LRA may indeed be associated with a slightly lower risk of stroke and mortality compared to carotid endarterectomy under GA [4,5].

The European Society for Vascular Surgery Management Guidelines of Atherosclerotic Carotid and Vertebral Artery Disease recommends that the choice of anesthesia (locoregional or general) should be made at the discretion of the surgeon and anesthesiologist performing the procedure, taking into account local experience, patient preferences, and the preferred antiplatelet strategy [6]. Consequently, in the absence of a medical contraindication for either approach, anesthesiologists and surgeons should mutually consider each others' preferences. Locoregional anesthesia should be performed under ultrasound guidance, as this can enhance the safety of this technique by providing visualization of cervical anatomical structures during infiltration [7]. However, the learnability of ultrasound-guided regional anesthesia remains poorly studied, and the number of blocks required to achieve proficiency is still a matter of debate [8].

Therefore, the implementation of CEA, performed by surgeons experienced in this procedure at a district hospital in Germany, provided an opportunity to retrospectively evaluate the learning curves of anesthesiologists inexperienced in ultrasound-guided cervical plexus blockades. Here, we report on the learnability and complication rates of ultrasound-guided LRA for CEA in a supervised setting for board-certified anesthesiologists newly performing LRA in this anatomical region. The primary endpoint was the incidence of insufficient block quality indicated by pain, restlessness, or the requirement for additional local or systemic anesthetics.

2. Materials and Methods

2.1. Study Design and Population

This is a retrospective, single-center study conducted at District Hospital Bergstrasse, Germany. All consecutive CEAs performed at District Hospital Bergstrasse from November 2013 to November 2017 were retrospectively reviewed. The surgical reports, anesthesia protocols, and medical records of the included patients were assessed. Cases were excluded if LRA was performed by an anesthesiologist experienced in LRA for CEA. The study was approved by the local ethics committee of the medical faculty at the University of Heidelberg, Germany (reference number: S-297/2017). Information that could identify individual patients was anonymized after data collection.

The primary endpoint of this study was the incidence of insufficient block quality from LRA, indicated by restlessness and pain (patient discomfort) or the need for additional analgesic medication during the procedure. Restlessness and pain represent relatively subjective parameters, both in the perception of patients and anesthesiologists. However, there is currently no generally accepted and more objective definition for regional anesthesia failure. The definition used in this document is based on a recommendation by Bottomley et al., recently published for peripheral nerve block failure [9]. Secondary endpoints were complications associated with LRA (e.g., Horner's syndrome, dysphagia) and the rate of intraoperative conversion to general anesthesia due to block failure. For this purpose, intraoperative recordings in anesthesiologic and surgical records were retrospectively analyzed. In particular, corresponding notes from anesthesiologists and surgeons, vital signs, additional pain medication administered during the procedure, and records from the post-anesthesia care unit were considered. Furthermore, postoperative complications were examined using physician notes in discharge summaries and follow-up records. Upon individual patient request, premedication with midazolam was administered prior to LRA.

2.2. Intervention

In this study, the learning curves of nine board-certified anesthesiologists were assessed to evaluate the learnability of ultrasound-guided combined superficial and deep cervical plexus blockades for CEA. All anesthesiologists were already familiar with regional anesthesia techniques, both with and without ultrasound guidance, in other anatomical regions, but none had prior experience with LRA for CEA. Initial theoretical training and practical supervision included the following:

- Introduction to the fundamentals of ultrasound-guided combined superficial and deep cervical plexus anesthesia, including the anatomy of the cervical plexus, techniques for visualizing the target anatomical structures using ultrasound, needle guidance during the blockades, the selection and dosage of local anesthetics, and potential complications, all through a two-hour theoretical training session.
- The first six ultrasound-guided cervical plexus blockades performed by each anesthesiologist were conducted under the supervision of an anesthesiologist with prior experience in this form of regional anesthesia for CEA to demonstrate practical feasibility.
- Additionally, some of the participating anesthesiologists independently chose to attend external training sessions to further enhance their proficiency in the procedure.

As recommended for cervical plexus anesthesia, 40 mL of 0.5% ropivacaine (Ropivacaine Hydrochloride 0.5%, Fresenius Kabi AG, Bad Homburg, Germany) was routinely administered, with 20 mL targeting the deep cervical plexus and 20 mL targeting the superficial cervical plexus [10–12]. For anesthesia of the deep cervical plexus, as recommended, the transverse processes of the C2 to C4 vertebrae were visualized using ultrasound, with the carotid bifurcation serving as an additional landmark. The anesthetic was deposited approximately 1 cm caudal to the bifurcation to ensure effective blockade of the deep cervical plexus branches. The needle was advanced in-plane under continuous ultrasound guidance toward the target area near the C3 transverse process to maintain precise visualization and maximize patient safety [13,14]. For anesthesia of the superficial cervical plexus, the posterior border of the sternocleidomastoid muscle was visualized using ultrasound in the region of the lateral cervical triangle. The goal was to infiltrate along the posterior border of the sternocleidomastoid muscle in a cranio-caudal direction to achieve anesthesia at the nerve point (punctum nervosum). The needle was guided in-plane to provide the highest possible level of patient safety [13,15].

In patients under LRA, neurological status was continuously monitored during the procedure through communication with them. Additionally, patients were instructed to squeeze a squeaky ball with the hand on the contralateral side of the operative area every 10 s during the clamping phase. If any new neurological symptoms occurred during the clamping phase, arterial shunting of the operative area was performed. The mean arterial blood pressure was kept above 100 mmHg during the clamping phase. After declamping, a systolic blood pressure below 140 mmHg was targeted. To maintain hemodynamics within the desired range, both during and after the procedure, urapidil hydrochloride, clonidine hydrochloride, norepinephrine, and Akrinor® were administered as needed. In cases of insufficient analgesia from the cervical plexus blockades, local anesthetics were administered by the surgeons and/or systemic anesthetics by the anesthesiologists, respectively, indicating block failure. If analgesia remained insufficient for the patient, conversion to GA was performed. In cases of general anesthesia, an arterial shunt was routinely placed intraoperatively. If LRA was contraindicated or rejected by the patient, GA was primarily performed with the same blood pressure targets. Technical neuromonitoring or cerebral oximetry were not available, which made LRA the preferred anesthesia technique for CEA in this setting.

2.3. Statistical Methods

The patients were divided into groups based on the experience of the attending anesthesiologist, with Group A including those who received LRA from anesthesiologists with experience in ≤ 3 cervical plexus blockades, Group B from those performing their 4th to 6th blockades, Group C from those performing their 7th to 9th blockades, and Group D from those with experience in more than 9 blockades. Groups A, B, and C were formed to represent three consecutive plexus blockades performed by each anesthesiologist. This number has proven sufficient in other studies to capture initial learning progress and was therefore adopted for our study [16]. Group D includes all LRA performed after an estimated learning phase of 9 blockades and is intended to represent the complication rate among experienced anesthesiologists, which remains above zero [9]. Baseline characteristics, block failure rates, and the frequency of anesthesia-associated complications were analyzed descriptively. Subsequently, statistical analysis was performed using the Pearson chi-square test for independence or Fisher's exact test if the sample size was smaller than five. To avoid a Type I error, the significance level was adjusted using the Bonferroni correction [17]. Findings were considered statistically significant if the p-value was <0.05 or <0.0083 after Bonferroni correction. Finally, the results were graphically presented using a dual-axis chart, displaying the cumulative number of LRA procedures performed alongside the continuously decreasing cumulative block failure rate.

The software used for data collection and analysis included Microsoft Excel (Microsoft Corporation, Redmond, WA, USA) and IBM SPSS Statistics 24 (IBM Corporation, Armonk, NY, USA).

3. Results

3.1. Baseline Characteristics of the Cohort

Over the 48-month study period, a total of 126 CEAs were performed at District Hospital Bergstrasse, Germany, and retrospectively analyzed. Thirty-eight cases were excluded because perioperative care was managed by an anesthesiologist experienced in locoregional anesthesia techniques for carotid surgery. In the remaining 88 cases, the attending anesthesiologists had no prior experience with these anesthesia techniques. These patients formed the cohort for our study. Of these, 83 CEAs were primarily performed under LRA and five under GA. Further epidemiological characteristics of the cohort are provided in Table 1.

Table 1. Baseline characteristics of the cohort: baseline characteristics (numbers and mean values) of all patients who were managed by anesthesiologists inexperienced in anesthesia techniques for carotid endarterectomy.

	Frequences
Total number of patients [n]	88
Age [years], mean (range)	71.9 (52; 86)
ASA classification, mean (range)	2.9 (2; 4)
Sex: male [n]	60 (68.2%)
Sex: female [n]	28 (31.8%)
Asymptomatic stenosis of carotid artery [n]	54 (61.4%)
Symptomatic stenosis of carotid artery [n]	34 (38.6%)
Premedication [n]	17 (19.3%)
Duration of procedure [min], mean (range)	107.3 (61; 181)
Eversion CEA [n]	38 (43.2%)
Conventional CEA [n]	50 (56.8%)
Primary intraoperative shunt [n]	18 (20.5%)
Secondary intraoperative shunt [n]	4 (4.5%)
Clamping time [min], mean (range)	26.0 (1; 59)
Primary locoregional anesthesia [n]	83 (94.3%)
Primary general anesthesia [n]	5 (5.7%)
Akrinor® [mL], mean (range)	1.3 (0; 5)
Norepinephrine [µg], mean (range)	0.0 (0; 200)
Clonidin [µg], mean (range)	62.2 (0;300)
Urapidil [mg], mean (range)	13.0 (0;150)

ASA: American Society of Anesthesiology; CEA: carotid endarterectomy; µg: microgram; ml: milliliters; min: minutes; n: number.

3.2. Complications During Locoregional Anesthesia for CEA

Insufficient block quality, indicated by restlessness and pain, or the requirement for additional intraoperative analgesic medication (locally administered by the surgeons or intravenously by the anesthesiologists, respectively), occurred in 15 patients. Three of these fifteen patients required conversion to GA during the procedure due to ongoing insufficient analgesia. Two patients reported dysphagia, while another developed Horner's syndrome following the cervical plexus blockade. Additionally, five patients experienced nausea during the surgical procedure (see Table 2).

Table 2. Complications during LRA for CEA: incidence of complications associated with locoregional anesthesia during carotid endarterectomy.

	Incidence of Complications [n]
Total number of patients with LRA	83
Insufficient block quality (restlessness and pain)	15 (18.1%)
Intraoperative conversion to general anesthesia	3 (3.6%)
Dyspnea	0
Nausea	5 (6.0%)
Horner's syndrome	1 (1.2%)
Dysphagia	2 (2.4%)

CEA: carotid endarterectomy; LRA: locoregional anesthesia; n: number.

3.3. Complication Rate in Relation to the Number of Previously Performed LRA Procedures

The patients were divided into groups (A, B, C, and D) based on the experience of the attending anesthesiologist. Group A included those who received LRA from anesthesiologists with experience in ≤ 3 cervical plexus blockades, Group B from those performing their 4th to 6th blockades, Group C from those performing their 7th to 9th blockades, and Group D from those with experience in 10 or more blockades. Group A included 21 patients, Group B included 12 patients, Group C included 9 patients, and Group D included 41 patients (see Table 3). As mentioned above, cervical plexus blockades for patients in Groups A and B were performed under the supervision of an anesthesiologist experienced in this technique. LRA for patients in Groups C and D was performed without supervision, with patients in Group C representing the first three independently performed blockades by anesthesiologists who had newly learned the LRA technique.

Table 3. Statistical analysis of the incidence of insufficient block quality and LRA-associated complications: incidence of insufficient block quality and LRA-associated complications across the groups and results of the statistical analysis, which revealed significant differences in the incidence of block failure. A significance level of $p < 0.05$, or $p < 0.0083$ after Bonferroni correction, was applied.

	Group A (≤3 LRA)	Group B (4–6 LRA)	Group C (7–9 LRA)	Group D (≥10 LRA)	Chi-Square (p-Value)	Post Hoc A vs. B (p-Value)	Post Hoc A vs. C (p-Value)	Post Hoc A vs. D (p-Value)
Number of patients [n]	21	12	9	41				
Number of anesthesiologists [n]	9	4	4	3				
Incidence of block failure [n]	42.9% [9]	0% [0]	0% [0]	14.6% [6]	0.003	0.008	0.019	0.014
Incidence of intraop. conversions to GA [n]	9.5% [2]	0% [0]	0% [0]	2.4% [1]	0.383			
Incidence of Horner´s syndrome [n]	0% [0]	8.3% [1]	0% [0]	0% [0]	0.112			
Incidence of dysphagia [n]	4.8% [1]	0% [0]	0% [0]	2.4% [1]	0.798			

GA: general anesthesia; intraop: intraoperative; LRA: locoregional anesthesia; n: number; vs.: versus.

When considering the frequency of complications in relation to the number of LRA procedures performed, the following was observed:

Insufficient block quality, indicated by restlessness and pain or the need for additional analgesic medication, occurred most frequently during the first three LRA procedures performed by each anesthesiologist (Group A; see Table 3). The statistical analysis revealed significant differences in the incidence of insufficient block quality among the groups ($p = 0.003$), with Group A showing the highest incidence (42.9%; see Table 3). After three LRA procedures, the incidence of block failure was significantly reduced (Group A vs. B, $p = 0.008$; see Table 3). Furthermore, the incidence of insufficient block quality did not increase again in Group C, representing the first three independently performed LRA procedures by each anesthesiologist after the supervision period.

In contrast, Group D showed a renewed increase in the incidence of insufficient block quality compared to Groups B and C. However, in relative terms, the increase was small and did not reach statistical significance. Correspondingly, a continuous overall decrease in the incidence of complications with the cumulative number of cervical plexus blockades performed was observed, as shown in Figure 1 (see Figure 1).

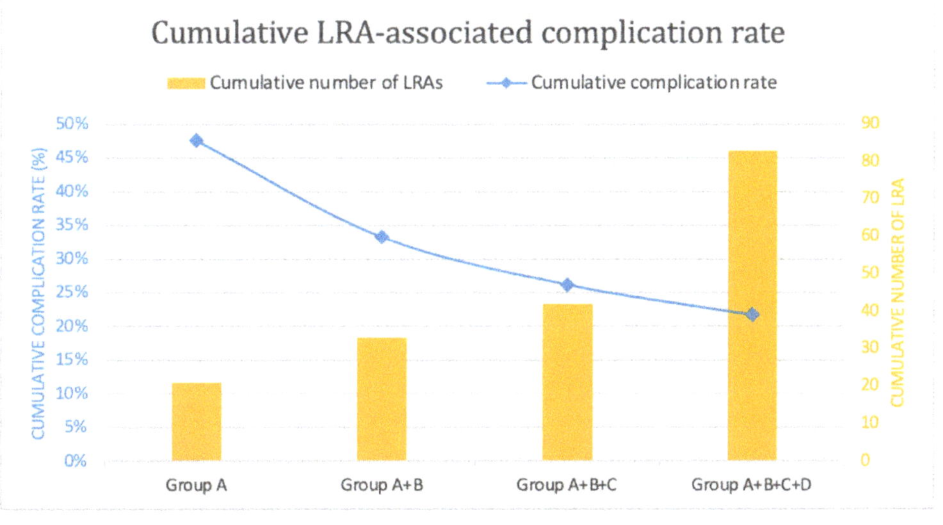

Figure 1. Locoregional anesthesia-associated complication rate.

The conversion rate from LRA to general anesthesia was highest in Group A, where the attending anesthesiologist had the least experience with the technique. Horner's syndrome and dysphagia, as additional complications related to locoregional anesthesia, occurred statistically independently of the number of previously performed LRA procedures (see Table 3).

Figure 1 illustrates the cumulative LRA-associated complication rate in our cohort plotted against the number of LRA procedures performed, categorized by the study groups A–D on a dual-axis chart. The x-axis represents the groups (A–D). The primary y-axis shows the cumulative complication rate as a line graph, while the secondary y-axis displays the cumulative number of LRA procedures as a bar graph. The complications considered in this illustration include insufficient block quality, dyspnea, dysphagia, and Horner's syndrome. Conversions to general anesthesia occurred due to insufficient block quality and are not counted additionally.

4. Discussion

In this study, we demonstrated, in 83 patients, that ultrasound-guided LRA (combined deep and superficial cervical plexus anesthesia) for CEA can be rapidly mastered by board-certified anesthesiologists. The overall complication rates were low, with insufficient block quality being the most frequent complication (n = 15, 18.1%), leading to conversions to GA in three cases. After three LRA procedures performed under supervision, we observed a significant reduction ($p = 0.008$) in the incidence of block failure, which did not increase during the first unsupervised blockades. Additional complications related to the locoregional anesthesia technique included dysphagia (n = 2) and Horner's syndrome (n = 1). However, the incidence of complications decreased continuously with the cumulative number of plexus blockades performed.

Our data, suggesting the rapid mastery of newly learned LRA under ultrasound guidance, are consistent with other findings. Helayel et al. demonstrated that, in inexperienced residents, only six practical exams were necessary after a theoretical introduction to reliably identify all structures of the axillary part of the brachial plexus using ultrasound, which forms the foundation of ultrasound-guided regional anesthesia [18]. In a phantom model of a peripheral nerve block, Kim et al. trained inexperienced medical students in hand–eye coordination, another key competence for safe and successful LRA. They found that five subsequent trials were sufficient to significantly improve hand–eye coordination for promising LRA outcomes [19]. These findings demonstrate the good learnability of key competencies for ultrasound-guided LRA, even for completely inexperienced examiners. In clinical practice, the application of these competencies may be complicated by factors such as anatomical variability in the target region and physician–patient interaction, which could increase the number of procedures needed for successful implementation [20,21]. Consistent with this, Morros et al. found that, in clinical scenarios, anesthesiologists with experience in nerve stimulator-guided regional anesthesia could successfully perform an independent ultrasound-guided blockade of the axillary plexus after 15 self-conducted blocks [22]. When compared to other procedures in anesthesiology, such as intubation—where approximately 200 intubations are required for safe mastery—ultrasound-guided LRA appears to be a rapidly learnable procedure [23]. In various studies, both nerve stimulator-guided and ultrasound-guided LRA have achieved favorable success rates, with ultrasound-guided techniques proving quicker to learn [8,24,25]. In line with these findings, we observed a rapid reduction in the incidence of insufficient block quality for cervical plexus blockades after only three supervised cervical plexus blockades performed by board-certified anesthesiologists with experience in LRA in other regions. This highlights the good learnability and transferability of ultrasound-guided LRA, particularly for the cervical plexus region, for anesthesiologists experienced in locoregional anesthesia techniques.

Following the rapid reduction in the incidence of block failure and other complications related to LRA in our cohort, we observed an interesting, though statistically non-significant, increase in incidence in Group D. Since this renewed increase in insufficient block quality did not occur in Group C (representing patients receiving the first three independently performed LRA procedures without supervision), the level of experience does not seem to provide a plausible explanation for this rise. Rather, the larger number of patients in Group D seems to offer a more accurate reflection of the average block failure and complication rates associated with LRA techniques, which evidently persist even among experienced anesthesiologists for various reasons [9,15,26,27]. This is further supported by the continuously decreasing overall complication rate we observed, calculated based on the cumulative number of LRA procedures performed.

In our cohort, no outcome-relevant complications associated with LRA were observed. Restlessness and pain, indicative of insufficient block quality, were the most frequent complications, occurring in 18.1% of patients and leading to conversions to GA in 3.6% of cases. Similarly, other studies report conversion rates to GA ranging from 0% to 4.3% [1,28–33]. As in our cohort, pain and restlessness were the most frequent causes of intraoperative conversions to GA [10,28]. Rates of insufficiency or failure of LRA, requiring supplementary intraoperative injections of local or systemic anesthetics, have been reported to range widely from 3% to 54% [10,30,34]. Since restlessness and pain represent the relatively subjective perceptions of both the patient and the attending anesthesiologists, these large differences can be explained well. Additionally, the lack of a clear definition of 'block failure' makes it a difficult outcome parameter to compare [9]. The definition of block failure used in our study—restlessness and pain or the need for additional analgesic medication during the procedure—represents a relatively subjective criterion too. Various definitions of peripheral nerve block failure have been used in recent years, each lacking purely objective criteria [9,26]. In their recently published work, Bottomley et al. defined block failure as the inability to perform the planned procedure due to insufficient analgesia. They proposed, alongside subjective patient comfort perception, the additional administration of local or systemic analgesics [9]. This approach was also adopted in our study, with the understanding that the generalizability of the results is limited by this potential bias. However, the similar rates of block failure and conversions to GA reported in other studies underline the plausibility of our findings.

Further LRA-related complications observed in our study were dysphagia and Horner's syndrome, likely due to accidental blockade of the stellate ganglion. In addition to these temporary complications, other studies report hemodynamic instability and respiratory insufficiency following the administration of local anesthetics in the cervical region, accidental puncture of vessels resulting in hematoma, or even intravascular injection of a local anesthetic, among others [15,35]. To reduce severe complications such as intravascular injections and vascular injuries, the ultrasound-guided technique has been shown to be superior to the neurostimulator-guided technique and is recommended by current guidelines [15,36]. Regarding different techniques for cervical plexus blockade, a systematic review of 69 observational studies found that superficial or intermediate blocks have the lowest risk of failure or complications and should therefore be the preferred techniques today [31]. These recommendations are supported by recent findings from Opperer et al., who demonstrated that the deep cervical plexus block, particularly due to its involvement of the phrenic nerve, negatively affects diaphragm motion and thus may pose a potential risk for respiratory impairment in patients with pre-existing pulmonary conditions [33]. Consequently, at our hospital, the superficial cervical plexus block has since been established as the standard technique for LRA in CEA. But even with these techniques, a certain complication rate persists among experienced LRA experts due to various reasons [9,26,27,37]. In particular, the significant interindividual anatomical variability and interconnections within the cervical plexus inherently seem to preclude a universally 'optimal application site' with 100% efficiency [15,20,21]. Furthermore, the inconsistent nomenclature of the cervical region and its fasciae in relation to the cervical plexus complicates the cross-study comparison of complication rates [38]. However, the overall complication rate of 22% and failure rate of 18% observed in our study align with reports in the literature on failure and complication rates, interestingly, despite the use of different cervical plexus block depths (superficial, intermediate, and deep) in various studies [9,26,37,39]. The cause of this appears to lie in the unique anatomy of the cervical fasciae, which allow good permeability for injected fluids [33,40]. Thus, the exact spread and, consequently, the specific blockade site of the cervical plexus can only be predicted to a limited extent by a specific injection depth. Consistent with this, clinically relevant complications appear with the same frequency even when explicitly comparing different block depths [33]. Therefore, it is primarily the ultrasound-guided technique, rather than the block depth of the plexus, that positively influences safety and success rates and is now considered the standard.

Looking at LRA from the patient's perspective, high satisfaction is evident. According to Davies et al., 92% of patients would choose LRA again for a subsequent procedure [41]. It is not only patients who prefer this technique; a preference for LRA, particularly the ultrasound-guided method, has also been demonstrated among residents [42]. Various curricula for learning LRA techniques have now been established [43,44].

Our study had several limitations. Firstly, due to the retrospective and single-center design, there was no standardized perioperative documentation of complications, and our data were not externally validated. Additionally, the relatively small sample size limits the validity of our data. Therefore, the present study design does not allow for generalization of the results or application to other medical settings or populations. Furthermore, every retrospective data analysis carries an inherent risk of bias regarding data completeness. Secondly, only board-certified anesthesiologists experienced in local anesthesia techniques were involved, which makes our results only partially transferable to other physicians. Due to the retrospective analysis, differences in group sizes (A-D) arose, as not every anesthesiologist performed the same number of LRA procedures. This may have obscured any effects of individual variations in learning curves. Thirdly, we used restlessness and pain as indicators of insufficient LRA, which are relatively subjective parameters. Additionally, preoperative anxiety influences pain levels and has been shown to be an independent risk factor for LRA failure [45,46]. Finally, the significant anatomical variation in the target region, such as interindividual sensory innervation by cranial nerves and peripheral nerves of the cervical plexus, contributes to varying individual responsiveness to LRA [15,20,21]. Therefore, prospective, multi-center studies with a larger number of participants and procedures are desirable to more accurately capture the learning curve of LRA techniques among anesthesiologists, as only such a design would allow for the generalization of the results, which is not feasible in our study. Additionally, a clear definition of 'insufficiency/failure of LRA' as an outcome parameter would be helpful to allow for better comparison between studies. Thus, our study should primarily be seen as an example and idea for conducting a suitably designed study that can generate transferable findings and be used to develop a curriculum.

5. Conclusions

Our study highlights the rapid learnability of ultrasound-guided cervical plexus blockades for board-certified anesthesiologists experienced in ultrasound-guided anesthesia techniques, demonstrating a low overall risk and supporting the training of anesthesiologists in this technique. It appears to require limited training effort in this specific setting, although no absolute conclusions can be drawn about the number of procedures needed to achieve proficiency due to the study design. However, this approach effectively integrates the advantages of ultrasound-guided LRA for CEA into clinical practice. While there appears to be a clear anesthesiologic advantage to LRA for CEA, the choice of anesthesia technique ultimately remains an interdisciplinary decision involving the entire treatment team.

Author Contributions: Conceptualization, A.K., N.G., B.S. and M.O.F.-K.; methodology, B.S. and A.K.; software, B.S. and A.K.; validation, B.S., N.G., A.K., A.O., D.B. and M.O.F.-K.; formal analysis, B.S. and A.K.; investigation, N.G., A.K. and B.S.; resources, A.K., A.O. and D.B.; data curation, N.G., B.S. and A.K.; writing—original draft preparation, B.S.; writing—review and editing, A.K., M.O.F.-K., A.O. and D.B.; visualization, B.S.; supervision, A.K. and M.O.F.-K.; project administration, A.K. and M.O.F.-K. All authors have read and agreed to the published version of the manuscript.

Funding: This research received no external funding.

Institutional Review Board Statement: The study was conducted in accordance with the Declaration of Helsinki and approved by the Ethics Committee of the medical faculty at the University of Heidelberg, Germany (protocol code S-297/2017, 19 June 2017).

Informed Consent Statement: Patient consent was waived due to the retrospective nature of the study and the anonymization of all data that could identify individual patients immediately after data collection.

Data Availability Statement: The original contributions presented in the study are included in the article; further inquiries can be directed to the corresponding author.

Conflicts of Interest: There is no relevant interests about Merck KGaA. The authors declare that they have any competing interests in this article.

References

1. Group, G.T.C.; Lewis, S.C.; Warlow, C.P.; Bodenham, A.R.; Colam, B.; Rothwell, P.M.; Torgerson, D.; Dellagrammaticas, D.; Horrocks, M.; Liapis, C.; et al. General anaesthesia versus local anaesthesia for carotid surgery (GALA): A multicentre, randomised controlled trial. *Lancet* **2008**, *372*, 2132–2142. [CrossRef]
2. Harky, A.; Chan, J.S.K.; Kot, T.K.M.; Sanli, D.; Rahimli, R.; Belamaric, Z.; Ng, M.; Kwan, I.Y.Y.; Bithas, C.; Makar, R.; et al. General Anesthesia Versus Local Anesthesia in Carotid Endarterectomy: A Systematic Review and Meta-Analysis. *J. Cardiothorac. Vasc. Anesth.* **2020**, *34*, 219–234. [CrossRef] [PubMed]
3. Hajibandeh, S.; Hajibandeh, S.; Antoniou, S.A.; Torella, F.; Antoniou, G.A. Meta-analysis and trial sequential analysis of local vs. general anaesthesia for carotid endarterectomy. *Anaesthesia* **2018**, *73*, 1280–1289. [CrossRef]
4. Hye, R.J.; Voeks, J.H.; Malas, M.B.; Tom, M.; Longson, S.; Blackshear, J.L.; Brott, T.G. Anesthetic type and risk of myocardial infarction after carotid endarterectomy in the Carotid Revascularization Endarterectomy versus Stenting Trial (CREST). *J. Vasc. Surg.* **2016**, *64*, 3–8.e1. [CrossRef] [PubMed]
5. Knappich, C.; Kuehnl, A.; Haller, B.; Salvermoser, M.; Algra, A.; Becquemin, J.P.; Bonati, L.H.; Bulbulia, R.; Calvet, D.; Fraedrich, G.; et al. Associations of Perioperative Variables With the 30-Day Risk of Stroke or Death in Carotid Endarterectomy for Symptomatic Carotid Stenosis. *Stroke* **2019**, *50*, 3439–3448. [CrossRef] [PubMed]
6. Naylor, R.; Rantner, B.; Ancetti, S.; de Borst, G.J.; De Carlo, M.; Halliday, A.; Kakkos, S.K.; Markus, H.S.; McCabe, D.J.H.; Sillesen, H.; et al. Editor's Choice—European Society for Vascular Surgery (ESVS) 2023 Clinical Practice Guidelines on the Management of Atherosclerotic Carotid and Vertebral Artery Disease. *Eur. J. Vasc. Endovasc. Surg.* **2023**, *65*, 7–111. [CrossRef]
7. AbuRahma, A.F.; Avgerinos, E.D.; Chang, R.W.; Darling, R.C., 3rd; Duncan, A.A.; Forbes, T.L.; Malas, M.B.; Murad, M.H.; Perler, B.A.; Powell, R.J.; et al. Society for Vascular Surgery clinical practice guidelines for management of extracranial cerebrovascular disease. *J. Vasc. Surg.* **2022**, *75*, 4S–22S. [CrossRef]
8. Luyet, C.; Schupfer, G.; Wipfli, M.; Greif, R.; Luginbuhl, M.; Eichenberger, U. Different Learning Curves for Axillary Brachial Plexus Block: Ultrasound Guidance versus Nerve Stimulation. *Anesthesiol. Res. Pract.* **2010**, *2010*, 309462. [CrossRef]
9. Bottomley, T.; Gadsden, J.; West, S. The failed peripheral nerve block. *BJA Educ.* **2023**, *23*, 92–100. [CrossRef]
10. Hakl, M.; Michalek, P.; Sevcik, P.; Pavlikova, J.; Stern, M. Regional anaesthesia for carotid endarterectomy: An audit over 10 years. *Br. J. Anaesth.* **2007**, *99*, 415–420. [CrossRef]
11. Telford, R.J.; Stoneham, M.D. Correct nomenclature of superficial cervical plexus blocks. *Br. J. Anaesth.* **2004**, *92*, 775. [CrossRef] [PubMed]
12. Kim, J.S.; Ko, J.S.; Bang, S.; Kim, H.; Lee, S.Y. Cervical plexus block. *Korean J. Anesthesiol.* **2018**, *71*, 274–288. [CrossRef] [PubMed]
13. Narouze, S. Sonoanatomy of the cervical spinal nerve roots: Implications for brachial plexus block. *Reg. Anesth. Pain Med.* **2009**, *34*, 616. [CrossRef] [PubMed]
14. Usui, Y.; Kobayashi, T.; Kakinuma, H.; Watanabe, K.; Kitajima, T.; Matsuno, K. An anatomical basis for blocking of the deep cervical plexus and cervical sympathetic tract using an ultrasound-guided technique. *Anesth. Analg.* **2010**, *110*, 964–968. [CrossRef] [PubMed]
15. Seidel, R. Cervical Plexus Blocks. *Anasthesiol. Intensivmed. Notfallmed Schmerzther.* **2017**, *52*, 806–813. [CrossRef]
16. Sites, B.D.; Gallagher, J.D.; Cravero, J.; Lundberg, J.; Blike, G. The learning curve associated with a simulated ultrasound-guided interventional task by inexperienced anesthesia residents. *Reg. Anesth. Pain Med.* **2004**, *29*, 544–548. [CrossRef]
17. Bland, J.M.; Altman, D.G. Multiple significance tests: The Bonferroni method. *BMJ* **1995**, *310*, 170. [CrossRef]
18. Helayel, P.E.; Conceicao, D.B.; Nascimento, B.S.; Kohler, A.; Boos, G.L.; Oliveira Filho, G.R. Learning curve for the ultrasound anatomy of the brachial plexus in the axillary region. *Rev. Bras. Anestesiol.* **2009**, *59*, 187–193. [CrossRef]
19. Kim, S.C.; Hauser, S.; Staniek, A.; Weber, S. Learning curve of medical students in ultrasound-guided simulated nerve block. *J. Anesth.* **2014**, *28*, 76–80. [CrossRef]
20. Shoja, M.M.; Oyesiku, N.M.; Griessenauer, C.J.; Radcliff, V.; Loukas, M.; Chern, J.J.; Benninger, B.; Rozzelle, C.J.; Shokouhi, G.; Tubbs, R.S. Anastomoses between lower cranial and upper cervical nerves: A comprehensive review with potential significance during skull base and neck operations, part I: Trigeminal, facial, and vestibulocochlear nerves. *Clin. Anat.* **2014**, *27*, 118–130. [CrossRef]
21. Shoja, M.M.; Oyesiku, N.M.; Shokouhi, G.; Griessenauer, C.J.; Chern, J.J.; Rizk, E.B.; Loukas, M.; Miller, J.H.; Tubbs, R.S. A comprehensive review with potential significance during skull base and neck operations, Part II: Glossopharyngeal, vagus, accessory, and hypoglossal nerves and cervical spinal nerves 1-4. *Clin. Anat.* **2014**, *27*, 131–144. [CrossRef] [PubMed]
22. Morros, C.; Perez-Cuenca, M.D.; Sala-Blanch, X.; Cedo, F. Ultrasound-guided axillary brachial plexus block: Learning curve and results. *Rev. Esp. Anestesiol. Reanim.* **2011**, *58*, 74–79. [CrossRef] [PubMed]
23. Bernhard, M.; Mohr, S.; Weigand, M.A.; Martin, E.; Walther, A. Developing the skill of endotracheal intubation: Implication for emergency medicine. *Acta Anaesthesiol. Scand.* **2012**, *56*, 164–171. [CrossRef] [PubMed]
24. Barrington, M.J.; Gledhill, S.R.; Kluger, R.; Clarke, A.L.; Wong, D.M.; Davidson, H.; Thomas, R. A Randomized Controlled Trial of Ultrasound Versus Nerve Stimulator Guidance for Axillary Brachial Plexus Block. *Reg. Anesth. Pain. Med.* **2016**, *41*, 671–677. [CrossRef]

25. Cataldo, R.; Carassiti, M.; Costa, F.; Martuscelli, M.; Benedetto, M.; Cancilleri, F.; Marinozzi, A.; Martinelli, N. Starting with ultrasonography decreases popliteal block performance time in inexperienced hands: A prospective randomized study. *BMC Anesthesiol.* **2012**, *12*, 33. [CrossRef]
26. Barrington, M.J.; Watts, S.A.; Gledhill, S.R.; Thomas, R.D.; Said, S.A.; Snyder, G.L.; Tay, V.S.; Jamrozik, K. Preliminary results of the Australasian Regional Anaesthesia Collaboration: A prospective audit of more than 7000 peripheral nerve and plexus blocks for neurologic and other complications. *Reg. Anesth. Pain Med.* **2009**, *34*, 534–541. [CrossRef]
27. Niazi, A.U.; Haldipur, N.; Prasad, A.G.; Chan, V.W. Ultrasound-guided regional anesthesia performance in the early learning period: Effect of simulation training. *Reg. Anesth. Pain Med.* **2012**, *37*, 51–54. [CrossRef]
28. Pasin, L.; Nardelli, P.; Landoni, G.; Cornero, G.; Magrin, S.; Tshomba, Y.; Chiesa, R.; Zangrillo, A. Examination of regional anesthesia for carotid endarterectomy. *J. Vasc. Surg.* **2015**, *62*, 631–634.e1. [CrossRef]
29. Andersen, C.A.; Rich, N.M.; Collins, G.J., Jr.; McDonald, P.T. Carotid endarterectomy: Regional versus general anesthesia. *Am. Surg.* **1980**, *46*, 323–327.
30. Sindjelic, R.P.; Vlajkovic, G.P.; Lucic, M.; Koncar, I.; Kostic, D.; Davidovic, L.B. Incidence of and indications for conversion of cervical plexus block to general anesthesia in patients undergoing carotid surgery: A single center experience. *J. Cardiovasc. Surg.* **2015**, *56*, 441–446.
31. Pandit, J.J.; Satya-Krishna, R.; Gration, P. Superficial or deep cervical plexus block for carotid endarterectomy: A systematic review of complications. *Br. J. Anaesth.* **2007**, *99*, 159–169. [CrossRef] [PubMed]
32. Hoefer, J.; Pierer, E.; Rantner, B.; Stadlbauer, K.H.; Fraedrich, G.; Fritz, J.; Kleinsasser, A.; Velik-Salchner, C. Ultrasound-guided regional anesthesia for carotid endarterectomy induces early hemodynamic and stress hormone changes. *J. Vasc. Surg.* **2015**, *62*, 57–67. [CrossRef] [PubMed]
33. Opperer, M.; Kaufmann, R.; Meissnitzer, M.; Enzmann, F.K.; Dinges, C.; Hitzl, W.; Nawratil, J.; Kokofer, A. Depth of cervical plexus block and phrenic nerve blockade: A randomized trial. *Reg. Anesth. Pain Med.* **2022**, *47*, 205–211. [CrossRef] [PubMed]
34. Sait Kavakli, A.; Kavrut Ozturk, N.; Umut Ayoglu, R.; Sagdic, K.; Cakmak, G.; Inanoglu, K.; Emmiler, M. Comparison of Combined (Deep and Superficial) and Intermediate Cervical Plexus Block by Use of Ultrasound Guidance for Carotid Endarterectomy. *J. Cardiothorac. Vasc. Anesth.* **2016**, *30*, 317–322. [CrossRef]
35. Stoneham, M.D.; Thompson, J.P. Arterial pressure management and carotid endarterectomy. *Br. J. Anaesth.* **2009**, *102*, 442–452. [CrossRef]
36. Delaunay, L.; Plantet, F.; Jochum, D. Ultrasound and regional anaesthesia. *Ann. Françaises D'Anesthésie Réanimation* **2009**, *28*, 140–160. [CrossRef] [PubMed]
37. Kokofer, A.; Nawratil, J.; Opperer, M. Regional anesthesia for carotid surgery: An overview of anatomy, techniques and their clinical relevance. *Anaesthesist* **2017**, *66*, 283–290. [CrossRef]
38. Scimia, P.; Gentili, L.; Sepolvere, G. Ultrasound-guided cervical plexus block: Understanding the cervical fasciae to clarify the nomenclature of this technique. *Minerva Anestesiol.* **2022**, *88*, 526–528. [CrossRef]
39. Ratnayake, A.; Abeysundara, A.; Samarasinghe, B.; Rathnayake, J.; Samarasinghe, S.; Perera, R.; Bandara, C. Use of intermediate cervical plexus block in carotid endarterectomy -an alternative to deep cervical plexus block: A case series. *BMC Anesthesiol.* **2024**, *24*, 288. [CrossRef]
40. Pandit, J.J.; Dutta, D.; Morris, J.F. Spread of injectate with superficial cervical plexus block in humans: An anatomical study. *Br. J. Anaesth.* **2003**, *91*, 733–735. [CrossRef]
41. Davies, M.J.; Murrell, G.C.; Cronin, K.D.; Meads, A.C.; Dawson, A. Carotid endarterectomy under cervical plexus block--a prospective clinical audit. *Anaesth. Intensive Care* **1990**, *18*, 219–223. [CrossRef] [PubMed]
42. Awad, I.T.; Sinclair, C.; Chen, E.W.; McCartney, C.J.; Cheung, J.J.; Dubrowski, A. Anesthesia residents' preference for learning interscalene brachial plexus block (ISBPB): Traditional Winnie's technique vs. ultrasound-guided technique. *Stud. Health Technol. Inform.* **2011**, *163*, 36–38. [PubMed]
43. Ouanes, J.P.; Schwengel, D.; Mathur, V.; Ahmed, O.I.; Hanna, M.N. Curriculum development for an advanced regional anesthesia education program: One institution's experience from apprenticeship to comprehensive teaching. *Middle East J. Anaesthesiol.* **2014**, *22*, 413–418. [PubMed]
44. Kim, T.E.; Tsui, B.C.H. Simulation-based ultrasound-guided regional anesthesia curriculum for anesthesiology residents. *Korean J. Anesthesiol.* **2019**, *72*, 13–23. [CrossRef]
45. Fuzier, R.; Lavidale, M.; Bataille, B.; Richez, A.S.; Magues, J.P. Anxiety: An independent factor of axillary brachial plexus block failure? *Ann. Françaises D'Anesthésie Réanimation* **2010**, *29*, 776–781. [CrossRef]
46. Kokofer, A.; Nawratil, J.; Opperer, M. Importance of instrument-based neuromonitoring during carotid surgery using regional anesthesia. *Anaesthesist* **2017**, *66*, 627–628. [CrossRef]

Journal of
Clinical Medicine

MDPI

Article

Sub-Tenon's Block in Patients with Previous Encircling Band Surgery—A Feasibility Study

Johannes Harte [1], Gesar Ugen [1], Joana Berger-Estilita [2,3], Andreas Ebneter [4] and Friedrich Lersch [1,*]

1 Department of Anesthesiology and Pain Medicine, Bern University Hospital, Inselspital, 3010 Bern, Switzerland
2 Institute for Medical Education, University of Bern, 3012 Bern, Switzerland
3 CINTESIS@RISE, Centre for Health Technology and Services Research, Faculty of Medicine, University of Porto, 4200-450 Porto, Portugal
4 Department of Ophthalmology, Cantonal Hospital St. Gallen, 9007 St. Gallen, Switzerland
* Correspondence: friedrich.lersch@insel.ch

Abstract: Introduction: During the COVID-19 pandemic, reducing aerosol-generating procedures became fundamental, particularly in ophthalmic surgeries traditionally performed under general anesthesia (GA). Regional anesthesia, such as sub-Tenon's block (STB), is widely used in vitreoretinal surgeries, offering a safer alternative by avoiding airway manipulation. However, the altered orbital anatomy in patients with previous scleral explant surgery creates unique challenges to STB application. This study aims to evaluate the effectiveness, safety, and feasibility of STB in patients after encircling band surgery. **Methods:** This retrospective analysis included 46 patients with a history of scleral explant surgery, undergoing vitreoretinal procedures at the Bern University Hospital. All procedures were conducted under STB with either analgosedation or GA for additional support when required. An ophthalmic surgeon or an experienced anesthesiologist performed the STBs. Data collected included block success rate, procedural difficulty, incidence of chemosis, and patient satisfaction. The Institutional Ethics Committee approved this study, and all participants provided informed consent. **Results:** STB was successfully administered in 93.5% of cases, with only three unsuccessful blocks. Block placement was rated as easy in 55% of cases, moderately difficult in 28%, and difficult in 17%. Chemosis was observed in 24% of patients, with severe cases in only 4%. Patient satisfaction scores were high, with most patients expressing satisfaction with the STB procedure. Conversion to GA was required in only one case due to alcohol withdrawal-related agitation. **Discussion:** The high success rate and minimal complications suggest that STB is a feasible and safe alternative to GA in patients with prior scleral buckling surgery. The altered orbital anatomy presents potential challenges, including scar tissue and compartmentalization, which may lead to patchy anesthesia. However, the use of STB avoids the risks associated with GA and may be especially beneficial for elderly or frail patients. Future studies should further investigate the hemodynamic implications of STB in these cases and the potential for ultrasound-guided techniques to improve accuracy and safety.

Keywords: sub-Tenon; buckling surgery; encircling band; regional anesthesia

1. Introduction

The COVID-19 pandemic prompted healthcare providers to adopt protocols that limit aerosol-generating procedures, particularly in surgeries where proximity to the respiratory tract increases the risk of viral transmission [1]. In ophthalmic surgery, this need translated into an increased emphasis on regional anesthesia to avoid general anesthesia (GA) where possible [2,3]. Sub-Tenon's block (STB) is a reliable and safe option for locoregional anesthesia in most vitreoretinal (VR) surgeries, providing excellent anesthesia and analgesia while eliminating the risks associated with airway manipulation in GA [4,5]. However, its use in patients with prior scleral explants in place is met with caution, as the altered orbital anatomy and presence of the encircling band can restrict the distribution of anesthetics and complicate block administration [6,7].

Traditionally, general anesthesia has been recommended in cases involving prior scleral buckling surgery due to concerns about complications from distorted ocular anatomy and the potential for ineffective blocks. The insertion of an encircling band often causes elongation or slight alteration in the structure of the eye, creating unique challenges for regional anesthesia, particularly when using sharp-needle techniques like retrobulbar or peribulbar blocks [8]. These blocks carry a heightened risk of globe perforation or other complications in elongated or scarred eyes [9]. STB, a blunt cannula technique that injects anesthetic into the sub-Tenon's space, is less invasive and may mitigate some of these risks. However, due to the mechanical obstruction posed by the encircling band, the procedure can become technically challenging, and it is unclear whether successful anesthesia can consistently be achieved in such cases.

Prior to the pandemic, STB was selectively employed for VR surgeries in elderly or medically frail patients, who would face higher risks under GA. This approach was guided by clinical judgment, balancing the need for adequate anesthesia against the patient's overall medical condition. During the pandemic, however, we began to extend this practice to a broader patient population with prior encircling scleral bands, aiming to minimize exposure to GA and reduce overall perioperative risk. In this feasibility study, we aimed to systematically evaluate the success rate, safety, and patient satisfaction associated with STB in patients who had previously undergone encircling band procedures. We hypothesized that STB could be a safe and effective alternative to GA, even in eyes with altered anatomy due to encircling bands. Our findings aim to inform future practice guidelines and contribute to expanding the application of regional anesthesia in complex ophthalmic cases, particularly in settings where GA poses additional risks.

2. Methods

2.1. Ethics

This study adhered the World Medical Association Declaration of Helsinki Ethical Principles for Medical Research Involving Human Subjects and complied with the Swiss Human Research Act. The Cantonal Ethics Committee of Bern (KEK Bern) Switzerland (Chairperson Prof. em. Dr. med. Christian Seiler) approved this study (BASEC-number: Req-2020-01360). Patients provided informed consent for both the sub-Tenon's block procedure under analgosedation and the ophthalmic surgery itself. Additionally, patients consented to the anonymised data analysis and the subsequent publication of the study results.

2.2. Study Design

This study is a retrospective cohort analysis that examines outcomes of patients with prior encircling band surgery who received sub-Tenon's block for vitreoretinal procedures. We included patients with a history of encircling scleral band placement who underwent various VR procedures, such as pars plana vitrectomy, oil removal, cryotherapy, and complex phacoemulsification, at the University Hospital of Bern, Switzerland.

Eligible Patients had a history of encircling scleral band placement. Participants were required to be scheduled for VR surgery, including procedures such as pars plana vitrectomy, oil removal, cryotherapy, and complex phacoemulsification, all of which necessitated a reliable anesthesia technique due to their complexity.

The ophthalmic surgeon and the anesthesiologist independently assessed the feasibility of performing STB. This evaluation considered factors such as the patient's orbital anatomy, any scarring from previous surgeries, and the specific requirements of the planned procedure. Additionally, patients were selected if their general health condition made them suitable for STB with or without analgosedation. Priority was given to individuals who could benefit from avoiding general anesthesia due to underlying comorbidities or frailty, thereby minimizing perioperative risk.

All patients with severe eye infections, systemic contraindications to regional anesthesia, and with extensive conjunctival or Tenon's capsule scarring were excluded due to the high likelihood of block failure or complications. Finally, we excluded all patients who were unable to provide informed consent.

The data for this study were collected retrospectively over two years, from March 2020 to April 2022, at the Department of Ophthalmology, University Hospital of Bern (Inselspital), Switzerland.

2.3. Outcome Measures

Primary Outcome: The success rate of STB, defined by adequate anesthesia during the procedure without the need for opioid administration in cases combined with GA.

Secondary Outcomes: Patient satisfaction rated on a scale, technical difficulty of block placement, incidence of adverse events, and overall effectiveness of the anesthesia.

2.3.1. Intervention

Given their prior encircling band surgery, each patient received an STB tailored to their specific surgical and anatomical needs. Depending on availability and expertise, the intervention was administered by either an ophthalmic surgeon or an experienced anesthesiologist. The STBs were administered either by a vitreoretinal surgeon or an experienced anesthesiologist. The surgeon had five years of experience as a consultant in vitreoretinal surgery, following specialized ophthalmology training. The anesthesiologist had six years of experience leading the ophthalmology anesthesiology team, with extensive daily expertise in performing and teaching ophthalmic regional anesthesia. The process involved several standardised steps to ensure consistency in the procedure and evaluate technical challenges. First, patients were positioned for optimal access to the eye undergoing surgery. The surgeon or anesthesiologist identified the area for block placement based on the presence of the encircling scleral band. Careful attention was paid to avoid interference from the band and any scar tissue from previous surgery.

After thorough disinfection, we opened the eye using a non-toothed forceps. Next, we lifted the conjunctiva with tweezers and made an incision in the conjunctiva and Tenon's capsule using scissors. We then advanced a blunt, pre-shaped 22G needle into the sub-Tenon space dorsally behind the eye, always following the contour of the globe. The sub-Tenon's space was typically accessed in the inferonasal quadrant to allow better distribution of the anesthetic while minimizing the risk of complications (watch the instructive video in the Supplement or consult Figure 1. For patients with scar tissue from previous surgeries, the clinician took additional time and care in positioning the cannula to avoid resistance or damage. Five mL of local anesthetic (a mixture of ropivacaine 1%, hyaluronidase 5 IU/mL, and clonidine 5 μg/mL) was injected into the sub-Tenon's space through the cannula, aiming at distribution behind the scleral buckle. This combination was selected based on its clinical benefits: ropivacaine 1% provides long-lasting anesthesia and analgesia, hyaluronidase 5 IU/mL facilitates the spread of the anesthetic within tissue planes, and clonidine 5 μg/mL prolongs the duration of analgesia through its α2-adrenergic agonist properties. During administration, the clinician monitored for any indications of restricted anesthetic spread, backflow, or excessive chemosis due to altered anatomy from the band or scar tissue. Adjustments were made if necessary, and top-up injections were applied when required.

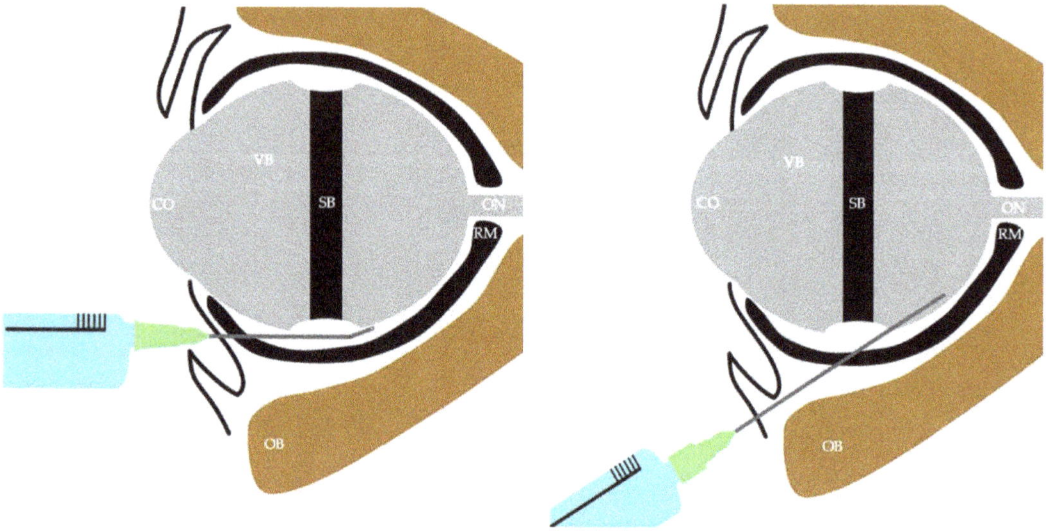

Figure 1. Comparing sub-Tenon block (STB) cannula trajectory vs. retrobulbar needle trajectory in a previously encircled, elongated eye; bulbar length is a serious risk for sharp-needle injury. The retrobulbar block, in contrast to the STB, penetrates the sclera. Legend: CO = cornea, VB = vitreous body, SB = scleral buckle, ON = optical nerve, RM = rectal muscle, OB = orbital bone.

Patients were continuously monitored using pulse oximetry, 3-lead ECG, and non-invasive blood pressure measurement. All patients received an intravenous line with a Ringer's acetate infusion. Analgosedation was administered to ensure patient comfort, with medications titrated as needed. These included propofol (10–20 mg boluses), dexmedetomidine (8–12 mcg boluses), fentanyl (25–50 mcg boluses), and ketamine (0.1–0.15 mg/kg bolus based on lean body weight), though their use was not standardised. In some cases, the STB was combined with GA to reduce postoperative opioid use and provide sustained analgesia. For general anesthesia, a premedication of 0.3 μg/kg bodyweight of dexmedetomidine iv was followed by propofol-alfentanil-ketamine induction, propofol TIVA maintenance (mg/kg/min) was used, and a laryngeal mask was placed to ensure airway patency in the majority of patients.

2.3.2. Assessment of Technical Difficulty

Following block placement, the clinician rated the technical difficulty encountered due to scar tissue on a standardised scale from 1 to 3 (1 = easy, 2 = moderate, 3 = difficult). Chemosis (swelling of the conjunctiva) post-STB was also rated on a scale from 1 to 3 (1 = no chemosis, 2 = intermediate, 3 = heavy chemosis), providing insights into potential complications from the procedure. Block success was evaluated at the start and end of the procedure, specifically noting whether adequate anesthesia was achieved without the need for opioid supplementation in patients under GA.

Patient satisfaction rate was measured the first time immediately after surgery capturing the patient's experience of anesthesia adequacy and comfort during the procedure, and again 6 to 24 h postoperatively on a scale from 1 to 5 (1 = very dissatisfied to 5 = completely satisfied). This satisfaction gauge was presumed to be reflective of postoperative analgesia.

2.4. Statistics

Descriptive statistics were used to summarize patient demographics, procedural details, and outcomes. Continuous variables, such as patient age and time since encircling band surgery, were presented as means with standard deviations (SDs) for normally distributed data or medians with interquartile ranges [IQRs] for non-normally distributed data. Categorical variables, including sex, STB success rates, and complication rates, were summarized as frequencies and percentages.

The primary outcome, the success rate of sub-Tenon's block, was calculated as the proportion of patients for whom the block provided sufficient anesthesia without requiring conversion to another form of anesthesia or additional opioid use in cases combined with GA.

Comparisons between groups based on the technical difficulty of block placement (easy, moderate, or difficult) were performed using appropriate statistical tests. For categorical variables, we used the chi-squared test or Fisher's exact test when expected cell counts were small. For continuous variables, the Kruskal–Wallis test was employed to compare non-normally distributed data across difficulty groups. Post hoc pairwise comparisons were conducted when significant differences were identified.

To assess the association between technical difficulty and block success, logistic regression analysis was performed, adjusting for potential confounders such as patient age and sex. Statistical significance was set at a p-value of <0.05. All analyses were conducted using SPSS, V.27 (IBM®, Armonk, NY, USA).

3. Results

We included 46 patients (37 males and 9 females) who underwent a total of 48 vitreoretinal surgeries (see Table 1). The average patient age was 61 years (range: 20–90 years). Surgical procedures included pars plana vitrectomy (PPV), oil removal, and complex phacoemulsification. The mean duration from encircling band surgery was 5.6 months, ranging from 6 days to 13 months, with one outlier at over 240 months.

Table 1. Patient characteristics and detailed analysis of factors influencing or associated with the difficulty level of STB.

	STB Difficulty			p-Value	Total
	1 = Easy (*n* = 25)	**2 = Moderate (*n* = 13)**	**3 = Difficult (*n* = 8)**		**46**
Male Sex	19 (51.4)	11 (29.7)	7 (18.9)	0.701	37 (80.4)
Age	63.0 [51.5–71.5]	66.0 [60.5–69.0]	64.5 [50.25–71.25]	0.591	65.5 [56.25–70.25]
STB Success	25 (100)	13 (100)	5 (62.5)	**<0.001**	43 (93.5)
Chemosis				**0.011**	
None	21 (84.0)	11 (84.6)	3 (37.5)		35 (47.9)
Intermediate	4 (16.0)	2 (15.4)	3 (37.5)		9 (12.3)
Heavy	0 (0.0)	0 (0.0)	2 (25.0)		2 (2.7)
Patient Satisfaction	5 [4–5]	5 [4–5]	3.5 [1–5]	**0.028**	5 [4–5]
VAS during STB	1 [1–2]	1 [1–2]	4.5 [2.25–5.0]	**<0.001**	1 [1–2]
Administration of systemic analgesia	7 (28.0)	4 (30.8)	6 (75.0)	**0.049**	17 (23.3)
Switch to PBB	0 (0.0)	0 (0.0)	2 (25.0)	**0.007**	2 (4.3)
Switch to GA	0 (0.0)	0 (0.0)	1 (12.5)	0.088	1 (2.2)

Acronyms: **GA**: General Anesthesia; **PBB**: Peribulbar Block; **STB**: Sub-Tenon's Block; **VAS**: Visual Analog Scale. Bold values significant for $p < 0.005$.

3.1. Primary Outcome

The STB was successful in most cases ($n = 43$, 93.5%), meeting the primary objective of the study. Two cases required conversion to peribulbar block (PBB) due to extensive scarring, and one patient necessitated general anesthesia (GA) because of alcohol withdrawal-related agitation. Among the successful cases, the block provided sufficient anesthesia to complete the procedure without additional opioid administration.

3.2. Secondary Outcomes

The safety objective was addressed through the analysis of complications. Chemosis was observed in 24% of patients, with severe cases reported in only 4%. No incidents of globe perforation or other major complications were recorded (consult Figure 2).

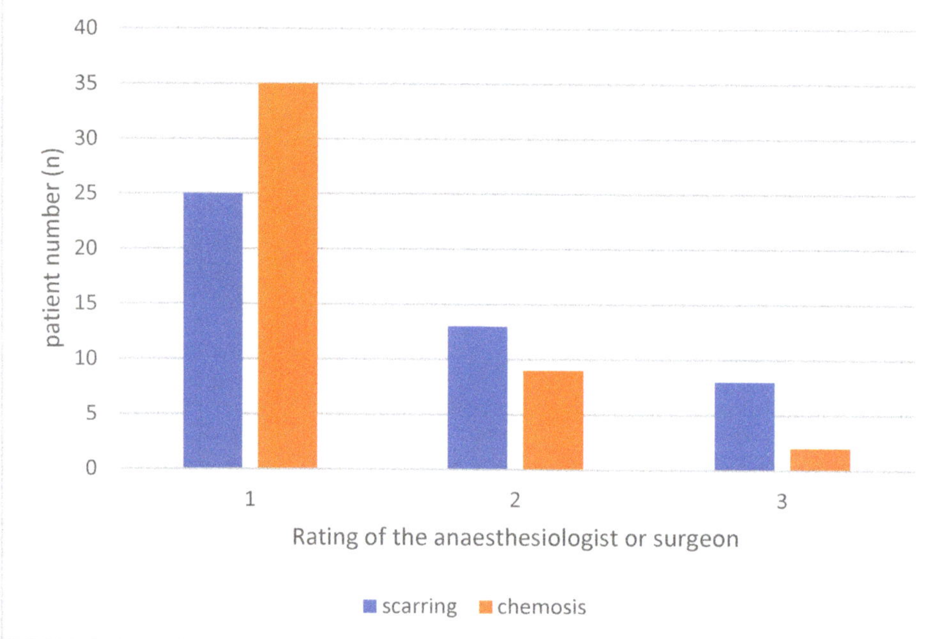

Figure 2. Scarring scaled from 1 to 3 (1 = easy, 2 = moderately difficult, 3 = difficult placement), chemosis after STB-administration also rated from 1 to 3 (1 = no chemosis, 2 = intermediate; 3 = heavy chemosis.

The surgeon performed the STB in 29 cases (63%), while an experienced anesthesiologist (FL) conducted the block in 19 cases (37%). Among these, the anesthesiologist independently administered the block in 17 cases, with the VR surgeon performing a top-up in 2 cases toward the end of the surgery. Clinician-reported technical difficulty ratings supported the feasibility objective. STB placement was rated as "easy" in 55% of cases, "moderately difficult" in 28%, and "difficult" in 17%. Higher difficulty ratings were associated with extensive scarring or band-related anatomical alterations. Chemosis occurred following block placement in 24% of cases, with severe chemosis observed in only two patients (4%). No statistical differences in performance were seen when the block was performed by the anesthetist vs. the surgeon ($p = 0.405$).

We also performed univariate regression analysis of the factors that influence block success. The results emphasize the importance of block difficulty and the absence of severe chemosis in determining the success of STB. Factors such as patient age and sex did not independently influence success, while the need for additional analgesia was indicative of reduced block efficacy (Table 2).

Table 2. Univariate logistic regression analysis of factors influencing sub-Tenon's block success. OR = Odds Ratio; CI = Confidence Interval; NS = Not Significant. Reference category for block difficulty is "Easy". Odds ratios represent the likelihood of block success compared to the reference group. A p-value of <0.05 indicates statistical significance. Predictors with "NS" were not significantly associated with block success.

Predictor		(OR)	95% (CI)	p-Value
Block Difficulty				
	Easy (ref)	--	--	--
	Moderate	0.85	0.55–1.30	**<0.001**
	Difficult	0.15	0.05–0.45	**<0.001**
Chemosis Severity		0.40	0.18–0.89	**0.02**
Patient Age		NS	NS	>0.1
Sex		NS	NS	>0.1
Need for Additional Analgesia		0.30	0.10–0.85	**0.01**

Bold values significant for $p < 0.005$.

A multivariate logistic regression model was not feasible due to the small sample size of 46 patients and the limited number of unsuccessful blocks ($n = 3$), which did not meet the requirement of at least 10 events per predictor variable. The skewed distribution of outcomes (93.5% success rate) further limited the model's ability to assess multiple predictors reliably. Sparse data in certain categories, such as "difficult" blocks and severe chemosis, compounded the issue by resulting in unstable estimates. To avoid overfitting and unreliable conclusions, we chose univariate logistic regression only to evaluate individual predictors.

Most patients (67%) received STB with analgosedation for both the block administration and the surgery, while 32% underwent general anesthesia (GA) in addition to the STB. A titrated approach was used for sedation, including propofol (mean dose 58 mg), fentanyl (mean 68 mcg), and dexmedetomidine (mean 11 mcg), with ketamine used in six cases (mean 16 mg). Only one patient required unplanned GA due to agitation from alcohol withdrawal; this case had a scar tissue rating of 3/3.

Overall, patient satisfaction with the anesthesia technique was high (Figure 3); patient satisfaction, a secondary objective, was high, with a median satisfaction score of 5 (on a scale of 1–5) reported immediately postoperatively. However, patients with more challenging blocks demonstrated slightly lower satisfaction scores, reflecting the impact of technical difficulties on patient experience.

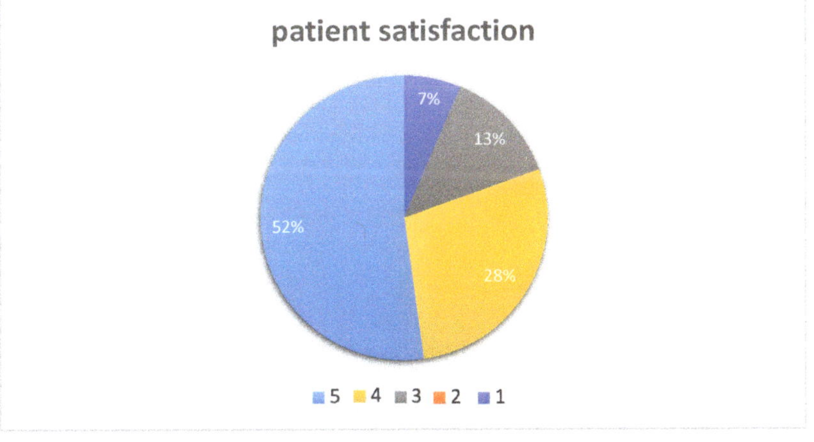

Figure 3. Patient satisfaction after surgery, 5 = completely satisfied, 4 = very satisfied, 3 = satisfied, 2 = dissatisfied, 1 = very dissatisfied.

Most patients reported being very satisfied or satisfied, affirming STB as a feasible and effective approach for this patient cohort.

4. Discussion

This study provides preliminary and descriptive data on the use of sub-Tenon's block (STB) in patients with prior encircling band surgery, highlighting its feasibility and safety. The STB effectively provided adequate anesthesia for vitreoretinal surgeries in most patients with prior encircling band surgery, with a low failure rate. Only two cases required additional intervention, and just one case needed unplanned conversion to general anesthesia. The administration of STB in patients with altered ocular anatomy due to scleral buckling was feasible, with 55% of cases rated as "easy" for block placement, 28% as "moderately difficult", and only 17% as "difficult". Severe chemosis was rare, occurring in just 4% of cases. The majority of patients expressed high satisfaction with the procedure, indicating that STB with or without sedation is a well-tolerated and preferred anesthesia option for this specific group, even with the anatomical complexities involved. These results suggest that STB is a viable alternative to GA, even in patients with altered ocular anatomy from prior surgery.

With regards to the primary outcome, we can state that a high success rate of STBs over indwelling encircling bands amounts to preliminary proof of feasibility. As for secondary outcomes, patient satisfaction was high with regards to intra- and postoperative pain. It was suggestive that patients with extensive scarring obtained insufficient analgesia. It can only be surmised that the two patients needing top-ups at the end of their surgery probably had patchy distributions of their blocks caused by encircling bands.

The use of STB in myopic eyes with previous scleral buckling poses unique challenges. Altered anatomy, particularly elongation of the globe, increases the risks associated with sharp-needle blocks, such as retrobulbar or peribulbar techniques. Dissection of scar tissue can lead to bulbar injury if strict visualization of ocular layers is not painstakingly pursued [9]. Increased bulbar length and the encircling band create technical difficulties, potentially raising the risk of complications like globe perforation. Compared to these sharp-needle methods, the blunt cannula used in STB allows for safer administration of local anesthetic, minimizing the risk of needle-related injuries (see Figure 1). STB can be thought of as the only intrafascial block providing sufficiently reliably regional anesthesia for surgery. The impediment of the encircling band to free intrafascial flow towards sensible nerves of the eye most likely favours patchy blocks, as they often occur in other intrafascial regional anesthesia [10].

In our cohort, STB administration was generally well-tolerated, with no incidences of apnea or bradycardia during liberal sedation. The only exception involved a patient in alcohol withdrawal who developed delirium, requiring a switch to GA. While the sedative requirements were slightly higher than usual, the surgery proceeded undisturbed in most cases. Importantly, this study emphasizes the need for careful patient selection and meticulous technique when applying STB in eyes with prior encircling surgery.

Despite the promising results, anatomical considerations merit further discussion. The encircling band can alter the distribution of local anesthetic, potentially creating "patchy" blocks in the sub-Tenon's space divided by scar tissue or the band itself. This highlights the importance of having a surgeon and anesthesiologist prepared to address intraoperative pain with systemic medications, top-up local anesthesia, or alternative techniques like PBB.

Additionally, when STB is used in combination with GA for postoperative analgesia, clinicians must monitor hemodynamic changes carefully. The transient increase in intraocular pressure (IOP) caused by the local anesthetic depot in the sub-Tenon's space could temporarily reduce retinal perfusion pressure, particularly in hypotensive patients [11]. Effective communication between anesthetists and surgeons is essential to identify and mitigate retinal perfusion deficits during surgery [12]. This hemodynamic concern may be more pronounced in previously encircled eyes due to their smaller sub-Tenon's compartments, warranting further investigation.

The role of ultrasound (US) in regional ophthalmic anesthesia, particularly in STB, warrants further exploration. While US is invaluable in sharp-needle techniques, such as retrobulbar and peribulbar blocks, for avoiding complications like scleral or staphyloma puncture in altered ocular anatomy, its benefits in STB remain debated [13,14]. The encircling band's contour is often visible under the conjunctiva and scar tissue, or it can be identified by tactile feedback using a conjunctival probe, negating the need for US guidance. Additionally, the band can be laid bare under a microscope in the surgical setting for further visualization. Incorporating US into STB poses unique challenges, including difficulty in visualizing the curved cannula, the thin tissue layer between the probe and cannula, and the risk of artifacts caused by metal and plastic components. These practical considerations, combined with the already high success rate of STB in this study, suggest that routine use of US may not be necessary. However, future research could evaluate whether US provides significant benefits in complex cases or for less experienced clinicians [5,15].

Overall, our findings suggest that STB is a feasible and safe alternative for patients with prior encircling band surgery. However, the technical challenges and physiological considerations underscore the importance of clinician expertise and real-time intraoperative management [16]. Further studies are needed to validate these findings and address the potential limitations posed by altered anatomy in this unique patient population.

The myopic eye poses distinct risks in the planning of locoregional anesthesia, especially sharp-needle blocks. Increased bulbar length is a significant limitation for retrobulbar blocks, as angulation of the needle with the orbital rim as a bevel point may increase the risk of bulbar perforation in the back of the eye.

Discussing our results in light of the preexisting literature is difficult given the prevailing scarcity of papers addressing this specific problem. Prior encircling is an independent risk factor for globe penetration, as found in a retrospective study evaluating this complication in patients undergoing retrobulbar and peribulbar blocks [7]. One case reported globe perforation during scissor-dissection of tissue while undertaking sub-Tenon's in a previously encircled eye [9].

This study had limitations: As a retrospective cohort study, it is subject to biases related to data collection and lacks the control over variables that a prospective study would offer. This limits the ability to draw definitive causal inferences. With only 46 patients included, the sample size is relatively small, which may reduce the generalizability of the findings and limits the power to detect rare complications or differences across subgroups. This study was conducted at a single institution, which may limit the applicability of the results to other settings with different patient populations, clinician expertise, or procedural protocols. The STB was performed by both vitreoretinal surgeons and anesthesiologists, which introduces variability in technique and experience. This may influence the observed success rates and complication rates of the procedure. This study primarily focuses on intraoperative outcomes and immediate postoperative satisfaction without assessing long-term outcomes or potential late complications associated with STB in patients with previous encircling band surgery.

These limitations suggest that further research, ideally through a larger, multicenter prospective study, would be beneficial to validate these findings and better understand the risks and benefits of STB in this patient population.

5. Conclusions

In conclusion, this study provides valuable preliminary data supporting the feasibility and safety of sub-Tenon's block (STB) as an effective anesthesia option for patients with prior scleral buckling surgery. Despite the anatomical challenges posed by scleral buckling, STB demonstrated a low failure rate, with the majority of patients experiencing successful block placement and high satisfaction with the procedure. The use of STB offers a viable alternative to general anesthesia (GA) with minimal complications.

However, the technical difficulties and potential for altered anesthetic distribution due to scar tissue or the encircling band highlight the importance of careful patient selection and expert execution. Additionally, while the STB technique was generally well-tolerated, clinicians must remain vigilant to the physiological challenges associated with altered ocular anatomy, particularly in managing intraoperative pain, hemodynamic changes, and retinal perfusion concerns.

Given this study's retrospective nature, small sample size, and the single-center design, further investigation through larger, multicenter, and prospective studies is desirable to validate these findings.

Author Contributions: Conceptualization, F.L. and J.H.; methodology, F.L.; software, J.B.-E.; validation, A.E., J.B.-E.; formal analysis, A.E., F.L. and J.H.; investigation, F.L. and J.H.; resources, A.E., J.B.-E. and F.L.; data curation, J.B.-E.; writing—original draft preparation, F.L. and J.H.; writing—review and editing, all authors; visualization, J.B.-E. and G.U. All authors have read and agreed to the published version of the manuscript.

Funding: This research received no external funding.

Institutional Review Board Statement: The study was conducted in accordance with the Declaration of Helsinki, and approved by the Institutional Review Board (or Ethics Committee) of the Cantonal Ethics Committee of Bern (KEK Bern) Switzerland (Chairperson Prof. em. Dr. med. Christian Seiler, BASEC-number: Req-2020-01360, approval date: 23 November 2020). Patients provided informed consent for both the sub-Tenon's block procedure under analgosedation and the ophthalmic surgery itself. Additionally, patients consented to the anonymised data analysis and the subsequent publication of the study results.

Informed Consent Statement: Informed consent was obtained from all subjects involved in the study.

Data Availability Statement: The data presented in this study are available on request from the corresponding author. The data are not publicly available due to data protection and ethical regulations, as patients were not specifically consented for data-analysis by third parties.

Conflicts of Interest: The authors declare no conflict of interest.

References

1. Hamilton, G.S. Aerosol-generating procedures in the COVID era. *Respirology* **2021**, *26*, 416. [CrossRef] [PubMed]
2. Nouvellon, E.; Cuvillon, P.; Ripart, J. Regional anesthesia and eye surgery. *Anesthesiology* **2010**, *113*, 1236–1242. [CrossRef] [PubMed]
3. Kumar, C.M.; Seet, E.; Chua, A.W.Y. Updates in ophthalmic anaesthesia in adults. *BJA Educ.* **2023**, *23*, 153–159. [CrossRef] [PubMed]
4. Chua, M.J.; Lersch, F.; Chua, A.W.Y.; Kumar, C.M.; Eke, T. Sub-Tenon's anaesthesia for modern eye surgery—Clinicians' perspective, 30 years after re-introduction. *Eye* **2021**, *35*, 1295–1304. [CrossRef] [PubMed]
5. Palte, H.D. Ophthalmic regional blocks: Management, challenges, and solutions. *Local Reg. Anesth.* **2015**, *8*, 57–70. [CrossRef] [PubMed]
6. Kumar, C.M.; Dowd, T.C. Complications of ophthalmic regional blocks: Their treatment and prevention. *Ophthalmologica* **2006**, *220*, 73–82. [CrossRef] [PubMed]
7. Hay, A.; Flynn, H.W.; Hoffman, J.I.; Rivera, A.H. Needle Penetration of the Globe during Retrobulbar and Peribulbar Injections. *Ophthalmology* **1991**, *98*, 1017–1024. [CrossRef] [PubMed]
8. Chronopoulos, A. Complications of Encircling Bands-Prevention and Management. *J. Clin. Exp. Ophthalmol.* **2015**, *6*, 440. [CrossRef]
9. Frieman, B.J.; Friedberg, M.A. Globe perforation associated with subtenon's anesthesia. *Am. J. Ophthalmol.* **2001**, *131*, 520–521. [CrossRef] [PubMed]
10. Juhl, C.S.; Rothe, C.; Støving, K.; Aasvang, E.K.; Rosenstock, C.V.; Lange, K.H.W.; Lundstrøm, L.H. Intraindividual variation of the transversus abdominis plane block: An exploratory study in healthy volunteers. *Reg. Anesth. Pain Med.* **2020**, *45*, 419–423. [CrossRef] [PubMed]
11. Kelly, D.J.; Farrell, S.M. Physiology and Role of Intraocular Pressure in Contemporary Anesthesia. *Anesth. Analg.* **2018**, *126*, 1551–1562. [CrossRef]
12. Sohn, H.J.; Moon, H.S.; Nam, D.H.; Paik, H.J. Effect of volume used in sub-Tenon's anesthesia on efficacy and intraocular pressure in vitreoretinal surgery. *Ophthalmologica* **2008**, *222*, 414–421. [CrossRef] [PubMed]
13. Luyet, C.; Eichenberger, U.; Moriggl, B.; Remonda, L.; Greif, R. Real-time visualization of ultrasound-guided retrobulbar blockade: An imaging study. *Br. J. Anaesth.* **2008**, *101*, 855–859. [CrossRef] [PubMed]
14. Sadler, A.; McLeod, G.; McHardy, P.G.; Wilkinson, T. Ultrasound detection of iatrogenic injury during peribulbar eye block: A cadaveric study. *Reg. Anesth. Pain Med.* **2020**, *45*, 740–743. [CrossRef] [PubMed]

15. Lersch, F.; Schnidrig, D.; Boemke, S.; Djonov, V.; Jaggi, D.; Heussen, F.M. Thiel cadaver eye as a training model for sub-Tenon's blocks: A feasibility study. *BMC Ophthalmol.* **2024**, *24*, 391. [CrossRef] [PubMed]
16. Mavrakanas, N.A.; Stathopoulos, C.; Schutz, J.S. Are ocular injection anesthetic blocks obsolete? Indications and guidelines. *Curr. Opin. Ophthalmol.* **2011**, *22*, 58–63. [CrossRef] [PubMed]

Journal of
Clinical Medicine

MDPI

Review

Simulation in Regional Anaesthesia: A Narrative Review of Its History, Evolution and Future Prospects

Ashish Ranjan Satapathy [1], Iskandar Bin Khalid [2] and Shahridan Mohd Fathil [2,3,*]

[1] Department of Anaesthesia, Ng Teng Fong General Hospital, Singapore 609606, Singapore; satapathyashish@gmail.com
[2] Department of Anaesthesiology and Intensive Care, Hospital Canselor Tuanku Muhriz, Universiti Kebangsaan Malaysia, Kuala Lumpur 56000, Malaysia
[3] Department of Anaesthesiology, Gleneagles Hospital Johor, Iskandar Puteri 79250, Malaysia
* Correspondence: cooldoc1971@gmail.com

Abstract: Regional anaesthesia has seen a resurgence of sorts since the widespread advent of ultrasound into clinical practice. The ability to access hitherto inaccessible nerves and fascial planes in the human body whilst ensuring visualisation of the needle tip during block performance has opened the proverbial floodgates leading to its widespread adoption, further supported by a growing body of evidence for its many benefits in a patient's perioperative journey and pain management. The concomitant advancement of technology and the development of powerful simulation and artificial intelligence tools has given a much-needed impetus towards improving training and safe practice in regional anaesthesia. Methods: We performed a detailed search of databases, including PubMed Medline, Web of Science, EBSCO, Embase and the Cochrane Library, up to October 2024. Our search was conducted using phrases including (but not limited to) "history of anaesthesia", "history of simulation", "regional anaesthesia and simulation", AI and "artificial intelligence and anaesthesia".

Keywords: regional anaesthesia; simulation; simulation in regional anaesthesia; AI and artificial intelligence

1. Introduction

Regional anaesthesia (RA) has long been the cornerstone of anaesthesia practice. RA, when used alone or in combination with GA, has been shown to provide improved perioperative analgesia [1–4], decreased post-operative complications [5–8], increased patient satisfaction [1,9] and an additional benefit of reduced cost [10,11]. In spite of these glaring advantages, RA, until fairly recently, has been an art practised by a dedicated and privileged few [12,13]. Limitations of ultrasound technology resulting in the inability to visualise the target nerve, the approaching needle and vital structures in the vicinity of the target had put this now invaluable asset on the backburner for decades.

This pendulum shifted in 1994 when Steven Kapral revealed the sonoanatomy of the brachial plexus using B mode ultrasound [14], inadvertently unleashing this powerful tool for the benefit of all anaesthesiologists and catapulting ultrasound-guided regional anaesthesia (UGRA) to the forefront of anaesthesia practice. Once the floodgates opened, there was no dearth of newer generations of ultrasound machines featuring superior resolution, features and portability, improved echogenic needles and enthusiastic clinicians who set out to stamp their authority in this emerging field [15].

Nevertheless, despite the widespread use of ultrasound in RA, the incidence of RA-related complications did not drastically decline as expected [16]. Conversely, there was an initial increase in case reports of unexpected complications [17–19], likely a consequence of the increasing number of blocks performed and the over-enthusiastic adoption and application of ultrasound for more challenging blocks.

Clinicians soon realised that attaining proficiency in UGRA requires a steep learning curve in comparison to traditional nerve-stimulation and landmark-based techniques due to the greater number of variables affecting successful block performance. In addition to sound anatomical knowledge, clinicians now needed to acquire an additional understanding of the sonoanatomy of each block, principles of practical ultrasonography, as well as the ability to mentally depict three-dimensional images from the two-dimensional picture seen on screen, recognize artefacts, and exclude background noise [20–23]. Furthermore, honing motor skills was required to improve hand-eye coordination, an essential skill for in-plane and out-of-plane needle alignment with the ultrasound probe whilst simultaneously maintaining focus on the target structure in the ultrasound image [24]. With ever-changing technology, the tools and techniques used in UGRA training have evolved to meet this required level of coordination between sensory and motor skills. Over the last decade or so, UGRA training has grown to incorporate high-fidelity simulation to ensure the next generation of RA practitioners are able to effectively use the powerful tools now at their disposal.

2. Why Do We Need Simulation in Healthcare

A 2013 patient-safety report from the United States revealed some alarming statistics: preventable medical errors have resulted in more than 400,000 yearly deaths, making it the third leading cause of mortality in the country [25]. Moreover, iatrogenic medical errors have resulted in 3.5 million per year experiencing permanent harm and disability in the United States [25]. The authors from the "Journal of Patient Safety" even went on to opine that:

> *"One of the main reasons for such alarming statistics may be related to the medical education culture. Since the Flexner report [26], many advances have been made in technology and teaching strategies; however, it is still not unusual for medical students to be taught almost the same way they were decades ago. Evidence-based methodology, patient safety, andragogy, accessible, high-quality media production, computers, smartphones, the Internet, 3D printers, high and low-fidelity mannequins—most of this is basically not taken into consideration when defining the curriculum and the pedagogical methods to shape and enhance the background of future health care professionals".*

The aerospace industry, where there is little margin for error akin to the healthcare industry, has quickly embraced many of the advances in simulation-based learning models, leading to a shift in safety rating of "risky" towards the end of the 1950s to "safer" in short period of several years [27]. Aviation simulation dates back to 1929 when Edwin Albert Link was the first to invent a flight simulator, a prototype model he coined the "Blue Box". This novel simulator was a fuselage-like device consisting of a cockpit and a control interface [28], which was later marketed as the "Pilot Maker". The simulator's ability to replicate flying motions and sensations enabled Link to train his own brother to pilot an aircraft within the same year. The year 1934 saw a series of American postal carriers' crashes attributed to pilot error in "poor meteorological conditions", which continued despite the contracting of the US Army Air Corps [29]. It was during this time that attention turned to the Link Pilot Maker, which, once utilised, produced results which were astounding, to say the least; pilot preparedness in the face of adverse weather conditions was significantly improved, and the number of accidents decreased dramatically. As a result, the simulator quickly became a mandatory component of pilot training in numerous countries [30,31]. The success of the Blue Box/Pilot Maker provided concrete evidence that simulation-based training (SBT) could be successfully applied in many human endeavours. It became apparent that simulated flight provided a controlled and protected environment where trainee pilots could be subjected to simulated high-risk scenarios that would not have been possible without endangering invaluable lives. In addition, the training was standardized, reproducible and could mimic real-world conditions with increasing levels of complexity, which allowed pilots with varying competence levels to attain flight proficiency and preparedness for adverse weather conditions. Repeated exposure to such situations in a simulated environment made the "learning objective" part of their subconscious, and they were able to spontaneously maintain a similar level of performance in live crisis situations. While the healthcare industry was slow to adopt simulation training as part of the curriculum, the aerospace industry, despite its relatively young age, has swiftly set SBT as the mandated standard for the training of pilots and other aviators [32].

3. Application of Simulation in Healthcare

It had become apparent from the damning 2013 patient safety report [18] that current pedagogical methods of training had become obsolete. Even before the aforementioned report, Choy et al. had remarked that the traditional concept of didactic teaching and the "see one- do one- teach one" approach had proven to be inconsistent, ineffective, time-consuming and an expensive model for teaching complex procedures to surgical trainees [33]. This belief has since been found to be equally applicable to all branches of medicine where complex procedural skills are required, including anaesthesia and intensive care.

In a BMJ article published in 2008 titled "Teaching Procedural skills", Grantcharav and Reznick aptly wrote [34]:

> *"See one, do one is no longer appropriate for educating health professionals to perform complex procedures. Graduated independence, the hallmark of the approach to teaching procedural skills, is being challenged by concerns for patient safety, the skyrocketing complexity of procedures, and a diminishing work week for trainees. Finding the balance between patient safety and physician training will require a more structured approach to our skills curriculum, including continuous assessment of skills, constructive feedback, and provision of opportunities for deliberate practice in the teaching environment."*

Simulation ensures delivery of this "teaching environment", which is safe, controlled, repeatable and reproducible, where problem-based learning is practised, and competences are developed to a high standard, ensuring the patient is protected from the novice learner. The authors further recommended that three sets of essential skills should be mandatory components as part of "Pre-Patient Training" in any high-procedural-skill speciality and that they should be done outside the clinical setting to protect patients. These include the following:

- Gaining a cognitive understanding of the specific procedure, including its steps, the function and the operation of the associated equipment.
- Receiving training in fundamental, generic enabling skills necessary for the procedure.
- Opportunity to carry out the procedure across multiple platforms, including virtual reality, bench model simulators, cadavers and live animal models.

The use of SBT in UGRA addresses the 3rd aspect of the required skill set described above by facilitating target image acquisition and identification and improving needling techniques via improved hand-eye coordination.

4. Why Do We Need Simulation in Regional Anaesthesia

RA, with its inherent procedural complexities, has not been immune to the deficiencies in teaching and training described above. The ASA Closed Claims Project, which serves as a reporting system that offers an indirect evaluation of anaesthesia practice safety in the United States, in its 1999 report, found that though the incidence of death and brain damage had started to decline from the 70s to the 90s, the incidence of non-fatal nerve injury had actually increased from 15 to 18% [35]. Though the Project represented a national quality-assurance system, albeit without a denominator, the closed claims data uncovered significant and previously overlooked aspects of adverse anaesthetic outcomes, including nerve injury. Focused teaching and training in airway techniques had led to a reduction in airway-related critical incidents and patient harm in the decades prior to the report, but the same outcome was not seen in the field of RA. This again highlighted the issue of lack of structured training in RA and the importance of practising blocks in simulated environments to reduce patient harm. The parallel advent of ultrasound at this time had necessitated the acquisition of a new set of skills with a steep learning curve, and educators soon realised that this had to be imparted at an early stage for anaesthesia trainees to have a meaningful impact on the quality of RA training and reducing patient harm. Hence, began the arduous task of identifying areas of RA training that anaesthesia trainees were lacking and where simulation could make a difference.

One such study from 2006 involved six anaesthesia residents who performed 520 peripheral nerve blocks on live patients over a one-month period [36]. Five quality-compromising behaviours were identified: (a) inability to recognize local anaesthetic maldistribution, (b) inability to detect an intramuscularly sited needle tip, (c) fatigue, (d) inability to synchronize patient and image laterality and (e) inappropriate selection of needle insertion site and angle relative to the probe, leading to poor needle visualisation. The two commonest errors identified in the study were the inability to achieve needle visualisation prior to needle advancement and non-intentional movements of the ultrasound probe. Based on the analysis of the committed errors and identification of quality-compromising behaviours, the authors identified key learning objectives for future training and simulation programs.

In a more recent review covering 28 studies from 2009 to 2023, Ashokka and colleagues looked specifically at the "educational outcomes related to the implementation of simulation in RA" [37]. Though the simulation platforms were heterogeneous, they discovered that two studies actually achieved reduced incidence of paraesthesia and clinical complications. What was even more encouraging to see was that the improvements in Lab settings and Clinical settings were seen in 12 and 11 studies, respectively, which accounted for 82% of the studies included. Furthermore, knowledge improvements and self-reported improvement in confidence were seen in 2 and 1 study, respectively. They have inferred from the available evidence that with the use of hybrid simulation techniques, we should be able to achieve sustained improvements beyond 6 months.

5. Simulators in Regional Anaesthesia Training

Simulators for the purposes of RA training have traditionally been classified into two groups based on fidelity, defined as the degree of exactness with which something is copied or reproduced [38]:

1. Low Fidelity: also called Part-task trainers. Models vary from simple homemade gelatin or agar constructs to fresh frozen cadavers. A prospective observational study comparing the commercial Blue Phantom model [39] with homemade gelatin and tofu models showed that after the costs of each model were considered, participants preferred the gelatin model despite the seemingly greater fidelity of the Blue Phantom [40].

Recently, with the introduction of 3D printing technology, it has been possible to print custom-made parts of the human body on which specific and simple tasks can be practiced and taught to trainees. Such models are invaluable for attaining spatial orientation to three-dimensional structures such as the deeper nerves and neuraxial blocks [41]. Another low fidelity but invaluable model available in recent times are Thiel cadavers, a form of flexible, soft-embalmed cadavers which feature acoustic and hydro dissection properties similar to that in vivo, yet with the advantage of greater durability compared to fresh frozen cadavers [42]. Widespread use of Thiel cadavers has been limited by cost, and there is evidence to suggest that meat-based phantom models are as effective as fresh frozen cadavers for teaching ultrasound-guided needling to novice practitioners [43]. This suggests that cheaper, cost-effective models can be used effectively for part-task training as long as the training objectives are suitably matched.

2. High Fidelity: also called Complex-task trainers. High-fidelity simulators usually involve multiple tasks and are either mannikin-based, screen-based, role-play or a hybrid system incorporating features of all three. The mannikin-based simulators can be used to run simulation scenarios for unanticipated adverse events related to RA, such as local anaesthetic systemic toxicity (LAST), with the scope to incorporate advanced life support while providing ample opportunity for observation and feedback. Screen-based simulators are used to teach anatomy, sonoanatomy and three-dimensional spatial orientation of complex structures. Currently, there are several high-fidelity simulators available on the market that can simulate the performance of central neuraxial blocks, intermediate and deep peripheral nerve blocks and even interfascial plane blocks (e.g., BlockSim®). Torrano et al. studied the utility of SBT as part of a 4-h RA training workshop where first-year anaesthesia residents were given two attempts on a high-fidelity erector spinae plane (ESP) block simulator, first without previous practice and second at the end of the course [44]. Their proficiency in UGRA appeared to be immediately enhanced as their second attempt yielded significant improvements in time to block performance, number of needle insertions and ability to accurately aim at the ESP.

High-fidelity simulators utilizing immersive virtual environments such as augmented reality (AR) and virtual reality (VR) have also significantly increased in popularity in recent years [45]. While AR complements and enhances the real world by overlaying digital objects onto the user's surroundings, VR immerses the user in an entirely separate digital environment, often with a head-mounted display unit and hand-held motion controllers, which allow interaction with the virtual environment. Proponents argue that VR-based simulators can facilitate RA training without geographic constraints and limitations, thus avoiding the financial, temporal and environmental costs of travel while presenting no safety risks to patients [46]. Additionally, data regarding the learner's performance can be easily stored and analysed for assessment and feedback at a later date. Nevertheless, Chuan et al., in a recent randomised controlled trial, found that RA novices who were trained using a program based on a virtual reality simulator designed and validated by the same team were not superior to those trained using a conventional teaching program in terms of a global rating or composite error score [47].

The use of high and low fidelity does not capture the entire gamut of available simulators. To mirror this sentiment, a new method of classification has been proposed [48]:

1. Physical fidelity: the simulator looks and feels real (e.g., an intravenous cannulation hand model)

2. Functional fidelity: the simulator might look different but achieves the purpose (is functional) of part-task training (e.g., using a banana to simulate loss of resistance during epidural insertion)
3. Psychological fidelity: produces an effect on the user identical to the actual experience and includes role play and hybrid simulation models.

High fidelity in all aspects is not required for effective simulation training. However, it is crucial to align the level of fidelity with the intended learning objectives. An alternative to an expensive high-fidelity model would be a series of part-task training models designed to teach a particular task along the continuum. When simulation training is more expensive and resource-intensive than traditional didactic teaching, a curriculum blending both educational modalities may offer the most cost-effective strategy. Available evidence strongly suggests the importance of incorporating simulation in RA training in some form or another to achieve a certain level of competence before its application to live patients [49]. A meta-analysis of simulation vs. non-simulation training by Cook et al. showed improvement in all measurable learning outcomes, such as time taken, procedural flow, and successful task completion. In this study, simulation was found to be most effective in developing technical and professional skills as opposed to enhancing theoretical knowledge [50]. Review articles and a systematic review have also confirmed the usefulness of simulation when integrated into RA teaching [51–53] with the advancement of technology and incorporation of artificial intelligence (AI) into all aspects of life, including healthcare, we should aim to take advantage of the opportunities to develop powerful but cost-effective tools to train our next generation of RA practitioners. We agree with Chen et al., who argued that the RA fraternity should come together to a consensus and adopt standardized 'core outcome sets', which will act as a framework for RA simulation research and ensure greater standardization of studies for systematic reviews in the future [53].

6. Artificial Intelligence in Regional Anaesthesia

Artificial intelligence (AI) is an area of computer science focusing on techniques that enable computers to mimic human intelligence [54]. With the development of quantum computing and exponential growth in computational speed, AI has evolved from its initial "replication" stage into being an autonomous, self-learning and adapting tool. Due to the ability of computers to process big data and breeze through millions of algorithms at a fraction of a second in real-time, these machines can perform complex tasks, identify and warn about deviations from the norm, suggest corrective measures that can aid decision-making whilst remaining indefatigable and ready to be used for the next task at the click of a button. There lies ample opportunity for the use of AI in RA to assist in training, pattern recognition, needle-tracking, haptic feedback, visualisation of LA spread, recognition of injection pressures and overall decision-making. The use of AI in RA has been studied in the following areas:

1. **Needle tip guidance systems**: Hand-eye coordination and real-time needle tip visualisation remain one of the most difficult aspects of RA to teach and master [24]. In a study conducted on anaesthetists and novice medical students, McLeod and colleagues demonstrated that the use of a novel needle-tip tracking system led to improved needle tip visualisation, needle alignment to the ultrasound transducer and needle advancement, with 75% of subjects showing enhanced performance over time with tracking technology [55]. More recent studies have added further credence to novel needle guidance systems and their utility in training [56–59].
2. **Augmented reality systems**:
    a. **Motion**: One of the most important aspects of RA training is gaining proficiency in the fine motor skills needed for safe needling. The Imperial College surgical

assessment device (ICSAD), a validated system to analyze hand motion, has been widely used for objective assessment of technical skills during surgical training. The use of this tool in performing ultrasound-guided supraclavicular brachial plexus blocks showed notable differences in performance between RA experts and novices, including variations in time taken, number of movements, and path length travelled by each hand. Additionally, it demonstrated tangible improvements in the novices' performances as they progressed through their RA fellowship [60]. A different group of investigators studying hand-motion analysis to assess needle tip tracking technology on a pork phantom noted a decrease in the number of hand movements and path length, but this was observed only for out-of-plane blocks [57]. A similar improvement in hand movements and path lengths was also seen in a study on volunteers performing a lumbar plexus block with needle tip tracking [58]. Although hand motion analysis does provide valuable information about the role of hand movements for specific tasks, as well as the economy of movements and efficiency, it does not provide a comparable evaluation of hand-eye coordination. Tools have been developed to evaluate hand-eye coordination in UGRA using self-assessment video-based methods [24], but without a metric for visual attention, these assessments remain somewhat subjective.

b. **Vision**: Correlating anatomy with sonoanatomy and forming a spatial orientation of identified structures is a requisite skill in UGRA that takes time to develop. Novice RA practitioners primarily depend on a selective visual processing pathway, utilizing limited top-down processing [61]. Their visual search is a slow process involving a sequential examination of one feature at a time that aligns with their explicit expectations. Moreover, this depends on the extent of background knowledge of the trainee, [62] hence the importance of didactic teaching methods in addition to simulation training. In contrast, experts can integrate top-down knowledge with holistic visual pattern recognition (i.e., bottom-up saliency), creating an implicit priority map that allows for quicker and more precise visual scanning [63]. This also allows them to direct more attention to task-relevant areas in accordance with the information reduction hypothesis [64]. Eye-tracking, which was first studied in laparoscopy, radiology and pathology [65], has now been applied to UGRA to assess decision-making and attention allocation objectively. This technology can help identify the difficulties encountered by individual trainees, thus allowing for more focused attention while also being used to cluster trainee performance levels and track their learning curve. Recent technological innovations in this field include neural network-linked automatic calibration of glasses and software that offers real-time performance updates, which can be monitored over multiple nerve blocks. UGRA studies utilizing eye-tracking technology [66–68] show that eye movements can differentiate experienced RA practitioners from novices. Additionally, reflective feedback based on real-time performance has the potential to expedite the UGRA learning process.

c. **Touch**: While the scanning phase of UGRA depends largely on visual attention, needling skills rely on haptic feedback. An example of a haptic simulator is the Simulator of Anaesthesia for Loco-Regional Procedures (SAILOR) system, which uses three-dimensional rendering on a desk-mounted virtual system controlled by a mouse and keyboard [69]. However, validation for this device was limited to self-reported satisfaction scores. The Regional Anaesthesia Simulator and Assistant (RASimAs) system is another tool that combines virtual feedback using MRI or CT images of real patients with haptic feedback through grounded haptics [70]. On a wider scale, grounded kinesthetic haptics have provided a more realistic feedback experience, although this has not always translated to improved performance in areas such as laparoscopy [71,72]. Further progress has been made with ungrounded cutaneous haptics, which uses vibration feedback, and this approach has been employed with the Intuitive Surgical Da Vinci Standard robot (Intuitive Surgical, Inc., Sunnyvale, CA, USA), showing some evidence of improvement in performance [73].

3. **Robotic technology:** the use of mechanical robots in anaesthesia is still in its early stages, primarily explored in tracheal intubation and RA. A notable application is the Robotic Endoscope Automated Laryngeal Imaging for Tracheal Intubation (REALITI), which provides real-time image recognition and automated orientation for intubation [74]. Initial tests on mannequins showed that untrained individuals performed better with REALITI's automated mode than with manual control. Another example is the use of the DaVinci system for performing single-shot nerve blocks and inserting perineural catheters under ultrasound guidance on a phantom model [75]. The Magellan robotic system, designed for semi-automated UGRA, features an arm that holds a nerve block needle at its tip, controlled by a joystick and software system [76]. Nevertheless, excessive reliance on robotic assistance for RA training should be avoided as although it may reduce performance variability among trainees, it could ultimately undermine overall competence. Overreliance on such technology could present risks in emergencies or during equipment malfunction. Therefore, it is important to integrate robotic technology in RA as feedback tools that support and complement, rather than replace, the learning process.

Cognitive robots, also known as clinical decision support (CDS) systems, serve to complement the RA operator's skills and can be valuable in both training and clinical application. These systems fall into two main categories: rule-based expert systems, which rely on algorithms developed by specialists in the field, and machine learning systems, which improve by identifying recurring patterns in data from patient procedures [77]. An example is the SAFer Injection for Regional Anaesthesia (SAFIRA), an innovative device that eliminates the need for an assistant during nerve blocks while allowing for syringe aspiration and cessation of injection if the pressure exceeds 15 psi [78]. As these systems continue to evolve, they hold the potential to enhance the practice and safety of RA.

7. Barriers to Implementation of AI in Regional Anaesthesia

It is apparent that AI has immense potential to influence the way we teach, assess and perform RA techniques. Nonetheless, it is important to recognise the limitations and barriers to its implementation in our day-to-day practice:

1. **Governance**: In addition to ensuring stability and transparency, AI governance is crucial to account for the rapid changes that technological innovation brings. This is akin to clinical research, where ethical considerations alleviate potential harm by providing values and principles that guide researchers. Governance procedures should be adopted for AI, similar to governance frameworks for clinical trials. The Alan Turing Institute provides guidance on artificial intelligence ethics and safety; its framework of ethical values is referred to as the 'SUM values' [79]. These embrace respectfulness, openness, inclusivity and justice. Because AI systems lack accountability, the institute has developed 'FAST track principles' based on fairness (data, design, implementation, outcome accountability, sustainability (safety, accuracy, reliability, security, and robustness), and transparency in order to gain public trust. AI governance may also ensure

compliance with the regulatory bodies involved in healthcare, which ultimately need to be convinced of the utility of emerging high-fidelity simulation systems.

2. **Cost:** A significant barrier to the implementation of AI platforms in RA is the potential costs involved. While the costs can be justified over the longer term, in terms of potentially improved safety and reduction in medicolegal fees, the initial investment required remains substantial at present time. Furthermore, current evidence is mixed in this context. Machine learning and robotic assistance do not necessarily increase procedural efficiency, and the evidence for reducing learning curves is varied across surgical contexts [80]. Therefore, more evidence is needed to support the use of AI in RA across a wide range of techniques and trainee populations, in addition to a robust validation tool to evaluate these novel simulation systems.

8. Evaluation of Novel Simulation Systems

It is now apparent that SBT has become essential for the adoption of new technologies in RA. Nonetheless, a well-established validation tool for the evaluation of simulation training is crucial to ensure that the limited resources at our disposal are optimally utilised. One such validation tool is the "Kirkpatrick Model", a widely used, four-level training evaluation method that benefits both learners and educators by elucidating the value and impact a specific training has had on a team.

It was in 1959 when Donald Kirkpatrick first published his ideas about training evaluation [81]; then, in 1975, he further defined them in his book *Evaluating Training Programmes*, which received widespread attention and adoption of his methodology. In 2016 James Kirkpatrick further refined and updated the methodology in a revised edition titled "*Kirkpatrick's Four Levels of Training Evaluation*" [82]. Since then, the Kirkpatrick model has become an invaluable tool for the learning and development community to evaluate new models of training.

The four levels of Kirkpatrick's Evaluation Model (Figure 1) are:

1. **Reaction**: this involves the trainees and measures the extent to which they find the training agreeable, relevant and engaging. Their satisfaction levels are usually assessed using a feedback form, often referred to as a 'Happy Sheet'. The biggest advantage of this level of assessment is that it is quick, simple, cheap and easy to conduct.
2. **Learning**: this level gauges the gain in knowledge and capability experienced by the trainee by conducting and comparing pre- and post-learning assessments. These assessments can be conducted via exams or an interview-style evaluation. Like the previous level, this level is relatively easy to set up and is useful for assessing quantifiable skills.
3. **Behaviour**: this level assesses the trainee's application of the acquired knowledge and skills in a working environment. Compared to Levels 1 and 2, Level 3 requires a greater level of participation from trainees as well as prolonged observation by assessors to identify any changes in behaviour and whether the change is relevant and sustained.
4. **Results**: this final level of the original model measures the direct and overall impact of the trainee's performance on the business or working environment. This involves individual assessments against agreed goals and is the toughest of the 4 levels.

An additional level, Level 5, **Return of Investment (ROI)**, was added by Jack Phillips in 2003 [83], which guides learning and development practitioners on how to calculate the ROI of training using data gathered from Kirkpatrick's Level 4 Evaluation in a more actionable format. It is a measure of the cost-effectiveness of the overall training.

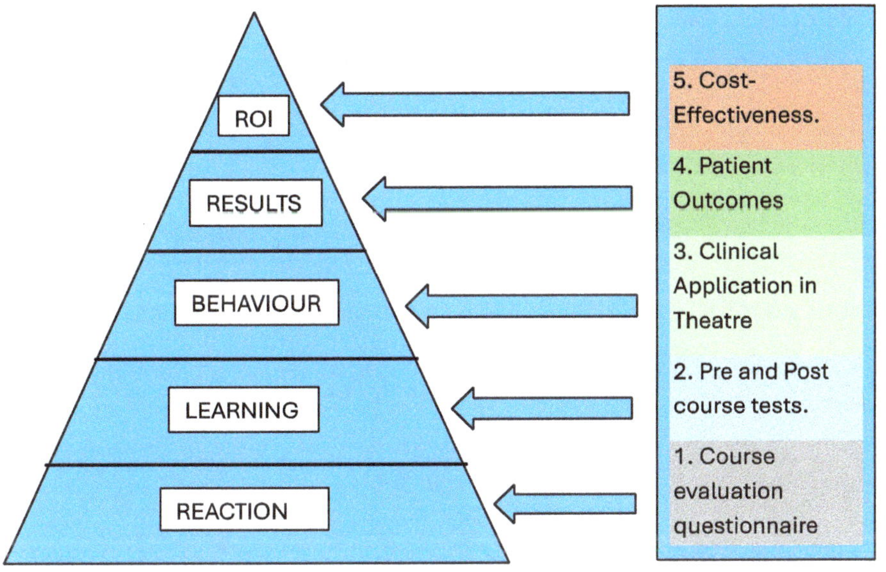

Figure 1. The Kirkpatrick Model as modified by Phillips.

9. Conclusions and Future Directions

With the innovations in simulation-based training, we currently bear witness to nothing short of another "industrial revolution" of sorts. Various branches of the sciences are amalgamating with digital technology to transform the field of medicine for the betterment of mankind. This transformation has already revolutionised the journey of medical trainees from the classroom to bedside patient care. Its implications for the advancement of education and training in regional anaesthesia are immense and may ultimately fulfil its promise of improving perioperative patient experiences and pain management.

Emerging evidence strongly suggests that AI platforms can be incorporated into tools not only for simulation training on cadavers, VR or AR models but also in actual performance of nerve blocks on patients to improve block outcomes as well as minimise injury and harm.

There exists concern that the skills acquired from SBT may not transfer to clinical practice; hence, further large-scale studies are vital to achieving ascension to level 5 of the Kirkpatrick Model (cost-effectiveness).

The need of the hour is wider acceptance, more multicentric trials and validation of AI training models to overcome the steep learning curve during RA training. We also need to recognise that technology is a double-edged sword for which we in the practice of medicine have been witness to time and again, hence the urgent need for a universal AI governance framework, akin to an ethics committee, to guide enthusiasts in the direction of "*primum non nocere*", our time-tested guiding principle.

We end this review with some pebbles of wisdom from Marhofer et al. [16]; "*There needs to be a balance between the evangelical fervour of the innovative enthusiast and the resistance of the clinical Luddite. Open minds, healthy scepticism, and a desire to work together are likely to benefit patients the most*".

Funding: This research received no external funding.

Institutional Review Board Statement: Not applicable.

Informed Consent Statement: Not applicable.

Data Availability Statement: Not applicable.

Conflicts of Interest: The authors declare no conflict of interest.

References

1. Hadzic, A.; Karaca, P.E.; Hobeika, P.; Unis, G.; Dermksian, J.; Yufa, M.; Claudio, R.; Vloka, J.D.; Santos, A.C.; Thys, D.M. Peripheral nerve blocks result in superior recovery profile compared with general anesthesia in outpatient knee arthroscopy. *Anesth. Analg.* **2005**, *100*, 976–981. [CrossRef] [PubMed]
2. Hadzic, A.; Arliss, J.; Kerimoglu, B.; Karaca, P.E.; Yufa, M.; Claudio, R.E.; Vloka, J.D.; Rosenquist, R.; Santos, A.C.; Thys, D.M. A comparison of infraclavicular nerve block versus general anesthesia for hand and wrist day-case surgeries. *Anesthesiology* **2004**, *101*, 127–132. [CrossRef] [PubMed]
3. Chelly, J.E.; David, B.; Williams, B.A.; Kentor, M.L. Anesthesia and postoperative analgesia: Outcomes following orthopedic surgery. *Orthopedics* **2003**, *26*, 865–871. [CrossRef] [PubMed]
4. Buist, R.J. A survey of the practice of regional anesthesia. *J. R. Soc. Med.* **1990**, *83*, 709–712. [CrossRef] [PubMed]
5. Moen, V.; Dahlgren, N.; Irestedt, L. Severe neurological complications after central neuraxial blockades in Sweden 1990–1999. *Anesthesiology* **2004**, *101*, 950–959. [CrossRef] [PubMed]
6. Borgeat, A.; Ekatodramis, G.; Kalberer, F.; Benz, C. Acute and nonacute complications associated with interscalene block and shoulder surgery: A prospective study. *Anesthesiology* **2001**, *95*, 875–880. [CrossRef] [PubMed]
7. Auroy, Y.; Narchi, P.; Messiah, A.; Litt, L.; Rouvier, B.; Samii, K. Serious complications related to regional anesthesia: Results of a prospective survey in France. *Anesthesiology* **1997**, *87*, 479–486. [CrossRef]
8. McCartney, C.J.; Brull, R.; Chan, V.W.; Katz, J.; Abbas, S.; Graham, B.; Nova, H.; Rawson, R.; Anastakis, D.J.; von Schroeder, H. Early but no long-term benefit of regional compared with general anesthesia for ambulatory hand surgery. *Anesthesiology* **2004**, *101*, 461–467. [CrossRef]
9. Hadzic, A.; Williams, B.A.; Karaca, P.E.; Hobeika, P.; Unis, G.; Dermksian, J.; Yufa, M.; Thys, D.M.; Santos, A.C. For outpatient rotator cuff surgery, nerve block anesthesia provides superior same-day recovery over general anesthesia. *Anesthesiology* **2005**, *102*, 1001–1007. [CrossRef] [PubMed]
10. Chan, V.W.; Peng, P.W.; Kaszas, Z.; Middleton, W.J.; Muni, R.; Anastakis, D.G.; Graham, B.A. A comparative study of general anesthesia, intravenous regional anesthesia, and axillary block for outpatient hand surgery: Clinical outcome and cost analysis. *Anesth. Analg.* **2001**, *93*, 1181–1184. [CrossRef] [PubMed]
11. Gonano, C.; Kettner, S.C.; Ernstbrunner, M.; Schebesta, K.; Chiari, A.; Marhofer, P. Comparison of economical aspects of interscalene brachial plexus blockade and general anaesthesia for arthroscopic shoulder surgery. *Br. J. Anaesth.* **2009**, *103*, 428–433. [CrossRef]
12. Grau, T.; Fatehi, S.; Motsch, J.; Bartusseck, E. Umfrage zur aktuellen Situation der Regionalanästhesie im deutschsprachigen Raum. Teil 2, Anwendung, Erfolgsraten und Techniken [Survey on current practice of regional anaesthesia in Germany, Austria, and Switzerland. Part 2, Use, success rates and techniques]. *Anaesthesist* **2004**, *53*, 847–855. [PubMed]
13. Smith, M.P.; Sprung, J.; Zura, A.; Mascha, E.; Tetzlaff, J.E. A survey of exposure to regional anesthesia techniques in American anesthesia residency training programs. *Reg. Anesth. Pain. Med.* **1999**, *24*, 11–16. [CrossRef]
14. Kapral, S.; Kraff, P.; Eibenberger, K.; Fitzgerald, M.; Gosh, R.; Weinstabl, C. Ultrasound guided regional anaesthesia approach for regional anaesthesia of the brachial plexus. *Anesth. Analg.* **1994**, *78*, 507–513. [CrossRef] [PubMed]
15. Sen, S.; Ge, M.; Prabhakar, A.; Moll, V.; Kaye, R.J.; Cornett, E.M.; Hall, O.M.; Padnos, I.W.; Urman, R.D.; Kaye, A.D. Recent technological advancements in regional anesthesia. *Best. Pract. Res. Clin. Anaesthesiol.* **2019**, *33*, 499–505. [CrossRef] [PubMed]
16. Marhofer, P.; Harrop-Griffiths, W.; Kettner, S.C.; Kirchmair, L. Fifteen years of ultrasound guidance in regional anaesthesia: Part 1. *Br. J. Anaesth.* **2010**, *104*, 538–546. [CrossRef] [PubMed]
17. Bigeleisen, P.E. Nerve puncture and apparent intraneural injection during ultrasound-guided axillary block does not invariably result in neurologic injury. *Anesthesiology* **2006**, *105*, 779–783. [CrossRef] [PubMed]
18. Bigeleisen, P.E. Ultrasound-guided infraclavicular block in an anticoagulated and anesthetized patient. *Anesth. Analg.* **2007**, *104*, 1285–1287. [CrossRef]
19. Borgeat, A.; Aguirre, J.; Neudorfer, C.; Jutzi, H. Severe brachial plexopathy after an ultrasound-guided single-injection nerve block for total shoulder arthroplasty in a patient with multiple sclerosis: What is the likely cause of this complication? *Anesthesiology* **2008**, *109*, 750–775. [CrossRef]
20. Niazi, A.U.; Haldipur, N.; Prasad, A.G.; Chan, V.W. Ultrasound-guided regional anesthesia performance in the early learning period: Effect of simulation training. *Reg. Anesth. Pain. Med.* **2012**, *37*, 51–54. [CrossRef] [PubMed]

21. Sites, B.D.; Chan, V.W.; Neal, J.M.; Weller, R.; Grau, T.; Koscielniak-Nielsen, Z.J.; Ivani, G.; American Society of Regional Anesthesia and Pain Medicine; European Society of Regional Anaesthesia and Pain Therapy Joint Committee. The American Society of Regional Anesthesia and Pain Medicine and the European Society of Regional Anaesthesia and Pain Therapy joint committee recommendations for education and training in ultrasound-guided regional anesthesia. *Reg. Anesth. Pain. Med.* **2010**, *35*, 74–80. [CrossRef] [PubMed]
22. Kim, S.; Hauser, S.; Staniek, A.; Weber, S. Learning curve of medical students in ultrasound-guided simulated nerve block. *J. Anesth.* **2014**, *28*, 76–80. [CrossRef]
23. de Oliveira Filho, G.R.; Helayel, P.E.; da Conceição, D.B.; Garzel, I.S.; Pavei, P.; Ceccon, M.S. Learning curves mathematical models for interventional ultrasound basic skills. *Anesth Analg.* **2008**, *106*, 568–573. [CrossRef] [PubMed]
24. Adhikary, S.D.; Hadzic, A.; McQuillan, P.M. Simulator for teaching hand-eye coordination during ultrasound-guided regional anaesthesia. *Br. J. Anaesth.* **2013**, *111*, 844–845. [CrossRef]
25. James, J.T. A new, evidence-based estimate of patient harms associated with hospital care. *J. Patient Saf.* **2013**, *9*, 122–128. [CrossRef] [PubMed]
26. Flexner, A. Medical Education in The United States and Canada. The Carnegie Foundation for the Advancement of Teaching. 1910. Available online: http://archive.carnegiefoundation.org/publications/pdfs/elibrary/Carnegie_Flexner_Report.pdf (accessed on 30 October 2024).
27. Bilotta, F.F.; Werner, S.M.; Bergese, S.D.; Rosa, G. Impact and implementation of simulation-based training for safety. *Sci. World J.* **2013**, *2013*, 652956. [CrossRef]
28. Edwin Link. Available online: http://www.nationalaviation.org/link-edwin (accessed on 10 August 2015).
29. Van der Linden, F. *Robert, Airlines and Air Mail: The Post Office and the Birth of the Commercial Aviation Industry*; University Press of Kentucky: Lexington, KY, USA, 2001.
30. Rosen, K.R. The history of medical simulation. *J. Crit. Care* **2008**, *23*, 157–166. [CrossRef] [PubMed]
31. Singh, H.; Kalani, M.; Acosta-Torres, S.; El Ahmadieh, T.Y.; Loya, J.; Ganju, A. History of simulation in medicine: From resusci annie to the ann myers medical center. *Neurosurgery* **2013**, *73* (Suppl. S4), 9–14. [CrossRef]
32. Cook, R.I.; Woods, D.D.; Miller, C. *A Tale of Two Stories: Contrasting Views of Patient Safety*; National Patient Safety Foundation: Chicago, IL, USA, 1997.
33. Choy, I.; Okrainec, A. Simulation in surgery: Perfecting the practice. *Surg. Clin. N. Am.* **2010**, *90*, 457–473. [CrossRef]
34. Grantcharov, T.P.; Reznick, R.K. Teaching procedural skills. *Br. Med. J.* **2008**, *336*, 1129–1131. [CrossRef] [PubMed]
35. Cheney, F.W. The American Society of Anesthesiologists Closed Claims Project: What Have We Learned, How Has It Affected Practice, and How Will It Affect Practice in the Future? *Anesthesiol. August* **1999**, *91*, 552–556. [CrossRef] [PubMed]
36. Sites, B.D.; Spence, B.C.; Gallagher, J.D.; Wiley, C.W.; Bertrand, M.L.; Blike, G.T. Characterizing novice behavior associated with learning ultrasound-guided peripheral regional anesthesia. *Reg. Anesth. Pain Med.* **2007**, *32*, 107–115. [CrossRef] [PubMed]
37. Ashokka, B.; Law, L.S.; Areti, A.; Burckett-St Laurent, D.; Zuercher, R.O.; Chin, K.J.; Ramlogan, R. Educational outcomes of simulation-based training in regional anaesthesia: A scoping review. *Br. J. Anaesth.* **2024**, *in press*. [CrossRef]
38. Fidelity. Merriam-Webster Dictionary. 2024. Available online: https://www.merriam-webster.com/dictionary/fidelity (accessed on 30 October 2024).
39. CAE Healthcare. Blue Phantom Ultrasound Training Medical Models. Available online: https://www.gtsimulators.com/collections/cae-blue-phantom-cae-healthcare/products/regional-anesthesia-ultrasound-training-block-bpnb150 (accessed on 2 June 2024).
40. Lahham, S.; Smith, T.; Baker, J.; Purdy, A.; Frumin, E.; Winners, B.; Wilson, S.P.; Gari, A.; Fox, J.C. Procedural simulation: Medical student preference and value of three task trainers for ultrasound guided regional anesthesia. *World J. Emerg. Med.* **2017**, *8*, 287–291. [CrossRef] [PubMed]
41. Bortman, J.; Baribeau, Y.; Jeganathan, J.; Amador, Y.; Mahmood, F.; Shnider, M.; Ahmed, M.; Hess, P.; Matyal, R. Improving clinical proficiency using a 3-dimensionally printed and patient specific thoracic spine model as a haptic task trainer. *Reg. Anesth. Pain Med.* **2018**, *43*, 819–824. [CrossRef] [PubMed]
42. Munirama, S.; Eisma, R.; Columb, M.; Corner, G.A.; McLeod, G.A. Physical properties and functional alignment of soft-embalmed Thiel human cadaver when used as a simulator for ultrasound guided regional anaesthesia. *Br. J. Anaesth.* **2016**, *116*, 699–707. [CrossRef] [PubMed]
43. Chuan, A.; Lim, Y.C.; Aneja, H.; Duce, N.A.; Appleyard, R.; Forrest, K.; Royse, C.F. A randomised controlled trial comparing meat-based with human cadaveric models for teaching ultrasound-guided regional anaesthesia. *Anaesthesia* **2016**, *71*, 921–929. [CrossRef]
44. Torrano, V.; Zadek, F.; Bugada, D.; Cappelleri, G.; Russo, G.; Tinti, G.; Giorgi, A.; Langer, T.; Fumagalli, R. Simulation-Based Medical Education and Training Enhance Anesthesia Residents' Proficiency in Erector Spinae Plane Block. *Front. Med.* **2022**, *9*, 870372. [CrossRef]

45. Tursø-Finnich, T.; Jensen, R.O.; Jensen, L.X.; Konge, L.; Thinggaard, E. Virtual Reality Head-Mounted Displays in Medical Education: A Systematic Review. *Simul. Healthc.* **2023**, *18*, 42–50. [CrossRef] [PubMed]
46. Orser, B.A.; Spadafora, S.M. Competence-Based Training and Immersion Virtual Reality: Paradigm-Shifting Advances in Medical Education. *Anesth. Analg.* **2022**, *135*, 220–222. [CrossRef] [PubMed]
47. Chuan, A.; Bogdanovych, A.; Moran, B.; Chowdhury, S.; Lim, Y.C.; Tran, M.T.; Lee, T.Y.; Duong, J.; Qian, J.; Bui, T.; et al. Using Virtual Reality to teach ultrasound-guided needling skills for regional anaesthesia: A randomised controlled trial. *J. Clin. Anesth.* **2024**, *97*, 111535. [CrossRef]
48. Stone, L.; Hellewell, S.A. Low cost simulation training in anaesthesia. *Update Anaesth.* **2014**, *29*, 44–46.
49. Maran, N.; Glavin, R. Low- to high-fidelity simulation—A continuum of medical education? *Med. Educ.* **2003**, *37*, 22–28. [CrossRef] [PubMed]
50. Cook, D.A.; Brydges, R.; Hamstra, S.J.; Zendejas, B.; Szostek, J.H.; Wang, A.T.; Erwin, P.J.; Hatala, R. Comparative effectiveness of technology-enhanced simulation versus other instructional methods: A systematic review and meta-analysis. *Simul. Healthc.* **2012**, *7*, 308–320. [CrossRef] [PubMed]
51. Udani, A.D.; Kim, T.E.; Howard, S.K.; Mariano, E.R. Simulation in teaching regional anesthesia: Current perspectives. *Local Reg. Anesth.* **2015**, *8*, 33–43.
52. Kim, T.E.; Tsui, B.C.H. Simulation-based ultrasound-guided regional anesthesia curriculum for anesthesiology residents. *Korean J. Anesthesiol.* **2019**, *72*, 13–23. [CrossRef] [PubMed]
53. Chen, X.X.; Trivedi, V.; AlSaflan, A.A.; Todd, S.C.; Tricco, A.C.; McCartney, C.J.L.; Boet, S. Ultrasound-guided regional anesthesia simulation training: A systematic review. *Reg. Anesth. Pain Med.* **2017**, *42*, 741–750. [CrossRef] [PubMed]
54. Bowness, J.; El-Boghdadly, K.; Burckett-St Laurent, D. Artificial intelligence for image interpretation in ultrasound-guided regional anaesthesia. *Anaesthesia* **2021**, *76*, 602–607. [CrossRef] [PubMed]
55. McLeod, G.A.; McKendrick, M.; Taylor, A.; Sadler, A.; Halcrow, J.; Mustafa, A.; Seeley, J.; Raju, P.; McKendrick, G. An initial evaluation of the effect of a novel regional block needle with tip-tracking technology on the novice performance of cadaveric ultrasound-guided sciatic nerve block. *Anaesthesia* **2020**, *75*, 80–88. [CrossRef]
56. McKendrick, M.; Sadler, A.; Taylor, A.; Seeley, J.; Filipescu, T.; Mustafa, A.; McKendrick, G.; Halcrow, J.; Raju, P.; McLeod, G.A. The effect of an ultrasound-activated needle tip tracker needle on the performance of sciatic nerve block on a soft embalmed Thiel cadaver. *Anaesthesia* **2020**, *76*, 209–217. [CrossRef] [PubMed]
57. Kåsine, T.; Romundstad, L.; Rosseland, L.A.; Ullensvang, K.; Fagerland, M.W.; Hol, P.K.; Kessler, P.; Sauter, A.R. Needle tip tracking for ultrasound-guided peripheral nerve block procedures—An observer blinded, randomised, controlled, crossover study on a phantom model. *Acta Anaesthesiol. Scand.* **2019**, *63*, 1055–1062. [CrossRef] [PubMed]
58. Kåsine, T.; Romundstad, L.; Rosseland, L.A.; Ullensvang, K.; Fagerland, M.W.; Kessler, P.; Bjørnå, E.; Sauter, A.R. The effect of needle tip tracking on procedural time of ultrasound-guided lumbar plexus block: A randomised controlled trial. *Anaesthesia* **2020**, *75*, 72–79. [CrossRef] [PubMed]
59. Mokhtar, M.N.; Suhaini, S.A.; Chan, W.K.; Khalid, I.; Tan, K.W.; Lim, A.C.C.; Budiman, M.; Samsudin, A.; Azizeh, A.; Madiman, V.V.S.; et al. Comparison of NeedleTrainer™ and ultrasound tissue simulator in a simulated environment among novice regional anaesthesia practitioners. *BMC Med. Educ.* **2024**, *24*, 1350. [CrossRef] [PubMed]
60. Chin, K.J.; Tse, C.; Chan, V.; Tan, J.S.; Lupu, C.M.; Hayter, M. Hand motion analysis using the imperial college surgical assessment device: Validation of a novel and objective performance measure in ultrasound-guided peripheral nerve blockade. *Reg. Anesth. Pain Med.* **2011**, *36*, 213–219. [CrossRef] [PubMed]
61. Wolfe, J.M.; Horowitz, T.S. What attributes guide the deployment of visual attention and how do they do it? *Nat. Rev. Neurosci.* **2004**, *5*, 495–501. [CrossRef] [PubMed]
62. Wolfe, J.M.; Vo, M.L.; Evans, K.; Greene, M. Visual search in scenes involves selective and nonselective pathways. *Trends Cogn. Sci.* **2011**, *15*, 77–84. [CrossRef] [PubMed]
63. Todd, R.M.; Manaligod, M.G.M. Implicit guidance of attention: The priority state space framework. *Cortex* **2018**, *102*, 121–138. [CrossRef]
64. Haider, H.; Frensch, P.A. Eye movement during skill acquisition: More evidence for the information reduction hypothesis. *J. Exp. Psychol. Learn. Mem. Cogn.* **1999**, *25*, 172–190. [CrossRef]
65. Ashraf, H.; Sodergren, M.H.; Merali, N.; Mylonas, G.; Singh, H.; Darzi, A. Eye-tracking technology in medical education: A systematic review. *Med. Teach.* **2018**, *40*, 62–69. [CrossRef] [PubMed]
66. Borg, L.K.; Harrison, T.K.; Kou, A.; Mariano, E.R.; Udani, A.D.; Kim, T.E.; Shum, C.; Howard, S.K.; ADAPT (Anesthesiology-Directed Advanced Procedural Training) Research Group. Preliminary experience using eye-tracking technology to differentiate novice and expert image interpretation for ultrasound-guided regional anesthesia. *J. Ultrasound Med.* **2018**, *37*, 329–336. [CrossRef] [PubMed]

67. Harrison, T.K.; Kim, T.E.; Kou, A.; Shum, C.; Mariano, E.R.; Howard, S.K.; ADAPT (Anesthesiology-Directed Advanced Procedural Training) Research Group. Feasibility of eye-tracking technology to quantify expertise in ultrasound-guided regional anesthesia. *J. Anesth.* **2016**, *30*, 530–533. [CrossRef]
68. McKendrick, M.-E.; Corner, G.; Tafili, T.; Obregón, M.; Kean, D.; Raju, P.; McLeod, G. Development of a progressive clinical expertise indicator for utrasound-guided regional anaesthesia. *Br. J. Anaesth.* **2016**, *116*, e938.
69. Bibin, L.; Lecuyer, A.; Burkhardt, J.; Delbos, A.; Bonnet, M. SAILOR: A 3-D medical simulator of loco-regional anaesthesia based on desktop virtual reality and pseudo-haptic feedback. In Proceedings of the VRST '08: 2008 ACM Symposium on Virtual Reality Software and Technology, Bordeaux, France, 27–28 October 2008; pp. 97–100.
70. Deserno, M.; D'Oliveira, J.; Grottke, O. Regional Anaesthesia Simulator and Assistant (RASimAs): Medical Image Processing Supporting Anaesthesiologists in Training and Performance of Local Blocks. In Proceedings of the IEEE 28th International Symposium on ComputerBased Medical Systems, Sao Carlos, Brazil, 22–25 June 2015; pp. 348–351.
71. Salkini, M.W.; Doarn, C.R.; Kiehl, N.; Broderick, T.J.; Donovan, J.F.; Gaitonde, K. The role of haptic feedback in laparoscopic training using the LapMentor II. *J. Endourol.* **2010**, *24*, 99–102. [CrossRef] [PubMed]
72. Våpenstad, C.; Hofstad, E.F.; Bø, L.E.; Kuhry, E.; Johnsen, G.; Mårvik, R.; Langø, T.; Hernes, T.N. Lack of transfer of skills after virtual reality simulator training with haptic feedback. *Minim. Invasive Ther. Allied Technol.* **2017**, *26*, 346–354. [CrossRef] [PubMed]
73. Pacchierotti, C.; Prattichizzo, D.; Kuchenbecker, K.J. Cutaneous feedback of fingertip deformation and vibration for palpation in robotic surgery. *IEEE Trans. Biomed. Eng.* **2016**, *63*, 278–287. [CrossRef] [PubMed]
74. Boehler, Q.; Gage, D.; Hofmann, P.; Gehring, A.; Chautems, C.; Spahn, D.; Biro, P.; Nelson, B. REALITI: A Robotic Endoscope Automated via Laryngeal Imaging for Tracheal Intubation. *IEEE Trans. Med. Robot. Bionics* **2020**, *2*, 157–164. [CrossRef]
75. Tighe, P.J.; Badiyan, S.J.; Luria, I.; Boezaart, A.P.; Parekattil, S. Robot-Assisted Regional Anesthesia: A Simulated Demonstration. *Anesth. Analg.* **2010**, *111*, 813–816. [CrossRef] [PubMed]
76. Hemmerling, T.M.; Taddei, R.; Wehbe, M.; Cyr, S.; Zaouter, C.; Morse, J. First Robotic Ultrasound-Guided Nerve Blocks in Humans Using the Magellan System. *Anesth. Analg.* **2013**, *116*, 491–494. [CrossRef]
77. Nair, B.G.; Gabel, E.; Hofer, I.; Schwid, H.A.; Cannesson, M. Intraoperative clinical decision support for anesthesia: A narrative review of available systems. *Anesth. Analg.* **2017**, *124*, 603–617. [CrossRef] [PubMed]
78. Bodhey, A.; Nair, A.; Seelam, S. SAFIRA pump: A novel device for fixed injection pressure and to control local anesthetic injection during peripheral nerve block. *J. Anaesthesiol. Clin. Pharmacol.* **2023**, *39*, 146–147. [CrossRef] [PubMed]
79. Leslie, D. *Understanding Artificial Intelligence Ethics and Safety: A Guide for the Responsible Design and Implementation of AI Systems in the Public Sector*; The Alan Turing Institute: London, UK, 2019. [CrossRef]
80. Park, J.J.; Tiefenbach, J.; Demetriades, A.K. The role of artificial intelligence in surgical simulation. *Front. Med. Technol.* **2022**, *4*, 1076755. [CrossRef] [PubMed]
81. Kirkpatrick, D.L. Techniques for Evaluation Training Programs. *J. Am. Soc. Train. Dir.* **1959**, *13*, 21–26.
82. Kirkpatrick, J.D.; Kirkpatrick, W.K. *Kirkpatrick's Four Levels of Training Evaluation*; Association for Talent Development: Alexandria, VA, USA, 2016; pp. 123–126.
83. Phillips, J.J. *Return on Investment in Training and Performance Improvement Programs*; Routledge: London, UK, 2003; pp. 25–32.

Journal of
Clinical Medicine

Systematic Review

Efficacy and Safety of Pericapsular Nerve Group Block (PENG) in Hip Surgery Under General Anaesthesia: A Systematic Literature Review and Meta-Analysis

Chryssoula Staikou [1], Martina Rekatsina [1,*], Matteo Luigi Giuseppe Leoni [2], Christos Chamos [3], Ioannis Kapsokalyvas [3], Giustino Varrassi [4] and Iosifina Karmaniolou [3]

1 Department of Anesthesia, Aretaieio University Hospital, 11528 Athens, Greece; c_staikou@yahoo.gr
2 Department of Medical and Surgical Sciences and Translational Medicine, Sapienza University of Rome, 00185 Rome, Italy; matteolg.leoni@gmail.com
3 Department of Anaesthetics, Guy's and St Thomas NHS Foundation Trust, London SE1 9RT, UK; christos.chamos@gstt.nhs.uk (C.C.); ioannis.kapsokalyvas@gstt.nhs.uk (I.K.); iosifina.karmaniolou@gstt.nhs.uk (I.K.)
4 Paolo Procacci Foundation, 00193 Rome, Italy; g.varrassi@fondazioneprocacci.org
* Correspondence: mrekatsina@gmail.com

Abstract: Background: The pericapsular nerve group (PENG) block is a novel ultrasound-guided regional technique that may provide analgesia to patients undergoing hip surgery. It has been extensively studied in recent years, but the evidence of superiority over other regional anaesthetic techniques is inconclusive. This review aimed to compare outcomes of the PENG block in patients undergoing hip surgery with standard techniques under general anaesthesia. **Methods**: PRISMA (Preferred Reporting Items for Systematic Reviews and Meta-Analyses) guidelines were followed throughout the preparation of this review. Randomised trials from electronic databases were included. We investigated postoperative pain scores, required analgesia, and adverse events associated with the block. **Results**: Ten studies satisfied the criteria to be included in the meta-analysis. Data from 646 patients were analysed, in which 321 patients received PENG block and 325 were included in the comparative groups. Pain scores at rest, at 24 h ($p = 0.04$) and 48 h ($p = 0.02$) were lower in patients who had received the PENG block. This group also required a smaller amount of opioids at 24 h after the procedure, but this difference was not statistically significant ($p = 0.53$); while a similar non-significant reduction in opioid consumption was also observed at 48 h. Although PENG seems to delay the time to the first analgesic request, we failed to prove a statistically significant difference ($p = 0.83$). Patient satisfaction also seems to be better in the PENG group, but not in a statistically significant way. No important side effects related to the block were described. **Conclusions**: PENG block for major hip surgery offers better postoperative analgesia, with possibly less opioid consumption. It seems to prolong the time to the first analgesic but does not significantly affect common side effects of anaesthesia/analgesia such as PONV or duration of hospital stay.

Keywords: pericapsular nerve group block; PENG block; general anaesthesia; meta-analysis

1. Introduction

Hip surgery, including hip arthroplasty and hip fracture surgery, is a common procedure with a high success rate, mainly performed in older adults and offers significant benefits to patients such as pain relief, increased active and passive mobility and ability to walk [1].

Nevertheless, hip surgery may be accompanied by postoperative pain that restricts early ambulation and increases the risk for adverse events (i.e., thromboembolism, cardiopulmonary complications), which prolongs hospital stay [1,2]. Opioid analgesia, despite being the mainstay of pain management after surgery, may incur multiple unwanted effects such as sedation, dizziness, lethargy, respiratory depression, or gastrointestinal complications [3].

Central neuraxial blocks [4], local analgesia (i.e., surgical site infiltration) [5,6] and a variety of peripheral nerve blocks have been proposed to offer better quality of analgesia and decrease opioid consumption [7–9]. Despite all the different available modalities, the optimal analgesic strategy remains undetermined [8]. The complexity of hip joint innervation [10], along with side effects of current regional techniques, such as quadriceps muscle weakness and consequent falls [11], require the development of new alternative methods.

The pericapsular nerve group (PENG) block is a novel, ultrasound-guided, regional technique that may provide effective and safe analgesia to patients undergoing hip surgery [12]. It targets the articular branches of the femoral, obturator and accessory obturator nerve that provide sensory innervation to the anterior hip capsule, offering high-quality analgesia without motor block [12]. Many investigators have highlighted the abovementioned benefits of the PENG block for different types of hip surgery [13,14]. Nevertheless, cases of motor weakness have also been reported [15,16].

Overall, the evidence has been inconclusive. This systematic review and meta-analysis aim to clarify the efficacy and safety of the PENG block in patients undergoing hip surgery under general anaesthesia.

2. Materials and Methods

2.1. Search Strategy

We adopted the Preferred Reporting Items for Systematic Reviews and Meta-Analyses (PRISMA) recommendations for the preparation of this review [17]. Randomised trials that investigated the efficiency of the PENG block for hip surgery under general anaesthesia were reviewed and evaluated using a predesigned protocol. The protocol was registered with the International Prospective Register of Systematic Reviews (PROSPERO-CRD42022335593).

Two authors (I.K. and M.R.) separately performed an exhaustive search for articles published from January 1990 until July 2024 in the electronic databases MEDLINE, Embase, PubMed, CINAHL, Cochrane Database of Systematic Reviews and clinicaltrials.gov. The search terms "pericapsular nerve block" or "PENG block" in combination with "hip surgery", "hip fracture surgery", "hip replacement", "hip prosthesis", "hip operation", "hip arthroplasty", "general anaesthesia" in all possible combinations, were used. The searches were re-run just before the final analyses and any further studies were identified. Additionally, manual searching for relevant publications of RTCs was conducted. The same two authors evaluated separately the abstracts retrieved; when agreement was not reached the opinion of a third author (C.S.) was obtained.

2.2. Eligibility Criteria

We included randomised trials studying the impact of PENG block for hip surgery (total hip arthroplasty and hip fracture) conducted under general anaesthesia in adult patients over 18 years old, published from January 1990 until July 2024. Only trials published in English, which clearly mentioned approval from the local ethics committee or the institutional review board, were considered eligible.

2.3. Data Extraction

A standardised data collection form was produced using Microsoft Excel 2016 (Microsoft Corp, Redmond, WA, USA). It was used for data extraction and entry by 3 authors (C.H., I.K., M.R.). Discrepancies in data extraction were resolved by a fourth author (C.S.). Data were sourced primarily from published tables or the manuscript text. If required data were missing, we attempted to contact the authors for clarification or extract from published figures using online plot digitiser software (WebPlotDigitizer 3.9, Ankit Rohatgi, 2015, Austin, TX, USA).

2.4. Outcomes Assessed

Our primary outcome was postoperative pain at 6, 24, and 48 h after surgery. Postoperative pain was assessed using both the resting pain score (static) and the pain score during movement (dynamic). Secondary outcomes were postoperative cumulative opioid consumption at 24 and 48 h after surgery, time to first analgesia request, duration of surgery and the occurrence of postoperative nausea and vomiting.

2.5. Risk of Bias Assessment in Included Studies

All studies were initially screened for bias using the JADAD scoring system. Trials with Jadad score < 4 were excluded. Studies with a Jadad score ≥ 4 were further assessed using the Cochrane Collaboration risk of bias assessment tool Version 2 (RoB2) [18]. The studies were independently assessed by I.K. and M.R. A score was assigned to each study by consensus; if an agreement could not be reached, the third author (C.S.) was again consulted. The risk of publication bias was assessed by visual examination of the funnel plot as well as by the Egger test [19].

2.6. Statistical Analysis

This meta-analysis was performed in line with recommendations from the Cochrane Collaboration and the PRISMA Statement [20]. The random effects model was used due to the different sets of studies (different control groups). As the overall effect estimate for continuous variables, we used the standardised mean difference (SMD) with 95% confidence intervals (CI). This approach was applied when the same outcome was measured using different units across studies when there were variations in the distribution of continuous variables, or when the possibility of non-normal data distribution across studies could not be ruled out. Mean difference with 95% confidence intervals was used to provide a direct comparison of outcomes measured on the same scale across studies, ensuring that the results reflect the absolute difference between groups. As an overall effect estimate of binary variables, we used the odds ratio. The heterogeneity was assessed using the I^2, the tau^2 and Cochran's Q-test along with the degrees of freedom and the corresponding p-value. An I^2 value higher than 50% or a statistically significant Cochran's Q-test were indicative of substantial heterogeneity [21]. Possible sources of heterogeneity within the outcome were identified in advance and included as covariates in the planned meta-regression analysis. The included covariates were skin infiltration for local analgesia, intraoperative opioid use and dose of local anaesthetic use for PENG block. For continuous variables reported as medians with interquartile ranges, these data were transformed into means and standard deviations following the guidelines provided by Wan et al. [22], as well as the Cochrane Handbook for systematic reviews of interventions [21]. Postoperative opioid use was converted to oral morphine equivalents (OME) to standardise the measurement across different types of opioids. Patient satisfaction scores not originally reported on a 10-point scale were converted to continuous values using linear transformation [23]. R software v4.3.2 (R Foundation for Statistical Computing, Vienna, Austria, www.r-project.org) was used for the analyses, and the level of statistical significance was set to 0.05.

3. Results

3.1. Study Characteristics

Of the 744 studies identified, 10 satisfied the inclusion criteria (Supplementary Figure S1). Data from 646 patients were analysed, in which 321 patients received PENG block and 325 were included in the comparative groups. A description of the included studies is summarised in Table 1.

3.2. Risk of Bias

The risk of bias table from the included studies is reported in Figure 1. Generally, included studies had an overall low risk of bias.

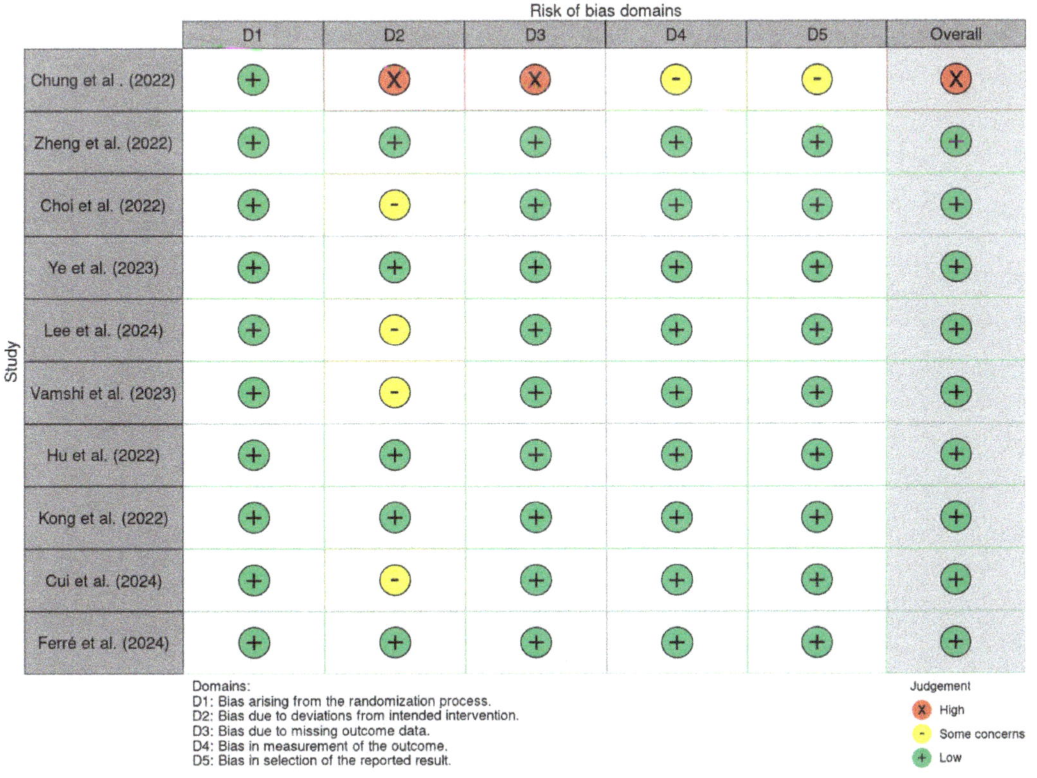

Figure 1. Summary of the risk of bias assessment for included studies across five domains using the Cochrane Risk of Bias 2.0 (RoB 2) tool [24–33]. Domains assessed include: D1 (bias arising from the randomisation process), D2 (bias due to deviations from the intended intervention), D3 (bias due to missing outcome data), D4 (bias in measurement of the outcome), and D5 (bias in the selection of the reported result). Judgments are categorised as low risk (green), some concerns (yellow), and high risk (red). The overall risk of bias for each study is also reported in the rightmost column.

3.3. Primary Outcomes

As previously reported, postoperative static and dynamic pain scores at 6, 24, and 48 h after surgery were considered as primary outcomes.

Table 1. Studies' characteristics.

Study (Year)	Patients (PENG/Control)	Type of Surgery	Type of Anaesthesia	PENG group: PENG only or PENG + LIA	Control Group	Local Anaesthetic Used (Concentration)	Dose of local Anaesthetic for the PENG Block	Adjuvants in PENG	Local Infiltration Analgesia Regimen	Intraoperative Opioid	Postoperative Opioids
Zheng et al. (2022) [24]	34/36	THA	GA	PENG + LIA	PENG saline	Ropivacaine 0.5%	100 mg		all patients: intra-articular infiltration 20 mL of 0.5% ropivacaine	Y (sufentanil 0.5–0.7 μg/kg)	Sufentanil (2.5 mcg increments), intravenous tramadol/butorphanol/meperidine allowed
Choi et al. (2022) [25]	27/27	THA	GA	PENG	Fascia iliaca compartment block	Ropivacaine 0.2%	40 mg	adrenaline 1:200,000	Not given	Y (fentanyl 1 mcg/kgl and remifentanil)	PCA Fentanyl
Ye et al., 2023 [26]	40/40	THA	GA	PENG	LIA	Ropivacaine 0.5%	100 mg	adrenaline 1:200,000	only control group infiltration of joint capsule with 0.33% ropivacaine, 1:200,000 adrenaline, total 30 mL	GA regimen not mentioned	Morphine PRN
Hu et al., 2023 [27]	45/45	THA	GA	PENG+LIA	Sham PENG block + LIA	Ropivacaine 0.2%	40 mg	adrenaline 1:200,000	LIA to both groups (patients in the PENG group received 20 mL of 0.5% ropivacaine with 1:200,000 epinephrine, while those in the Sham group received 40 mL.)	Y (sufentanil 0.3 mg/kg and remifentanil)	Morphine SC (rescue)
Kong et al., 2022 [28]	25/25	THA	GA	PENG+LIA	Fascia iliaca compartment block	Ropivacaine 0.375%	112.5 mg		all patients received 15 mL of 0.375% ropivacaine for local infiltration anaesthesia before suturing	Y (fentanyl 1 mcg/kg and remifentanil)	PCA Fentanyl
Cui et al., 2024 [29]	36/36	Hip arthroplasty	GA	PENG	Supra-inguinal fascia iliaca	Ropivacaine 0.3%	60 mg		Not mentioned	Y (sufentanil 0.4 mcg/kg + extra sufentanil 0.05 mcg/kg if needed + sufentanil 0.1 mcg/kg before end of surgery and remifentanil)	PCA Sufentanil
Chung et al. (2022) [30]	25/25	THA	GA	PENG+LIA	PENG saline	Ropivacaine 0.5%	125 mg		All patients received wound infiltration of 20mL ropivacaine 0.375% from the surgeon at the end of the surgical procedure	Y (fentanyl 0.9 mcg/kg))	PCA Fentanyl

Table 1. *Cont.*

Study (Year)	Patients (PENG/Control)	Type of Surgery	Type of Anaesthesia	PENG group: PENG only or PENG + LIA	Control Group	Local Anaesthetic Used (Concentration)	Dose of local Anaesthetic for the PENG Block	Adjuvants in PENG	Local Infiltration Analgesia Regimen	Intraoperative Opioid	Postoperative Opioids
Lee et al., 2023 [31]	30/30	Hip fracture	GA	PENG+LIA	Lumbar Plexus Block + LIA	Ropivacaine 0.5%	100 mg		All patients (wound infiltration and a periarticular injection of 20 mL of 0.25% ropivacaine with ketorolac (30 mg) at the end of the surgical procedure)	GA regimen not mentioned	PCA Fentanyl
Vamshi et al., 2023 [32]	30/30	THA	GA	PENG	Suprainguinal fascia iliaca block	Bupivacaine 0.25%	75 mg	1 mcg/kg clonidine diluted in bupivacaine solution	Not mentioned	Y (fentanyl 2 microgram/kg + additional bolus of 0.5 mcg/kg as needed)	PCA Morphine
Ferré et al., 2024 [33]	29/31	THA	GA	PENG+LIA	LIA	Ropivacaine 0.475%	95 mg		All patients received 80 mL of ropivacaine 2 mg/mL (for a total dose of 160 mg	Y (sufentanil if necessary 2.5–7.5 mcg)	Oxycodone PRN

PENG = pericapsular nerve group, LIA = local infiltration analgesia, THA = total hip arthroplasty, GA = general anaesthesia, PCA = Patient Control Analgesia, SC = subcutaneously, Y = YES, N = NO, PRN= pro re nata (as needed).

3.4. Pain Score at Rest (Static)

The cumulative pain scores at rest at 6, 24, and 48 h post-surgery were examined in five studies [24–29] (n = 416) for the 6 and 24 h time points, while four studies [24–28] (n = 344) reported data on pain intensity at 48 h post-surgery. Globally, the analysis indicated lower pain intensity in patients treated with the PENG block (Figure 2A). At 6 h, there was a non-significant reduction in pain of 0.46 on a 0–10 pain scale (MD, −0.46; 95% CI, −1.21 to 0.30; $p = 0.23$, $I^2 = 93\%$). However, at 24 h, the pain reduction became statistically significant, with a decrease of 0.53 (MD, −0.53; 95% CI, −1.03 to −0.02; $p = 0.04$, $I^2 = 87\%$). The pain scores during rest at 6 and 24 h after surgery were characterised by substantial heterogeneity. Sensitivity analysis showed that when the study of Ye et al. [26] was removed, the pooled results at 6 h follow-up were improved (MD, −0.72; 95% CI, −1.37 to −0.07; $p = 0.03$) while the heterogeneity was only slightly reduced ($I^2 = 78.6\%$), (Supplementary Figure S2). Meta-regression analysis for pain intensity at 6 h revealed no role for skin infiltration for local analgesia ($p = 0.85$), for the dose of local anaesthetic used for the block ($p = 0.67$), while intraoperative opioid use was statistically significant ($p = 0.04$).

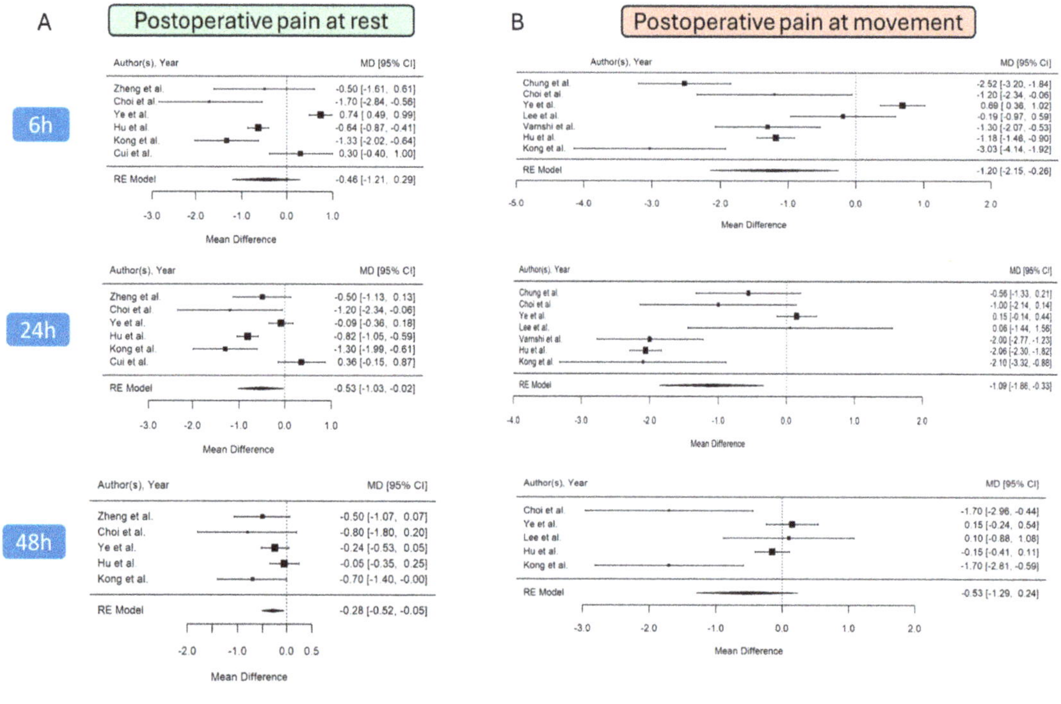

Figure 2. Forest plot displaying pooled effect sizes for postoperative VAS scores at rest (**A**) and dynamic pain scores (**B**), measured at 6, 24, and 48 h after surgery [24–33].

Similar findings were observed at the 24 h follow-up, where the sensitivity analysis confirmed the significant influence of the study by Ye et al. [26] on the pooled results (MD, −0.64; 95% CI, −1.23 to −0.05; $p = 0.03$), (Supplementary Figure S2). However, heterogeneity was not significantly reduced ($I^2 = 83\%$). The meta-regression analysis revealed no significant effect of skin infiltration for local analgesia ($p = 0.70$), the dose of local anaesthetic used for the block ($p = 0.99$), or intraoperative opioid use ($p = 0.42$). The VAS at 24 h follow-up should be interpreted cautiously, as the random effects model, sensitivity analysis, and meta-regression did not account for the variability in the effect size of the PENG block at 24 h post-surgery. Therefore, this outcome can be considered unstable. By 48 h, the pain reduction remained significant, though smaller, at 0.28 (MD, −0.28; 95% CI, −0.52 to −0.05; $p = 0.02$), with no evidence of heterogeneity ($I^2 = 25\%$).

No publication bias was observed through visual inspection of funnel plots and confirmed by Egger's regression tests (6 h follow-up, Egger's regression test: $p = 0.21$; 24 h follow-up, Egger's regression test: $p = 0.34$; 48 h follow-up, Egger's regression test: $p = 0.23$).

3.5. Pain Score at Movement (Dynamic)

The post-surgical dynamic pain score at 6 and 24 h was reported by seven studies [26–32] with a total of 444 patients. Data on pain intensity during movement at 48 h post-surgery were provided by five studies [25–28,31] involving 334 patients. Overall pain scores showed significant improvement at both 6 and 24 h after surgery. The reduction in pain intensity at 6 h was 1.20 (MD, −1.20; 95% CI, −2.15 to −0.26; $p = 0.013$, $I^2 = 95\%$), and at 24 h, it was 1.09 (MD, −1.09; 95% CI, −1.86 to −0.33; $p = 0.005$, $I^2 = 92\%$). However, no significant improvement was observed at the 48 h follow-up (MD, -0.53; 95% CI, −1.29 to 0.24; $p = 0.18$, $I^2 = 88\%$), as shown in Figure 2B. Similar to the pain scores at rest, the dynamic pain scores were affected by high heterogeneity. Sensitivity analysis did not alter the overall estimates of the dynamic pain score, indicating that the effect size was consistent across all studies, even though the overall heterogeneity remained high. Meta-regression analysis revealed a significant impact of intraoperative opioid use on pain intensity at both 6 h ($p < 0.001$) and 24 h ($p = 0.003$) post-surgery. However, no significant effects were found for skin infiltration for local analgesia or the dose of local anaesthetic used for the block.

3.6. Secondary Outcomes

Postoperative cumulative opioid consumption at 24 and 48 h after surgery

The amount of opioid analgesia required after surgery at 24 h was reported by eight studies [25–28,30–33] (n = 504), while a similar set of eight studies reported the 48 h opioid consumption [24–28,31–33] (n = 524). Overall, the analysis indicated lower cumulative opioid consumption at 24 h in patients treated with the PENG block even if not statistically significant (SMD, -0.19; 95% CI, -0.80 to 0.41; $p = 0.53$, $I^2 = 91\%$), (Figure 3A). Sensitivity analysis did not change the overall estimates of the cumulative opioid consumption at 24 h, indicating that the effect size is similar across all studies. Meta-regression analysis revealed a significant role in intraoperative opioid use ($p = 0.002$), while no significant effect was observed for skin infiltration for local analgesia ($p = 0.64$) and the dose of local anaesthetic used for the block ($p = 0.47$).

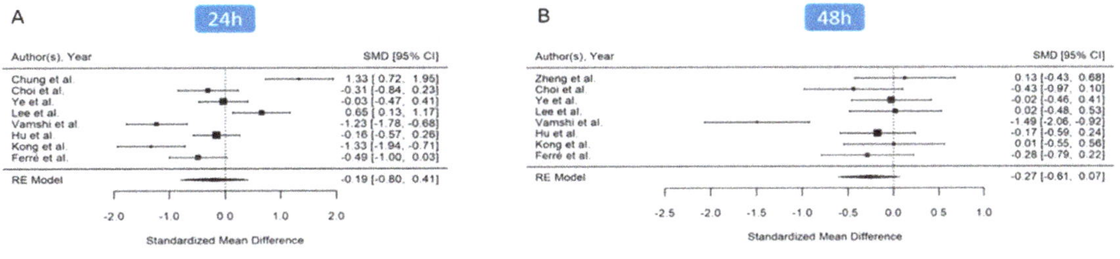

Figure 3. Forest plot displaying pooled effect sizes for postoperative cumulative opioid consumption at 24 and 48 h after surgery [24–28,30–33]. (**A**) At 24 h post-surgery, the PENG block group showed a reduction in cumulative opioid consumption, though this reduction did not reach statistical significance. (**B**) By 48 h, the reduction in opioid consumption remained non-significant. Substantial heterogeneity was present among studies.

At 48 h, the same non-significant reduction in opioid consumption was observed (SMD, −0.27; 95% CI, −0.61 to 0.07; p = 0.12, I^2 = 73%) (Figure 3B). The sensitivity analysis did not alter the overall estimates of cumulative opioid consumption at 48 h. Meta-regression analysis demonstrated a non-significant effect for the following variables: intraoperative opioid use (p = 0.14), skin infiltration for local analgesia (p = 0.59), and the dose of local anaesthetic used for the block (p = 0.36).

3.7. Time to First Analgesia Request

Time to first analgesia request was reported by only two studies [27,31], while Chung et al. [30] only provided data on the incidence of analgesic requests within a specific time range, which did not allow for effect size calculation. As a result, pooling the results from the two studies [27,31] showed a reduction in the time to the first analgesic request in the PENG group compared to the control group. However, this reduction was not statistically significant (SMD, −0.11; 95% CI, −1.08 to 0.87; p = 0.83, I^2 = 88%), (Figure 4). Given that only two studies were included, neither sensitivity analysis nor meta-regression was possible.

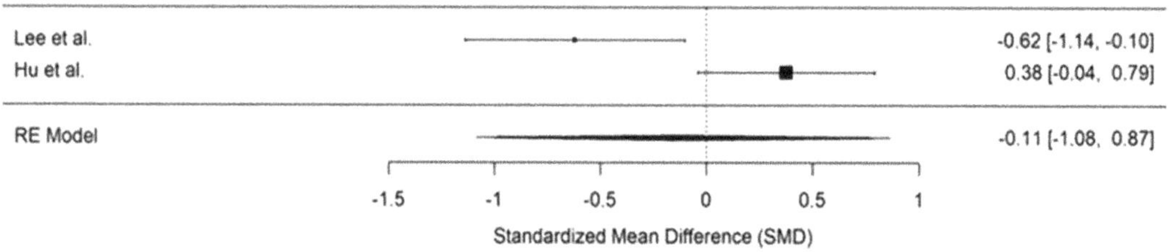

Figure 4. Forest plot displaying pooled effect sizes for time to first analgesia request post-surgery [27,31].

3.8. Duration of Surgery

The duration of surgery was reported by eight articles [24,25,27–32] and averaged 88 ± 20 min. No significant difference in the duration of surgery was observed in the overall analysis between patients who received the PENG block and controls (SMD, −0.11; 95% CI, −0.28 to 0.07; p = 0.23, I^2 = 0%), (Figure 5).

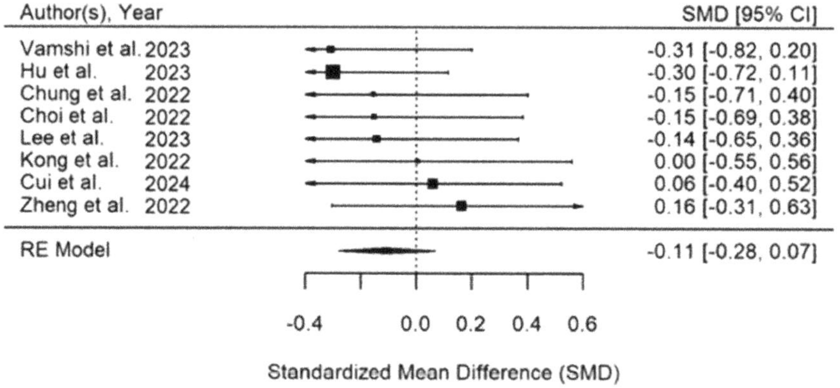

Figure 5. Forest plot displaying pooled effect sizes for the duration of surgery in patients receiving PENG block versus control. The analysis included eight studies [24,25,27–32] and showed no significant difference in the duration of surgery between the PENG block group and controls.

3.9. Patient Satisfaction

Patient satisfaction was assessed in three studies [25,28,31], though using different rating scales. After standardising the data to a common scale (0 to 10), the overall effect size indicated higher satisfaction levels among patients who received the PENG block. However, this increase in satisfaction did not reach statistical significance (SMD, 0.90; 95% CI, −0.30 to 2.09; $p = 0.14$), and there was considerable heterogeneity among the studies ($I^2 = 92\%$), (Figure 6).

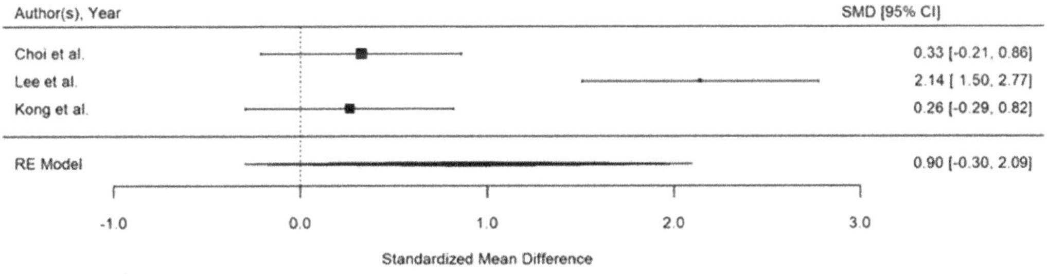

Figure 6. Forest plot displaying the pooled effect sizes for patient satisfaction [25,28,31]. The satisfaction data were standardised to a common scale (0 to 10) for comparison. Although there was an increase in satisfaction levels among patients who received the PENG block, this improvement did not reach statistical significance.

3.10. Length of Hospital Stay

Five studies reported the length of hospital stay [25–27,31,33]. To enable a direct comparison between studies, the length of stay was standardised to hours across all reports. All patients demonstrated a similar length of hospital stay, and the PENG block treatment did not significantly affect this outcome (SMD −0.15; 95% CI, −0.36 to 0.06, $p = 0.16$, $I^2 = 0\%$) (Figure 7). There was no observed heterogeneity among the studies.

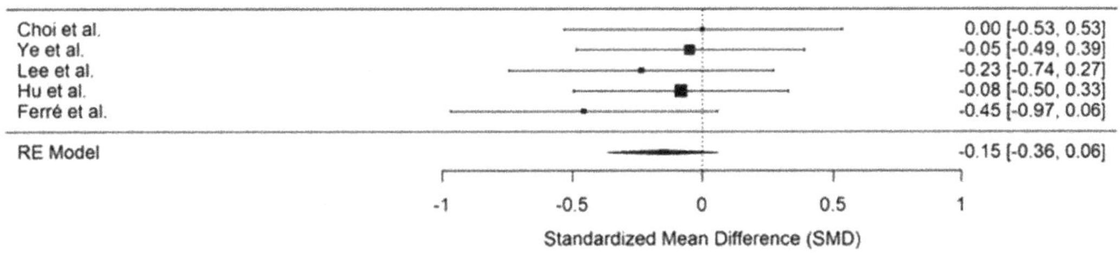

Figure 7. Forest plot displaying pooled effect sizes for the length of hospital stay (in hours) [25–27,31,33]. The PENG block group showed a slight reduction in the length of hospital stay compared to the control group, but this reduction was not statistically significant.

3.11. Occurrence of Postoperative Nausea and Vomiting

Occurrence of postoperative nausea was reported in five studies [24,27,28,30,31]. No significant reduction in the odds of nausea was observed in the PENG block group compared to controls (OR 0.02, 95% CI −0.63 to 0.66; $p = 0.96$, $I^2 = 0\%$), (Figure 8A). Similarly, four studies [24,27,30,32] reported the occurrence of vomiting, and no significant reduction was observed in the PENG block group (OR 0.61, 95% CI 0.26 to 1.41; $p = 0.25$, $I^2 = 23.3\%$), (Figure 8B).

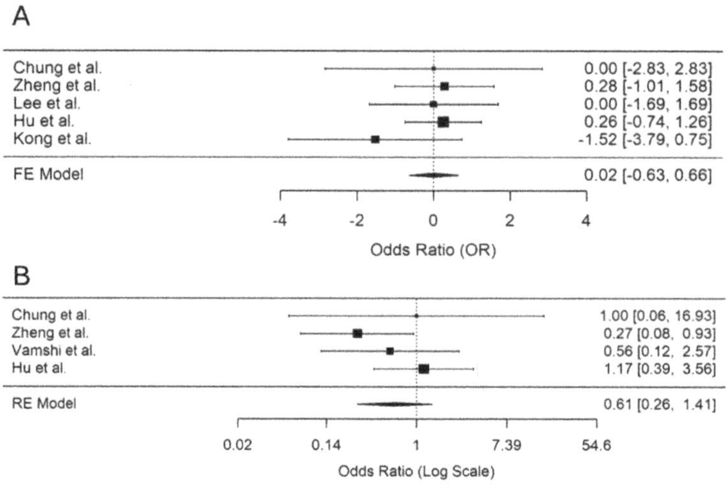

Figure 8. Forest plots displaying the pooled odds ratios (OR) for postoperative nausea (**A**) and vomiting (**B**) in patients receiving PENG block versus control [24,27,28,30–32].

4. Discussion

The PENG block has been favoured in hip surgery for its analgesic efficacy and purported motor-sparing properties [34]. This meta-analysis included data from 10 randomised trials regarding the efficacy and safety of this recently introduced block for patients undergoing hip surgery. According to our results, PENG block is beneficial in terms of reducing postoperative pain intensity at 24 and 48 h. Specifically, pain at rest was significantly reduced at 24 and 48 h after surgery in patients treated with the PENG block, with significant heterogeneity at earlier time points but reduced variability at 48 h. Dynamic pain scores showed significant improvement at both 6 and 24 h post-surgery; however, this benefit was not sustained at 48 h, with high heterogeneity persisting across all time points.

Opioid consumption was one of the secondary outcomes of our study; the meta-analysis did not show a statistically significant difference among groups, even though the overall consumption of opioids was higher in the non-PENG block groups, both at 24 and at 48 h. PENG block was not associated with a significant prolongation of time to the first analgesic request postoperatively. However, the meta-regression analysis identified a significant role of intraoperative opioid use in influencing several outcomes: static pain scores at 6 h, dynamic pain scores at 6 and 24 h post-surgery, as well as postoperative cumulative opioid consumption at 24 and 48 h after surgery. The incidence of postoperative nausea and vomiting was similar between the groups. Similarly, the length of hospital stay was not affected. Patient satisfaction was only mentioned in three studies. Higher satisfaction was reported by patients who received a PENG block; however, this did not reach statistical significance.

As a novel modality, PENG block has been compared to other locoregional analgesic techniques, such as lumbar plexus block [31], fascia iliaca [13,14,25,29,32], or other mini-invasive analgesic methods (i.e., periarticular infiltration) [26,33]. Importantly, this block has been described to be performed under ultrasound guidance [12] so that the iliopubic eminence, the iliopsoas muscle and tendon, the femoral artery, and the pectineus muscle are observed. The local anaesthetic is administered in the musculofascial plane between the psoas tendon anteriorly and the pubic ramus posteriorly in increments under ultrasound vision [12]. In the future, technological advancements such as three-dimensional reconstruction imaging and magnetic resonance microscopy of peripheral nerves may play a significant role in peripheral nerve blocks and plane blocks [35].

The results of this meta-analysis showed that compared to other blocks or conventional opioid-based analgesia, PENG block was associated with better postoperative analgesia at 24 and 48 h. At 6 h after the surgical procedure pain at rest did not show a significant difference, but pain at movement was significantly reduced. The abovementioned findings on pain intensity differ from those reported by Huda et al. [36] in their meta-analysis. The authors found that PENG block offered no significant pain relief compared to other methods up to 24 h postoperatively. Since we have no results regarding pain during the immediate postoperative period, we cannot compare our findings to those of Farag et al. [37], who reported in their meta-analysis that at 30 min postoperatively dynamic pain was significantly lower using PENG block compared to other blocks or parenteral analgesia. Interestingly, these authors found that the analgesic superiority of the block did not last and faded quickly; there was no difference in analgesia compared to the other methods at 6 h postoperatively or later. This result is also different from the findings of our research. The differences may be at least partly attributed to the different characteristics of the studies included in the two meta-analyses, such as type of surgery or setting (i.e., arthroscopy, scheduled or emergency cases, use of PENG in the emergency department), type of anaesthesia, and comparison of PENG block with different modalities (i.e., lumbar plexus block and other locoregional techniques) [13,14,25,26,29,31–33]. Still, despite the above discrepancies, both meta-analyses agree with our results that PENG block is associated with reduced opioid consumption in the first 24 postoperative hours [36,37]. Moreover, we found that this beneficial effect may last up to 48 h. Our results showed that even at 48 h, the analgesic consumption was less in patients who had a PENG block, even though the difference was not significant ($p = 0.12$).

In contrast to Huda et al. [36], we did not find that PENG block prolongs intraoperative analgesia, i.e., the time of request of the first analgesic dose after the procedure did not differ among the groups. This is in accordance with our finding that the PENG block did not reduce the cumulative opioid consumption 48 h after the procedure. However, this finding does not undermine the importance of better analgesia in the PENG group, especially when considering the growing evidence of postoperative pain chronification in patients with poor acute postoperative pain management [38,39].

Similar to previous results, we found no significant statistical difference in PONV [36]. Farag et al. [37], on the other hand, found no significant difference in nausea, pruritus, and dizziness, while patients who received a PENG block had significantly less vomiting. The small number of studies that reported this side effect might have prevented us from finding a difference between the groups.

Regarding hospital stay, the results of this meta-analysis are in accordance with previous findings, suggesting no effect of PENG block on time to patient discharge from hospital [36]. Also, we had no clear result on the possible superiority of the PENG block with regards to patient satisfaction, although according to previous meta-analyses, the PENG block was associated with higher scores of patient satisfaction [36,37].

Limitations

This meta-analysis has a few limitations, mainly due to the small sample sizes of most studies and the different research protocols. The PENG block was compared to other blocks or analgesic methods. The included studies differed in their methodology regarding the comparator groups since a few used active comparator groups (i.e., different blocks), while others used non-block control groups or sham control groups. Also, the studies differed in the local anaesthetic used as well as the doses/volumes and concentrations of the injected solution.

Moreover, the type of surgery (total hip arthroplasty and hip fracture surgery), as well as the surgical teams, were not the same in all studies. Nevertheless, we consider that the severity of the procedures was similar since only studies with hip fracture surgery and total hip arthroplasty were included in the analysis. The heterogeneity of studies is a common limitation in most meta-analyses. To minimise data variability, we applied strict inclusion criteria in our search strategy and study evaluation process. Additionally, meta-regression analyses were conducted to further investigate the potential sources of heterogeneity. Finally, we had no adequate data to analyse analgesia in the immediate and early postoperative period.

5. Conclusions

In conclusion, according to our meta-analysis, the PENG block used in major hip surgery offers better postoperative analgesia; however, less opioid consumption is not warranted. It does not prolong the time to the first analgesic, and it does not seem to affect significantly common side effects of anaesthesia/analgesia such as PONV, or the duration of hospital stay. As a novel technique, PENG block can be described as a safe and effective regional block technique for patients undergoing hip fracture surgery. However, the existing evidence is not adequate to draw firm conclusions. More high-quality data from large, well-designed randomised clinical trials, as well as cadaveric and anatomical trials, will be needed and further analyses are required to confirm the superiority of the PENG block over other locoregional techniques or conventional analgesic modalities used in hip surgery.

Supplementary Materials: The following supporting information can be downloaded at: https://www.mdpi.com/article/10.3390/jcm14020468/s1, Figure S1. PRISMA 2020 flow diagram for new systematic reviews which included searches of databases, registers and other sources; Figure S2. Sensitivity analysis of mean differences (MD) in pain scores during rest at 6 hours (A) and 24 hours (B) post-surgery.

Funding: This research received no external funding.

Institutional Review Board Statement: Ethical review and approval were waived for this study as it is based on previously conducted clinical trials.

Informed Consent Statement: Patient Informed Consent were waived for this study as it is based on previously conducted clinical trials.

Data Availability Statement: Data are available upon request to the corresponding author.

Conflicts of Interest: The authors declare no conflicts of interest.

References

1. Patel, N.; Golwala, P. Approaches for Total Hip Arthroplasty: A Systematic Review. *Cureus* **2023**, *15*, e34829. [CrossRef]
2. Hwang, S.K. Experience of Complications of Hip Arthroplasty. *Hip Pelvis* **2014**, *26*, 207–213. [CrossRef]
3. Rekatsina, M.; Theodosopoulou, P.; Staikou, C. Effects of Intravenous Dexmedetomidine Versus Lidocaine on Postoperative Pain, Analgesic Consumption and Functional Recovery After Abdominal Gynecological Surgery: A Randomized Placebo-controlled Double Blind Study. *Pain Physician* **2021**, *24*, E997–E1006. [PubMed]
4. Vītola, E.; Buraka, N.; Erts, R.; Golubovska, I.; Miscuks, A. Effect of different low doses of intrathecal morphine (0.1 and 0.2 mg) on pain and vital functions in patients undergoing total hip arthroplasty: A randomised controlled study. *BMC Anesthesiol.* **2022**, *22*, 377. [CrossRef] [PubMed]
5. Yang, Q.; Wang, H.; Xiao, Q.; Luo, Z.; Zhou, Z. Analgesic effect of a new "cocktail" of local infiltration analgesia after total hip arthroplasty-A prospective randomized controlled study. *Zhongguo Xiu Fu Chong Jian Wai Ke Za Zhi Zhongguo Xiufu Chongjian Waike Zazhi Chin. J. Reparative Reconstr. Surg.* **2022**, *36*, 1485–1491. [CrossRef] [PubMed] [PubMed Central]

6. Peng, X.Q.; Fei, Z.G.; Sun, C.G.; Zhou, Q.J. Efficacy and safety of local infiltration analgesia for pain management in total knee and hip arthroplasty: A meta-analysis of randomized controlled trial. *Medicine* **2020**, *99*, e20640. [CrossRef]
7. Gianakos, A.L.; Romanelli, F.; Rao, N.; Badri, M.; Lubberts, B.; Guss, D.; DiGiovanni, C.W. Combination Lower Extremity Nerve Blocks and Their Effect on Postoperative Pain and Opioid Consumption: A Systematic Review. *J. Foot Ankle Surg.* **2021**, *60*, 121–131. [CrossRef]
8. Jackson, T.J. Editorial Commentary: The Optimal Nerve Block for Hip Arthroscopy Is Undetermined. *Arthroscopy* **2023**, *39*, 298–299. [CrossRef] [PubMed]
9. Flaviano, E.; Bettinelli, S.; Assandri, M.; Muhammad, H.; Benigni, A.; Cappelleri, G.; Mariano, E.R.; Lorini, L.F.; Bugada, D. Erector spinae plane block versus fascia iliaca block after total hip arthroplasty: A randomized clinical trial comparing analgesic effectiveness and motor block. *Korean J. Anesthesiol.* **2023**, *76*, 326–335. [CrossRef] [PubMed]
10. Birnbaum, K.; Prescher, A.; Hessler, S.; Heller, K.D. The sensory innervation of the hip joint--an anatomical study. *Surg. Radiol. Anat.* **1997**, *9*, 371–375. [CrossRef] [PubMed]
11. Johnson, R.L.; Kopp, S.L.; Hebl, J.R.; Erwin, P.J.; Mantilla, C.B. Falls and major orthopaedic surgery with peripheral nerve blockade: A systematic review and meta-analysis. *Br. J. Anaesth.* **2013**, *110*, 518–528. [CrossRef] [PubMed]
12. Girón-Arango, L.; Peng, P.W.H.; Chin, K.J.; Brull, R.; Perlas, A. Pericapsular Nerve Group (PENG) Block for Hip Fracture. *Reg. Anesth. Pain Med.* **2018**, *43*, 859–863. [CrossRef] [PubMed]
13. Aliste, J.; Layera, S.; Bravo, D.; Jara, Á.; Muñoz, G.; Barrientos, C.; Wulf, R.; Brañez, J.; Finlayson, R.J.; Tran, D.Q. Randomized comparison between pericapsular nerve group (PENG) block and suprainguinal fascia iliaca block for total hip arthroplasty. *Reg. Anesth. Pain Med.* **2021**, *46*, 874–878. [CrossRef]
14. Mosaffa, F.; Taheri, M.; Manafi Rasi, A.; Samadpour, H.; Memary, E.; Mirkheshti, A. Comparison of pericapsular nerve group (PENG) block with fascia iliaca compartment block (FICB) for pain control in hip fractures: A double-blind prospective randomized controlled clinical trial. *Orthop. Traumatol. Surg. Res.* **2022**, *108*, 103135. [CrossRef]
15. Yu, H.C.; Moser, J.J.; Chu, A.Y.; Montgomery, S.H.; Brown, N.; Endersby, R.V.W. Inadvertent quadriceps weakness following the pericapsular nerve group (PENG) block. *Reg. Anesth. Pain Med.* **2019**, *44*, 611–613. [CrossRef]
16. Endersby, R.V.W.; Moser, J.J.; Ho, E.C.Y.; Yu, H.C.; Spencer, A.O. Motor blockade after iliopsoas plane (IPB) and pericapsular nerve group (PENG) blocks: A little may go a long way. *Acta Anaesthesiol. Scand.* **2021**, *65*, 135–136. [CrossRef]
17. Page, M.J.; McKenzie, J.E.; Bossuyt, P.M.; Boutron, I.; Hoffmann, T.C.; Mulrow, C.D.; Shamseer, L.; Tetzlaff, J.M.; Akl, E.A.; Brennan, S.E.; et al. The PRISMA 2020 statement: An updated guideline for reporting systematic reviews. *BMJ* **2021**, *372*, n71. [CrossRef] [PubMed]
18. Sterne, J.A.C.; Savović, J.; Page, M.J.; Elbers, R.G.; Blencowe, N.S.; Boutron, I.; Cates, C.J.; Cheng, H.Y.; Corbett, M.S.; Eldridge, S.M.; et al. RoB 2: A revised tool for assessing risk of bias in randomised trials. *BMJ* **2019**, *366*, l4898. [CrossRef] [PubMed]
19. Egger, M.; Davey Smith, G.; Schneider, M.; Minder, C. Bias in meta-analysis detected by a simple, graphical test. *BMJ* **1997**, *315*, 629–634. [CrossRef]
20. Liberati, A.; Altman, D.G.; Tetzlaff, J.; Mulrow, C.; Gøtzsche, P.C.; Ioannidis, J.P.A.; Clarke, M.; Devereaux, P.J.; Kleijnen, J.; Moher, D. The PRISMA statement for reporting systematic reviews and meta-analyses of studies that evaluate health care interventions: Explanation and elaboration. *PLoS Med.* **2009**, *6*, e1000100. [CrossRef]
21. Higgins, J.P.T.; Thomas, J.; Chandler, J.; Cumpston, M.; Li, T.; Page, M.J.; Welch, V.A. (Eds.) *Cochrane Handbook for Systematic Reviews of Interventions Version 6.4 (Updated August 2023)*; Cochrane: London, UK, 2023. Available online: www.training.cochrane.org/handbook (accessed on 15 October 2024).
22. Wan, X.; Wang, W.; Liu, J.; Tong, T. Estimating the sample mean and standard deviation from the sample size, median, range, and/ or interquartile range. *BMC Med. Res. Methodol.* **2014**, *14*, 135. [CrossRef] [PubMed]
23. Harwell, M.R.; Gatti, G.G. Rescaling ordinal data to interval data in educational research. *Rev. Educ. Res.* **2001**, *71*, 105–131. [CrossRef]
24. Zheng, J.; Pan, D.; Zheng, B.; Ruan, X. Preoperative pericapsular nerve group (PENG) block for total hip arthroplasty: A randomized, placebo-controlled trial. *Reg. Anesth. Pain Med.* **2022**, *47*, 155–160, Erratum in *Reg. Anesth. Pain Med.* **2022**, *47*, e4. [CrossRef]
25. Choi, Y.S.; Park, K.K.; Lee, B.; Nam, W.S.; Kim, D.H. Pericapsular Nerve Group (PENG) Block versus Supra-Inguinal Fascia Iliaca Compartment Block for Total Hip Arthroplasty: A Randomized Clinical Trial. *J. Pers. Med.* **2022**, *12*, 408. [CrossRef] [PubMed] [PubMed Central]
26. Ye, S.; Wang, L.; Wang, Q.; Li, Q.; Alqwbani, M.; Kang, P. Comparison between Ultrasound-Guided Pericapsular Nerve Group Block and Local Infiltration Analgesia for Postoperative Analgesia after Total Hip Arthroplasty: A Prospective Randomized Controlled Trial. *Orthop. Surg.* **2023**, *15*, 1839–1846. [CrossRef] [PubMed] [PubMed Central]
27. Hu, J.; Wang, Q.; Hu, J.; Kang, P.; Yang, J. Efficacy of Ultrasound-Guided Pericapsular Nerve Group (PENG) Block Combined With Local Infiltration Analgesia on Postoperative Pain After Total Hip Arthroplasty: A Prospective, Double-Blind, Randomized Controlled Trial. *J. Arthroplast.* **2023**, *38*, 1096–1103. [CrossRef] [PubMed]

28. Kong, M.; Tang, Y.; Tong, F.; Guo, H.; Zhang, X.L.; Zhou, L.; Ni, H.; Wang, B.; Liu, Y.; Liu, J. The analgesic efficacy of pericapsular nerve group block in patients with intertrochanteric femur fracture: A randomized controlled trial. *PLoS ONE* **2022**, *17*, e0275793. [CrossRef] [PubMed] [PubMed Central]
29. Cui, X.; Cheng, Z.; Zhang, T.; Xu, H.; Luan, H.; Feng, J.; Zhang, X.; Zhu, P. Effect of pericapsular nerve group block and suprainguinal fascia iliaca block on postoperative analgesia and stress response in elderly patients undergoing hip arthroplasty: A prospective randomized controlled double-blind trial. *BMC Anesthesiol.* **2024**, *24*, 220. [CrossRef] [PubMed] [PubMed Central]
30. Chung, C.J.; Eom, D.W.; Lee, T.Y.; Park, S.Y. Reduced Opioid Consumption with Pericapsular Nerve Group Block for Hip Surgery: A Randomized, Double-Blind, Placebo-Controlled Trial. *Pain Res. Manag.* **2022**, *2022*, 6022380. [CrossRef] [PubMed] [PubMed Central]
31. Lee, T.Y.; Chung, C.J.; Park, S.Y. Comparing the Pericapsular Nerve Group Block and the Lumbar Plexus Block for Hip Fracture Surgery: A Single-Center Randomized Double-Blinded Study. *J. Clin. Med.* **2023**, *13*, 122. [CrossRef] [PubMed] [PubMed Central]
32. Vamshi, C.; Sinha, C.; Kumar, A.; Kumar, A.; Kumari, P.; Kumar, A.; Kumar, S.; Arun, S.K. Comparison of the efficacy of pericapsular nerve group block (PENG) block versus suprainguinal fascia iliaca block (SFIB) in total hip arthroplasty: A randomized control trial. *Indian J. Anaesth.* **2023**, *67*, 364–369. [CrossRef] [PubMed] [PubMed Central]
33. Ferré, F.; Rey, J.; Bosch, L.; Menut, R.; Ferrier, A.; Ba, C.; Halimi, C.; Collinson, I.; Tissot, B.; Labaste, F.; et al. Pericapsular nerve group (PENG) block combined with local infiltration analgesia is not superior to local infiltration analgesia for the management of postoperative pain after primary elective total hip arthroplasty: A prospective, randomized, controlled, single-blind trial. *Heliyon* **2024**, *10*, e33766. [CrossRef] [PubMed] [PubMed Central]
34. DEL Buono, R.; Padua, E.; Pascarella, G.; Costa, F.; Tognù, A.; Terranova, G.; Greco, F.; Perez, M.F.; Barbara, E. Pericapsular nerve group block: An overview. *Minerva Anestesiol.* **2021**, *87*, 458–466. [CrossRef]
35. Pušnik, L.; Lechner, L.; Serša, I.; Cvetko, E.; Haas, P.; Jengojan, S.A.; Snoj, Ž. 3D fascicular reconstruction of median and ulnar nerve: Initial experience and comparison between high-resolution ultrasound and MR microscopy. *Eur. Radiol. Exp.* **2024**, *8*, 100. [CrossRef] [PubMed] [PubMed Central]
36. Huda, A.U.; Ghafoor, H. The Use of Pericapsular Nerve Group (PENG) Block in Hip Surgeries Is Associated With a Reduction in Opioid Consumption, Less Motor Block, and Better Patient Satisfaction: A Meta-Analysis. *Cureus* **2022**, *14*, e28872. [CrossRef]
37. Farag, A.; Hendi, N.I.; Diab, R.A. Does pericapsular nerve group block have limited analgesia at the initial post-operative period? Systematic review and meta-analysis. *J. Anesth.* **2023**, *37*, 138–153. [CrossRef] [PubMed]
38. Camilloni, A.; Nati, G.; Maggiolini, P.; Romanelli, A.; Carbone, G.; Giannarelli, D.; Terrenato, I.; De Marinis, M.G.; Rossi, A.; D'Angelo, D.; et al. Chronic non-cancer pain in primary care: An Italian cross-sectional study. *Signa Vitae* **2021**, *17*, 54–62. [CrossRef]
39. Montero Matamala, A.; Hanna, M.; Perrot, S.; Varrassi, G. Avoid Postoperative Pain to Prevent Its Chronification: A Narrative Review. *Cureus* **2022**, *14*, e22243. [CrossRef]

Journal of
Clinical Medicine

MDPI

Review

Rebound Pain—Management Strategies for Transitional Analgesia: A Narrative Review

Kevin J. Murphy * and Brian O'Donnell

Department of Anaesthesiology and Intensive Care Medicine, Cork University Hospital, T12DC4A Cork, Ireland; brian.odonnell@hse.ie
* Correspondence: kevinjmurphy9@gmail.com; Tel.: +353-(021)-492-2000

Abstract: Peripheral nerve blocks (PNBs), while effective in reducing postoperative opioid use and side effects, are often associated with rebound pain (RP), a significant clinical issue requiring proactive management. Methods: A systematic search of electronic databases (e.g., PubMed, EMBASE, Cochrane Library) was conducted for studies investigating rebound pain following regional anaesthesia. Recent findings: RP has a high incidence in ambulatory patients and is influenced by patient, surgical, and anaesthetic factors. Preoperative education, multimodal analgesia, continuous nerve blocks, and intravenous dexamethasone may mitigate RP. Although RP does not typically affect overall opioid use, recovery, or patient satisfaction, the majority of patients experiencing RP would still choose PNBs for future surgery.

Keywords: peripheral nerve blocks; postoperative pain; rebound pain; regional anaesthesia; multimodal analgesia

1. Introduction

Several definitions of rebound pain (RP) exist in the literature. A marked increase in pain intensity upon dissipation of a peripheral nerve block (PNB) is a common feature in all RP definitions [1]. Other common defining features include pain categorised as 'severe' and/or causing despair following regression of PNB [2]. Rebound pain can have a profound negative impact on quality of recovery following surgery and reduced activities of daily living for a protracted period of time [1].

The aetiology of RP remains uncertain. It is unclear whether rebound pain is simply a subjective patient experience upon transiting from 'complete regional analgesia' to 'no regional analgesia'; a reflection of the under-treatment of pain with appropriate, 'round the clock dosing' of multimodal systemic analgesia; or if RP is mechanistically related to transient nociceptive afferent blockade using sodium channel-blocking local anaesthetic agents. Some authors suggest that rebound pain and hyperalgesia share similar mechanisms [3]. Animal experiments may contribute to understanding transient hyperalgesia that can follow the resolution of a nerve block. Kolarczyk and Williams investigated behavioural changes after a single-shot ropivacaine sciatic nerve block in rats and found modest heat hyperalgesia after block resolution, without hyperalgesia to mechanical stimuli. The authors postulate the abnormal hyperactivity of C-fibers as causative [4]. Janda et al. also found evidence of transient thermal hyperalgesia in rats, approximately two hours following block resolution [5]. These experiments are of particular importance as they potentially isolate the nerve block as a principal contributing factor to RP. While bupivacaine can induce Schwann cell degeneration and demyelination, leading to transient neurotoxicity [6], this is likely not the primary cause of RP as the associated neurogenic pain is typically of longer duration [1]. Mechanical trauma from the regional anaesthesia needle insertion and local anaesthetic injectate barotrauma may also contribute to perineural inflammation [7].

In the last decade, the practice of regional anaesthesia has advanced significantly, particularly following the introduction of ultrasound-guided regional anaesthesia (UGRA). The benefits of regional anaesthesia have been well documented, and include reduced perioperative opioid use, shorter hospital stays, and the prevention of persistent post-surgical pain (PPSP) [8–10]. Unfortunately, rebound pain is an increasingly recognised adverse event [11]. Poorly controlled postoperative pain is associated with short-term consequences such as cardiovascular and respiratory complications, as well as long-term issues such as persistent post-surgical pain, opioid use disorder, and increased healthcare costs [12–14]. Although there is insufficient evidence to attribute these negative outcomes directly to RP, patient dissatisfaction and unanticipated healthcare resource utilisation have been independently associated with RP [15,16].

There is a wide variance in the incidence of rebound pain, but it is reported as being as high as 50% in patients who receive a PNB [17]. Patient risk factors associated with RP include severe pre-operative pain, female sex, and psychosocial factors such as depression [3,17]. Older patients may also experience less severe and less frequent rebound pain. A study by Sort et al. found that patients >65 years old undergoing emergency ankle fracture surgery reported lower levels of rebound pain compared to those aged between 20 and 60 years old [18]. This may be explained by age-related changes in nociceptive perception, such as a decreased sensitivity to pressure pain [19].

For procedural risk factors, patients undergoing boney surgery are 6.5 times more likely to develop rebound pain compared to those who undergo soft tissue surgery. There is a high incidence of RP in ambulatory surgery [17]. Prior to performing regional anaesthesia, the above risk factors should be considered in line with strategies for mitigation, which will be the focus of the remainder of this article.

2. Strategies for Mitigation

2.1. Patient Education

Rebound pain can occur irrespective of local anaesthetic type, volume, or concentration [20]. Thus, other factors besides the choice of local anaesthetic must be considered. Avoidance of the phenomenon of RP through prevention is the ideal objective. Patient education and management of expectations is an important factor in this. Patients expect post-surgical pain, and it is one of their most commonly reported surgical concerns [21]. It is unknown how those expectations are modified when they receive regional anaesthesia. Studies have demonstrated that individuals who expect effective pain relief often experience reduced pain perception and altered brain activity in response to painful stimuli [22]. Conversely, if these expectations are not met, it may lead to increased pain perception and reporting. This is important to consider for patients undergoing PNBs, who are often informed of significant postoperative pain relief [23]. Patients should be given a realistic expectation of block duration and understanding of the signs associated with block resolution. Educational initiatives such as pre-procedural classes and meetings with anaesthesiologists have been shown to increase the rates at which patients accept regional anaesthesia options [24,25]. Although patient education materials surrounding peripheral nerve blocks can be highly variable [26], providing written or multimedia information in addition to verbal instructions can help patients improve compliance with multimodal analgesia prior to block regression, and reduce anxiety and uncertainty before and after surgery [27].

2.2. Continuous PNB Catheters

The use of PNB catheters and continuous infusions of local anaesthetics might significantly reduce the occurrence of rebound pain by prolonging the effects of PNBs beyond the time point of significant nociceptive input. The prolongation of the sensory block might circumvent the abrupt end to the sensory blockade, thereby facilitating a tapering of the local anaesthetic effect [28].

Salviz et al. randomised patients undergoing arthroscopic rotator cuff repair surgery into three groups receiving general anaesthesia (GA) alone, GA combined with a single-shot interscalene block, and GA combined with a perineural interscalene catheter. The catheter group reported significantly lower pain scores than the other two groups at all time points, with a lower incidence of rebound pain [29]. Kim et al. randomised patients undergoing rotator cuff repair to receive single-shot or patient-controlled bolus analgesia via a continuous brachial plexus catheter. They report a lesser incidence in rebound pain in patients who received interscalene continuous nerve catheters at 12 h, when compared with a single-shot block [30].

Ganta and colleagues studied 50 patients who received either a single-shot infraclavicular PNB versus a continuous infusion of local anaesthetic for distal radius fractures. Although not statistically significant, the continuous infusion group had lower pain scores and had lower opioid requirements at each interval post operatively [31].

A recent study by Lee et al. found that continuous infraclavicular catheters reduced both the intensity and duration of rebound pain when compared to a single shot infraclavicular block for distal radius fixation. However, there was no difference in opioid consumption between the two groups. A potential limitation of this study is the use of intravenous dexmedetomidine for patient sedation, which may have influenced acute postoperative pain and subsequent analgesic requirements [32].

While continuous nerve blocks are effective and have become widely adopted, they are limited by certain practical considerations. Catheter migration can occur in both upper and lower extremities. Previous studies have reported catheter dislodgement rates of 21.7%, 9.1%, and 4.5% after continuous popliteal sciatic, infraclavicular, and interscalene blocks, respectively [29,32,33].

Careful patient follow-up is required to ensure both quality and safety, as delayed recovery of sensory and motor function is an inevitable consequence of continuous nerve block techniques. Previous studies have highlighted the risk of falls and pressure injuries in patients receiving continuous femoral nerve catheters [34]. Although the concentration, volume, and infusion rate of the local anesthetic may impact the preservation of motor function and proprioception, the precise relationship between these factors and clinical outcomes is uncertain and may vary depending on the specific anatomic location [35].

Perineural catheters also incur a small additional risk of block site complications [6]. The effective insertion of a PNB catheter requires a high level of expertise, and the safe use of continuous local anaesthesia infusions is both labour and material intensive. These cost and management factors have particularly hampered their use for ambulatory surgery.

2.3. Adjuvants

The prolongation of the effects of a PNB can be achieved through various adjuvants, which can be combined with local anaesthetic agents and administered perineurally. These include clonidine, dexmedetomidine, dexamethasone, buprenorphine, midazolam, epinephrine, tramadol, magnesium, morphine, and others [36,37]. In addition to prolonging the duration of analgesia, these adjuvants help to reduce overall dose requirements for local anaesthetics [36]. However, concerns for potential neural side effects and the toxicity of these adjuvants exist [37]. Many of these agents are not licensed for perineural use.

Dexamethasone, when given perineurally, has been shown to reduce rebound pain. Fang et al. investigated the effect of dexamethasone added to ropivacaine in patients undergoing upper limb fracture surgery. Patients who received perineural dexamethasone and ropivacaine had a five-hour mean prolongation of block, and less peak pain scores after block regression as compared to those who received ropivacaine alone [38]. It is not known how perineurally administered dexamethasone prolongs the effect of local anaesthetic agents. In mouse models of PNB, axonal degeneration and demyelination seen with the perineural administration of bupivacaine alone were significantly lessened with the admixture of perineural bupivacaine and dexamethasone [39].

Dexamethasone can also be effective in reducing RP when given intravenously. In patients undergoing ankle fracture surgery with regional anaesthesia, Gao et al. reported a reduction in rebound pain and increased PNB block duration in patients who received IV dexamethasone when compared to a control group who did not receive IV dexamethasone [40]. Interestingly, in a study by Barry et al., the absence of the intraoperative use of IV dexamethasone was cited as an independent risk factor for developing rebound pain [17]. While individual studies have indicated that perineurally administered dexamethasone may extend the duration of PNB compared to intravenous administration [41,42], a recent meta-analysis by Singh and colleagues found that both routes of administration have been shown to be equally efficacious in prolonging the duration and analgesic effect of peripheral nerve blocks. The same study also showed that the time to onset of rebound pain was also significantly delayed in the dexamethasone group compared with the control group. The optimal dose of prophylactic dexamethasone was not investigated. While the meta-analysis was limited by substantial clinical heterogeneity, the findings may be generalisable across diverse surgical populations and various nerve blocks [43].

When compared, IV and perineural dexamethasone exhibit similar safety profiles, particularly regarding postoperative nausea and vomiting and perioperative glucose levels. No long-term neurological adverse events have been associated with perineural dexamethasone, however its use remains off label [42].

The mechanism for rebound pain reduction by dexamethasone is unclear, but its role as an analgesic agent is well evidenced. It is thought to attenuate pain sensitisation by inhibiting nociceptive C-fiber transmission at the dorsal root ganglion and reducing prostaglandin production, thereby mitigating hyperalgesia [44]. As a potent anti-inflammatory agent, dexamethasone may reduce the inflammatory cascade triggered by surgical trauma and potentially modulate electrical impulses in afferent nerves supplying the injured site [45].

Ketamine offers potential to attenuate rebound pain when given perineurally. Ketamine is an NMDA antagonist which possesses anti-nociceptive and local anaesthetic properties. A recent meta-analysis of 12 RCTs examined the analgesic efficacy of perineural ketamine. The authors found that perineural ketamine was associated with a longer duration of analgesia, and lesser opioid requirement without influencing the duration of the sensory and motor block [46]. Intravenous ketamine has, however, been shown consistently to be ineffective in preventing RP. It is unclear whether perineurally administered ketamine influences RP.

Dexmedetomidine and clonidine are both centrally acting alpha-2 receptor agonists. Knight et al. found that perineurally administered dexmedetomidine, as a local anaesthetic adjuvant, appears to improve analgesia without increasing the risk of local anaesthetic neurotoxicity [36]. Dexmedetomidine is, however, associated with bradycardia and sedation when administered in this fashion [47]. This may significantly limit any potential utility. Clonidine has been shown to prolong block duration when given perineurally, without influencing the rebound pain phenomenon [47]. Both drugs carry the risk of unwanted side effects of dizziness, pruritis, headaches, and blurred vision [48].

Buprenorphine, when given perineurally, exerts its effects by blocking synaptic transmission [36]. Williams and colleagues found that buprenorphine doses exceeding 300 μg were linked to a decrease in rebound pain following PNBs for hip and knee arthroplasty, but lower doses had no such effect [47]. A further study by Tulsyan et al. found that both 150 and 300 μg doses of buprenorphine, when added to levobupivacaine for a lumbar plexus block, provided similar levels of postoperative pain relief. A dose of 300 μg, however, resulted in significant sedation and respiratory depression [49]. Hence, although buprenorphine 150 μg appears to be an optimal dose providing prolonged postoperative analgesia and minimal sedation, it has not been shown to mitigate rebound pain.

2.4. Multimodal Analgesia

It can be argued that a relatively abrupt unmasking of the typical nociceptive pain trajectory is purely a consequence of the inadequate pre-emptive administration of multimodal analgesia [50]. Many studies investigating rebound pain after PNB do not routinely incorporate perioperative systemic multimodal analgesia. Patients undergoing ambulatory outpatient surgery usually receive significantly less analgesic medication prior to discharge than those for whom inpatient accommodation is planned [1]. The transition of postoperative clinical care pathway oversight from anaesthesiologists to surgeons should be actively planned and managed. A collaborative multidisciplinary approach has been described by Saminiemi and colleagues as proven successful in avoiding excessive pain on block resolution [51].

Oral pain medications can start immediately after surgery, with the intent of achieving a steady state before regional anaesthesia wears off. A postoperative pain regimen for adult patients receiving a peripheral nerve block for ambulatory surgery has been proposed by Dawson et al. [52], but there are no studies to support its effectiveness in preventing RP.

Pre-emptive analgesia, where opioid medications are administered prior to block regression, has also been suggested as a means to provide a smooth transition to as-needed oral analgesics. One study demonstrated superior pain control with a lumbar plexus block compared to a fascia iliaca block for up to two hours post-arthroscopic hip surgery. Both groups received a standard dose of oxycodone postoperatively, resulting in similar opioid consumption and discharge times. The absence of postoperative rebound pain in both groups may be attributed to the preemptive analgesic effect of the opioid medication [53].

The optimal timing and dosing of postoperative analgesia is challenging due to factors such as the variable onset of rebound pain. For instance, rebound pain may occur 12–24 h after extremity fracture fixation [31,33] or 1–2 days after shoulder arthroscopy [54]. A recent study by Uppal and colleagues investigated giving 2 mg of hydromorphone six hours after an interscalene block to patients undergoing arthroscopic shoulder surgery. Although they did not find any difference in the worst pain score at 24 h compared with the placebo, it is likely that the peak effect of the study drug may not have coincided with the worst pain intensity, due to a large discrepancy between their hypothesised sensory block duration (6 h) and recruitment data (12 h) [55].

It should be noted that patients may also be reluctant to start taking pain medications, especially opioids, before experiencing pain. Additionally, these medications can have side effects like dizziness, nausea, and sedation, which can be problematic for ambulatory patients [56].

2.5. Pain Mechanisms

Recent advances in neuroscience and biotechnology have led to an increased understanding of the neuronal circuits and molecular mechanisms involved in pain modulation. These include genetic mutations, epigenetic and posttranslational modification, inflammasomes, signaling pathways, and microbiota [57]. This progress has facilitated the identification of novel diagnostic and therapeutic targets for different pain mechanisms [58].

Nociceptive pain, the most prevalent form of pain, originates from actual or threatened damage to non-neural tissue, leading to the activation of nociceptors. This transient response to noxious stimuli triggers protective and evasive actions. Nociplastic pain describes chronic pain conditions not attributable to direct nociceptor activation or neuropathy, but characterised by clinical and psychophysical evidence of altered nociceptive processing. Neuropathic pain is pain caused by a lesion or disease of the somatosensory nervous system. It can result from sources as varied as nerve compression, channelopathies, autoimmune disease, and incision.

Understanding the neurobiological basis of pain is key to developing mechanism-based analgesia, contingent on improved diagnostics. Elucidating neuroadaptive changes in rebound pain will enable targeted therapies. Continued translational research is essential, focusing on molecular mechanisms, targeted pharmaceutical strategies (including mechanisms of action and clinical applications), sensory phenotypes, patient clusters, and predictors of analgesic efficacy in rebound pain.

3. Conclusions

Peripheral nerve blocks (PNBs) have revolutionised postoperative pain management by reducing opioid exposure and associated side effects. However, PNBs are often linked to rebound pain, a common issue that requires proactive management to prevent short-term discomfort, long-term complications, and increased resource utilisation. Recent studies have shown that the incidence of this could be as high as 50% in ambulatory patients, and is influenced by patient, surgical, and anaesthetic factors [13].

Preoperative education is crucial for managing patient expectations and encouraging the early use of systemic multimodal pain management. A collaborative effort between anaesthesiologists and surgeons may optimise patient outcomes in this regard [13]. Continuous nerve block techniques can provide extended pain relief during the postoperative period, and intravenous dexamethasone may be a protective factor in preventing rebound pain. More research is needed into the use of pre-emptive analgesia as a means of mitigating against rebound pain.

Although rebound pain may occur with regional anaesthesia, no influence on cumulative postoperative opioid use, patient recovery outcomes, and patient satisfaction has been identified. Interestingly, despite the occurrence of rebound pain, 96% of patients expressed a preference for nerve blocks in future surgical procedures [17].

Rebound pain is a problem that requires active management to mitigate negative effects on the patient experience.

Funding: This research received no external funding.

Conflicts of Interest: The authors declare no conflicts of interest.

References

1. Muñoz-Leyva, F.; Cubillos, J.; Chin, K.J. Managing rebound pain after regional anesthesia. *Korean J. Anesthesiol.* **2020**, *73*, 372–383. [CrossRef] [PubMed]
2. Henningsen, M.J.; Sort, R.; Møller, A.M.; Herling, S.F. Peripheral nerve block in ankle fracture surgery: A qualitative study of patients' experiences. *Anaesthesia* **2018**, *73*, 49–58. [CrossRef]
3. Dada, O.; Gonzalez Zacarias, A.; Ongaigui, C.; Echeverria-Villalobos, M.; Kushelev, M.; Bergese, S.D.; Moran, K. Does rebound pain after peripheral nerve block for orthopedic surgery impact postoperative analgesia and opioid consumption? A narrative review. *Int. J. Environ. Res. Public Health* **2019**, *16*, 3257. [CrossRef]
4. Kolarczyk, L.M.; Williams, B.A. Transient heat hyperalgesia during resolution of ropivacaine sciatic nerve block in the rat. *Reg. Anesth. Pain Med.* **2011**, *36*, 220–224. [CrossRef] [PubMed]

5. Janda, A.; Lydic, R.; Welch, K.B.; Brummett, C.M. Thermal hyperalgesia after sciatic nerve block in rat is transient and clinically insignificant. *Reg. Anesth. Pain Med.* **2013**, *38*, 151–154. [CrossRef]
6. Morita, S.; Oizumi, N.; Suenaga, N.; Yoshioka, C.; Yamane, S.; Tanaka, Y. Dexamethasone added to levobupivacaine prolongs the duration of interscalene brachial plexus block and decreases rebound pain after arthroscopic rotator cuf repair. *J. Shoulder Elb. Surg.* **2020**, *29*, 1751–1757. [CrossRef] [PubMed]
7. Lavand'homme, P. Rebound pain after anesthesia in the ambulatory patient. *Curr. Opin. Anaesthesiol.* **2018**, *31*, 679–684. [CrossRef] [PubMed]
8. Kwon, S.K.; Yang, I.H.; Bai, S.J.; Han, C.D. Periarticular injection with corticosteroid has an additional pain management effect in total knee arthroplasty. *Yonsei Med. J.* **2014**, *55*, 493–498. [CrossRef] [PubMed]
9. Eroglu, M.; Er, M.S.; Altinel, L.; Kokulu, S.; Yucehan, M. The efficacy of subcutaneous local analgesic infusion in the early post-operative period after bilateral total knee arthroplasty. *Eklem Hastalik. Cerrahisi Jt. Dis. Relat. Surg.* **2015**, *26*, 158–163. [CrossRef]
10. Andreae, M.H.; Andreae, D.A. Regional anaesthesia to prevent chronic pain after surgery: A Cochrane systemic review and meta-analysis. *Br. J. Anaesth.* **2013**, *111*, 711–720. [CrossRef]
11. Nicholson, T.; Maltenfort, M.; Getz, C.; Lazarus, M.; Williams, G.; Namdari, S. Multimodal Pain Management Protocol Versus Patient Controlled Narcotic Analgesia for Postoperative Pain Control after Shoulder Arthroplasty. *Arch. Bone Jt. Surg. ABJS* **2018**, *6*, 196–202. [PubMed]
12. de Oliveira, R.M.; Tenório, S.B.; Tanaka, P.P.; Precoma, D. Control of pain through epidural block and incidence of cardiac dysrhythmias in postoperative period of thoracic and major abdominal surgical procedures: A comparative study. *Braz. J. Anesthesiol.* **2012**, *62*, 10–18. [CrossRef]
13. Shea, R.A.; Brooks, J.A.; Dayhoff, N.E.; Keck, J. Pain intensity and postoperative pulmonary complications among the elderly after abdominal surgery. *Heart Lung* **2002**, *31*, 440–449. [CrossRef] [PubMed]
14. Fletcher, D.; Stamer, U.M.; Pogatzki-Zahn, E.; Zaslansky, R.; Tanase, N.V.; Perruchoud, C.; Kranke, P.; Komann, M.; Lehman, T. Chronic postsurgical pain in Europe: An observational study. *Eur. J. Anaesth.* **2015**, *32*, 725–734. [CrossRef] [PubMed]
15. Hade, A.D.; Okano, S.; Pelecanos, A.; Chin, A. Factors associated with low levels of patient satisfaction following peripheral nerve block. *Anaesth. Intensive Care* **2021**, *49*, 125–132. [CrossRef]
16. Jen, T.T.; Ke, J.X.; Wing, K.J.; Denomme, J.; McIsaac, D.I.; Huang, S.-C.; Ree, R.M.; Prabhakar, C.; Schwarz, S.K.; Yarnold, C.H. Development and internal validation of a multivariable risk prediction model for severe rebound pain after foot and ankle surgery involving single-shot popliteal sciatic nerve block. *Br. J. Anaesth.* **2022**, *129*, 127–135. [CrossRef] [PubMed]
17. Barry, G.S.; Bailey, J.G.; Sardinha, J.; Brousseau, P.; Uppal, V. Factors associated with rebound pain after peripheral nerve block for ambulatory surgery. *Br. J. Anaesth.* **2021**, *126*, 862–871. [CrossRef]
18. Sort, R.; Brorson, S.; Gögenur, I.; Nielsen, J.K.; Møller, A.M. Rebound pain following peripheral nerve block anaesthesia in acute ankle fracture surgery: An exploratory pilot study. *Acta Anaesthesiol. Scand.* **2019**, *63*, 396–402. [CrossRef] [PubMed]
19. Lautenbacher, S.; Kunz, M.; Strate, P.; Nielsen, J.; Arendt-Nielsen, L. Age effects on pain thresholds, temporal summation and spatial summation of heat and pressure pain. *Pain* **2005**, *115*, 410–418. [CrossRef]
20. Abdallah, F.W.; Halpern, S.H.; Aoyama, K.; Brull, R. Will the real benefits of single shot interscalene block please stand up? A sys-temic revie wand meta-analysis. *Anesth. Analg.* **2015**, *120*, 1114–1129. [CrossRef]
21. Berkowitz, R.B.; Vu, J.; Brummett, C.; Waljee, J.; Englesbe, M.; Howard, R. The Impact of Complications and Pain on Patient Satisfaction. *Ann. Surg.* **2021**, *273*, 1127–1134. [CrossRef] [PubMed]
22. Büchel, C.; Geuter, S.; Sprenger, C.; Eippert, F. Placebo analgesia: A predictive coding perspective. *Neuron* **2014**, *81*, 1223–1239. [CrossRef] [PubMed]
23. Sunderland, S.; Yarnold, C.H.; Head, S.J.; Osborn, J.A.; Purssell, A.; Peel, J.K.; Schwarz, S.K. Regional versus general anesthesia and the incidence of unplanned health care resource utilization for postoperative pain after wrist fracture surgery: Results from a retrospective quality improvement project. *Reg. Anesth. Pain Med.* **2016**, *41*, 22–27. [CrossRef]
24. Brooks, B.S.; Barman, J.; Ponce, B.; Sides, A.; Vetter, T.R. An electronic surgical order, undertaking patient education, and obtaining informed consent for regional analgesia before the day of surgery reduce block-related delays. *Local Reg. Anesth.* **2016**, *9*, 59–64. [CrossRef] [PubMed]
25. Elkassabany, N.M.; Abraham, D.; Huang, S.; Kase, B.; Pio, F.; Hume, E.; Israelite, C.; Liu, J. Patient education and anesthesia choice for total knee arthroplasty. *Patient Educ. Couns.* **2017**, *100*, 1709–1713. [CrossRef]
26. Kumar, G.; Howard, S.K.; Kou, A. Availability and Readability of Online Patient Education Materials Regarding Regional An-esthesia Techniques for Perioperative Pain Management. *Pain Med.* **2017**, *18*, 2027–2032. [PubMed]
27. Jlala, H.; French, J.; Foxall, G.; Hardman, J.; Bedforth, N. Effect of preoperative multimedia information on perioperative anxiety in patients undergoing procedures under regional anaesthesia. *Br. J. Anaesth.* **2010**, *104*, 369–374. [CrossRef]
28. Nobre, L.V.; Cunha, G.P.; de Sousa, P.C.C.B.; Takeda, A.; Ferraro, L.H.C. Peripheral nerve block and rebound pain: Literature review. *Braz. J. Anesthesiol. Engl. Ed.* **2019**, *69*, 587–593. [CrossRef]

29. Salviz, E.A.; Xu, D.; Frulla, A. Continuous interscalene block in patients having outpatient rotator cuff repair surgery: A pro-spective randomized trial. *Anesth. Analg.* **2013**, *117*, 1485–1492. [CrossRef]
30. Kim, J.H.; Koh, H.J.; Dong, K.K. Interscalene brachial plexus bolus block versus patient-controlled interscalene indwelling catheter analgesia for the first 48 hours after arthroscopic rotator cuff repair. *J. Shoulder Elb. Surg.* **2018**, *27*, 1243–1250. [CrossRef] [PubMed]
31. Ganta, A.; Ding, D.; Fisher, N. Continuous infraclavicular brachial plexus block versus single-shot nerve block for distal radius surgery: A prospective randomized control trial. *Orthop. Trauma.* **2018**, *32*, 22–26.
32. Lee, J.-H.; Kim, H.-J.; Kim, J.K.; Cheon, S.; Shin, Y.H. Does intravenous patient-controlled analgesia or continuous block prevent rebound pain following infraclavicular brachial plexus block after distal radius fracture fixation? A prospective randomized controlled trial. *Korean J. Anesthesiol.* **2023**, *76*, 559–566. [CrossRef] [PubMed]
33. Ding, D.Y.; Manoli, A.; Galos, D.K.; Jain, S.; Tejwani, N.C. Continuous popliteal sciatic nerve block versus single injection nerve block for ankle fracture surgery: A prospective randomized comparative trial. *J. Orthop. Trauma* **2015**, *29*, 393–398. [CrossRef] [PubMed]
34. Aguirre, J.; Del Moral, A.; Cobo, I.; Borgeat, A.; Blumenthal, S. The role of continuous peripheral nerve blocks. *Anesthesiol. Res. Pract.* **2012**, *2012*, 560879. [CrossRef]
35. Le, L.T.; Loland, V.J.; Mariano, E.R.; Gerancher, J.; Wadhwa, A.N.; Renehan, E.M.; Sessler, D.I.; Shuster, J.J.; Theriaque, D.W.; Maldonado, R.C.; et al. Effects of local anesthetic concentration and dose on continuous interscalene nerve blocks: A dual-center, randomized, observer-masked, controlled study. *Reg. Anesth. Pain Med.* **2008**, *33*, 518–525. [CrossRef]
36. Knight, J.B.; Schott, N.J.; Kentor, M.L.; Williams, B.A. Neurotoxicity of common peripheral nerve block adjuvants. *Curr. Opin. Anaesthesiol.* **2015**, *28*, 598–604. [CrossRef]
37. Kirksey, M.A.; Haskins, S.C.; Cheng, J.; Liu, S.S. Local anesthetic peripheral nerve block adjuvants for prolongation of analgesia: A systematic qualitative review. *PLoS ONE* **2015**, *10*, e0137312. [CrossRef] [PubMed]
38. Fang, J.; Shi, Y.; Du, F. The effect of perineural dexamethasone on rebound pain after ropivacaine single-injection nerve block: A randomized controlled trial. *BMC Anesthesiol.* **2021**, *21*, 47. [CrossRef] [PubMed]
39. An, K.; Elkassabany, N.M.; Liu, J. Dexamethasone as adjuvant to bupivacaine prolongs the duration of thermal antinociception and prevents bupivacaine-induced rebound hyperalgesia via regional mechanism in a mouse sciatic nerve block model. *PLoS ONE* **2015**, *10*, e0123459. [CrossRef] [PubMed]
40. Gao, M.; Li, Y.; Yu, J.; Li, W.; Qin, S.; Zhang, Y.; Zhu, L.; Hou, Z.; Wang, Q. The Effects of Intravenous Dexamethasone on Rebound Pain After Nerve Block in Patients with Ankle Fracture: A Randomized Controlled Trial. *J. Pain Res.* **2023**, *16*, 1127–1136. [CrossRef] [PubMed]
41. Heesen, M.; Klimek, M.; Imberger, G. Co-administration of dexamethasone with peripheral nerve block: Intravenous vs perineural application: Systematic review, meta-analysis, meta-regression and trial-sequential analysis. *Br. J. Anaesth.* **2018**, *120*, 212–227. [CrossRef]
42. Hussain, N.; Langenbergh, T.V.D.; Sermer, C.; Fontes, M.L.; Atrey, A.; Shaparin, N.; Sawyer, T.R.; Vydyanathan, A. Equivalent analgesic effectiveness between perineural and intravenous dexamethasone as adjuvants for peripheral nerve blockade: A systematic review and meta-analysis. *Can. J. Anaesth.* **2017**, *65*, 194–206. [CrossRef]
43. Singh, N.P.; Makkar, J.K.; Chawla, J.K.; Sondekoppam, R.V.; Singh, P.M. Prophylactic dexamethasone for rebound pain after peripheral nerve block in adult surgical patients: Systematic review, meta-analysis, and trial sequential analysis of randomised controlled trials. *Br. J. Anaesth.* **2024**, *132*, 1112–1121. [CrossRef] [PubMed]
44. Zell, V.; Juif, P.E.; Hanesch, U. Corticosterone analgesia is mediated by the spinal production of neuroactive metabolites that enhance GABAergic inhibitory trans- mission on dorsal horn rat neurons. *Eur. J. Neurosci.* **2015**, *41*, 390.e7. [CrossRef]
45. Maagaard, M.; Stormholt, E.R.; Nielsen, L.F. Perineural and systemic dexamethasone and ulnar nerve block duration: A random-ized, blinded, placebo-controlled trial in healthy volunteers. *Anesthesiology* **2023**, *138*, 625.e33. [CrossRef] [PubMed]
46. Xiang, J.; Cao, C.; Chen, J.; Kong, F.; Nian, S.; Li, Z.; Li, N. Efficacy and safety of ketamine as an adjuvant to regional anesthesia: A systematic review and meta-analysis of randomized controlled trials. *J. Clin. Anesth.* **2024**, *94*, 111415. [CrossRef] [PubMed]
47. Williams, B.A.; Ibinson, J.W.; Mangione, M.P.; Modrak, R.T.; Tonarelli, E.J.; Rakesh, H.; Kmatz, A.M.; Cohen, P.Z. Research priorities regarding multimodal peripheral nerve blocks for postoperative analgesia and anesthesia based on hospital quality data extracted from over 1,300 cases (2011–2014). *Pain Med.* **2015**, *16*, 7–12. [CrossRef]
48. El-Boghdadly, K.; Brull, R.; Sehmbi, H. Perineural dexmedetomidine is more efective than clonidine when added to local anesthetic for supraclavicular brachial plexus block: A systemic revie wand meta-analysis. *Anesth. Analg.* **2017**, *124*, 2008–2020. [CrossRef] [PubMed]
49. Tulsyan, V.; Singh, J.; Thakur, L.; Verma, V.; Minhas, A. A comparative study of buprenorphine in two different doses as an adjuvant to levobupivacaine in US-guided lumbar plexus block for postoperative analgesia. *Ain-Shams J. Anesthesiol.* **2021**, *13*, 7. [CrossRef]
50. Hamilton, D.L. Rebound pain: Distinct pain phenomenon or nonentity? *Br. J. Anaesth.* **2021**, *126*, 761–763. [CrossRef] [PubMed]

51. Samineni, A.V.; Seaver, T.; Sing, D.C. Peripheral nerve blocks associated with shorter length of stay without increasing readmission rate for ankle open reduction internal fixation in the outpatient setting: A propensity-matched analysis. *J. Foot Ankle Surg.* **2021**, *62*, 1165–1169.
52. Dawson, S.; Loewenstein, S. Severe Rebound pain after peripheral nerve block for ambulatory extremity surgery is an underappreciated problem. Comment on Br J Anaesth 2021; 126: 862-71. *Br. J. Anaesth.* **2021**, *126*, e204–e205. [CrossRef] [PubMed]
53. Wolff, A.B.; Hogan, G.W.; Capon, J.M.; Napoli, A.M.; Smith, H.J.; Gaspar, P.S. Pre-operative lumbar plexus block provides superior post-operative analgesia when compared with fascia iliaca block or general anesthesia alone in hip arthroscopy. *J. Hip Preserv. Surg.* **2016**, *3*, 338–345. [CrossRef] [PubMed]
54. Stiglitz, Y.; Gosselin, O.; Sedaghatian, J.; Sirveaux, F.; Molé, D. Pain after shoulder arthroscopy: A prospective study on 231 cases. *Orthop. Traumatol. Surg. Res.* **2011**, *97*, 260–266. [CrossRef] [PubMed]
55. Uppal, V.; Barry, G.; Ke, J.X.C.; Kwofie, M.K.; Trenholm, A.; Khan, M.; Shephard, A.; Retter, S.; Shanthanna, H. Reducing rebound pain severity after arthroscopic shoulder surgery under general anesthesia and interscalene block: A two-centre randomized controlled trial of pre-emptive opioid treatment compared with placebo. *Can. J. Anaesth.* **2024**, *71*, 773–783. [CrossRef] [PubMed]
56. Bruhn, J. Pain rebound in day surgery: How can we avoid it? *Reg. Anesth. Pain Med.* **2019**, *44*, A8–A10.
57. Cai, H.; Ao, Z.; Tian, C.; Wu, Z.; Kaurich, C.; Chen, Z.; Gu, M.; Hohmann, A.G.; Mackie, K.; Guo, F. Engineering human spinal microphysiological systems to model opioid-induced tolerance. *Bioact. Mater.* **2023**, *22*, 482–490. [CrossRef] [PubMed]
58. Souza Monteiro de Araujo, D.; Nassini, R.F. TRPA1 as a therapeutic target for nociceptive pain. *Expert Opin. Ther. Targets* **2020**, *24*, 997–1008. [CrossRef]

Journal of
Clinical Medicine

MDPI

Article

Adaptation and Validation of the Survey of Pain Attitudes (SOPA-Brief Scale (30 Items)) in Greek

Ioannis Dalakakis [1], Nadia Malliou [1,*], Despoina Sarridou [1], Eleni Moka [2] and Aikaterini Amaniti [1]

1 Department of Anesthesiology and Intensive Care, School of Medicine, Aristotle University of Thessaloniki, 54124 Thessaloniki, Greece; idalakakis@gmail.com (I.D.); dsarridou@auth.gr (D.S.); aamaniti@auth.gr (A.A.)
2 Department of Anesthesiology, Creta Interclinic Hospital, Hellenic Healthcare Group (HHG), 71304 Heraklion Crete, Greece; mokaeleni@hotmail.com
* Correspondence: kmallio@auth.gr; Tel.: +30-6973731380

Abstract: Background: The attitudes and beliefs of patients with chronic pain significantly affect their response to treatment. The Survey of Pain Attitudes (SOPA) scale was developed to identify pain-related beliefs. The aim of the present study was to adapt and validate the short version (30 items) of the Survey of Pain Attitudes in 200 Greek patients living with chronic pain, mainly due to rheumatic and musculoskeletal diseases (RMDs). **Method**: In addition to the SOPA-Brief scale (30 items), the participants completed the Pain Beliefs, Perceptions and Attitudes Inventory (PBAPI) and also the Chronic Pain Coping Inventory (CPCI). **Results**: Data analysis revealed that the internal reliability coefficient of the scale in the Greek language was Cronbach's a = 0.773 for the individual items, and for the subscales, it ranged from Cronbach's a = 0.56 (for the SOPAMedication scale) to Cronbach's a = 0.78 (for the SOPASolicitude scale). Similarly, the SOPA-Brief subscales in Greek showed positive correlations with subscales of both the PBAPI and the CPCI. Finally, an exploratory factor analysis was performed on the dataset and confirmed the structure of the original scale (Eigenvalues > 1), with 71.54% of variance explained. **Conclusions**: Overall, the psychometric properties of the short version of the Attitudes Towards Pain Scale (30 items) in Greek show acceptable internal reliability and validity for the scale to be used in daily clinical and research practice.

Keywords: chronic pain; attitudes towards pain; survey of pain attitudes-brief; perceptions of pain; beliefs about pain

1. Introduction

In recent years, research has increasingly been focusing on the psychosocial factors that influence pain and, by extension, affect the outcomes of treatment. The aim is to generate more data on the parameters of pain that may influence decision making on chronic pain management so that treatment planning can become even more effective [1]. An individual's beliefs and attitudes towards pain can influence the likelihood of them developing long-term pain or disability associated with it [2]. It has been found that patients who adopt passive coping strategies, such as "rest and medication", use three times as many healthcare appointments and have twice the level of disability due to their pain compared to those who adopt active strategies (e.g., exercise) [3]. Changing patients' attitudes towards pain can reduce their level of pain and its impact on their quality of life [4].

It is not uncommon that patients who have experienced pain for prolonged periods of time try to avoid any activity that could potentially exacerbate their pain. This is a coping strategy that can become maladaptive when used repeatedly, leading to an avoidant behavior based on fear [5,6]. The assessment and use of coping strategies are the cornerstones of pain management. A patient may use cognitive and behavioral resources to manage specific external and/or internal demands that are assessed as stressful or go beyond the individual's resources [7]. Pain coping strategies employ cognitive processes that involve an internal appraisal of the pain and then the mobilization of the coping resources available for managing the pain. This is followed by responses to pain and its effects based on the initial appraisals. Responses have been classified as active (e.g., remaining in employment) and passive (e.g., continued rest), depending on whether the response involves performing a task versus avoiding activity as a means of dealing with pain. Current pain adaptation paradigms do not account for the numerous patients that do not show signs of the effects of chronic pain. Resilience is the integrative perspective illuminating the traits and mechanisms underlying the ability to recover and the sustainability of quality of life in individuals recovering from trauma and distress [8]. Maladaptive pain coping and beliefs may eliminate any positive benefits of adaptive coping responses [7].

A person's attitudes and beliefs have a significant impact on their response to pain treatment [9]. Multidisciplinary approaches to pain typically focus on cognitive interventions aimed at changing unhelpful or dysfunctional cognitive attitudes and beliefs about pain, such as avoidance and fear of activity, catastrophizing and the belief that pain is necessarily the result of tissue damage [10]. Studies have shown that these approaches lead to increased functional performance, induce positive changes in pain experience (i.e., measures of sensation and ratings of pain as "unpleasant"), increase cognitive coping and appraisal (positive coping measures) and decrease behavioral expressions of pain [11]. Several scales exist to assess patients' attitudes and beliefs about pain. The Survey of Pain Attitudes (SOPA) is one of them, and it was developed to identify pain-related beliefs. It has been proven to be useful in the management of chronic pain [12,13]. Previous results of SOPA use beliefs of associating disability with pain and both psychological and physical dysfunction. A strong belief that pain equals physical injury in association with greater physical dysfunction and that emotions affect pain which is associated with psychosocial dysfunction [14].

This scale, which assesses a range of attitudes towards pain, was originally developed by Jensen et al. (1987) [13–15] to assess patients' attitudes towards five pillars of the chronic pain experience: pain control, pain-related disability, medical treatment of pain, caring for others and medication for pain. In its original version, it consisted of 57 items and had seven subscales. Its factorial structure was not distinct or confirmed, and its completion time was quite prolonged. For these reasons, Tait and Chibnall (1997) [16] proceeded to create the short version, with 30 items, which was translated and evaluated for its psychometric characteristics in Greek in the present study. The reliability of the 30-item version of the scale was satisfactory (with a Cronbach's range of a = 0.7 to 0.83; however, a was 0.5 in some subscales). The correlations of the final subscales with the subscales of the original version were high, and in addition, the corresponding correlations with other psychometric scales were also high. The SOPA-Brief (30 items) [16] consists of 30 questions with the possibility of a single response on a 5-point Likert-type scale, from 0 to 4, where 0 means completely wrong and 4 means completely right. The questionnaire can be completed either by the participant, the researcher or a health professional, if necessary. There are some additional scales that assess pain-related beliefs, such as the Pain Beliefs and Perceptions Inventory [17], the Pain Catastrophizing scale [18] and also the Fear–Avoidance Beliefs Questionnaire (FABQ) [19]. In the present study, we tried to adapt and validate the psychometric characteristics of the SOPA-Brief (30 items) [16] in Greek patients with chronic pain, mainly due to rheumatic and musculoskeletal diseases (RMDs).

2. Materials and Methods

For the use of SOPA Brief in this study, including the process of translation, adaptation and validation in Greek, permission was obtained from Professor Tait. The translation process lasted one month. The translation from the original language into the Greek language was performed by an independent translator. A bilingual translator adapted the questionnaire into Greek, his native language, in order to better reflect the local expressions. The first translator was aware of the specific concepts the questionnaire intended to measure, so that the Greek version would more closely reflect the original tool. The second translation was produced by a "naïve translator" who did not know the aim of the questionnaire, so that subtle differences with the original questionnaire could be identified [15]. Discrepancies between the two translators were discussed with the researcher and an expert in order for them to be resolved. The initial translation was performed independently to ensure the accuracy of the translation. Similarly, the reverse translation was performed by two independent translators, in their native language, to avoid any form of bias. Finally, the expert and the researcher cross-checked the result before proceeding to the pilot phase of weighting. For the process of the cross-cultural adaption of questionnaires, there are numerous guidelines, and several best practices have been suggested, but no one "gold standard" has, as of yet, been clearly defined [20]. Therefore, in this process, we followed the guidelines of Tsang et al. [21].

The questionnaires were distributed to a total of 200 patients with a diagnosis of chronic pain and a primary diagnosis of an RMD (68.5%), without any restriction or exclusion criteria relative to a specific diagnosis in the validation process. These were patients in the outpatient clinic of the Chronic Pain Clinic of the AHEPA University General Hospital of Thessaloniki, during the period June–December 2018 for the pilot phase (n = 50). Then, during the period January–June 2019, data collection from the remaining participants (n = 150) followed. Finally, during the period December–May 2023, the first 30 patients were recruited to complete the questionnaires again, in order to conduct test reliability checks for repeated measures.

The sampling method was convenience sampling. The chronic pain diagnosis criterion had to be met, and the researcher had to have easy access to a high enough number of patients. Although this is a non-probability sampling method, it is the most applicable and widely used method in clinical research. In this method, researchers approach participants according to their availability and accessibility. Therefore, it is quick, cheap and convenient for its accessibility and proximity to the participants [22]. Even though non-probability sampling methods are practical and cost-effective, they do present some disadvantages and biases, like selection bias because participants are not randomly chosen. This could result in some groups not being present in the sample and hence in the researcher not being able to achieve the necessary representativeness. This could limit the ability to generalize outcomes. Still, in our target population, this method is preferred due to the specific criterion that needs to be present [23].

In Chronic Pain Units, patients are referred for chronic-pain-specific follow-up regardless of their baseline diagnosis, which makes them suitable participants in this validation study. Still, this Pain Unit mainly treats patients with non-malignant chronic pain, due to fibromyalgia, osteoarthritis, rheumatoid arthritis and several other, rarer chronic pain syndromes.

During recruitment, participants were informed about the purposes of this study verbally and written consent was obtained, according to which they were informed (a) on the principles of the protection of their personal data and (b) that their personal data would be safeguarded. The principal researcher also had to keep records until the end of this study. Then, the consent form informed participants of the ways in which they could withdraw their participation at any time and contact the researcher by phone or email. An adequate time frame was kept in order to avoid response from memory for test–retest reliability.

Psychometric Properties and Statistical Analysis

Each scale and questionnaire was evaluated based on two properties: reliability and validity. Questionnaire reliability was assessed through internal consistency and test–retest reliability. Internal consistency assesses the extent to which the questions that make up a scale measure the same concept. It is calculated by means of Cronbach's alpha, which assesses the degree of correlation between the questions in the questionnaire. Values greater than or equal to 0.7 are acceptable; however, in the use of new scales and questionnaires, values between 0.5 and 0.6 could also be acceptable. Indeed, there is much debate, especially for scales and questionnaires undergoing weighting, whether researchers derive more information about the internal reliability of the new instrument by looking at Cronbach's for all individual items or only for subscales when they exist [24]. In this study, item internal consistency was calculated for each question. Test–retest reliability was calculated using Spearman's rho correlation coefficient, which is able to adopt values between −1 and 1, where 1 indicates a perfect correlation and −1 indicates a perfect negative correlation. In this study, a correlation was interpreted as very strong ($r > \pm 0.8$), moderately strong ($r \pm 0.6$–0.8), fair ($r \pm 0.3$–0.6) and poor ($r < \pm 0.3$) [25].

Exploratory factor analysis (EFA) was performed on the data to examine the covariance of variables by groups in order to interpret the correlations between them. Most importantly, this was to check whether the tool adapted to the Greek language follows the original structure of Tait and Chibnall [16] with 7 factors. If not, some structural adaptation, better suited for the Greek population, would be needed. The Kaiser–Meyer–Olkin (KMO) test and Bartlett's global test were used to test the suitability of the collected data in applying the factor analysis. KMO values > 0.5 indicate the correct choice of method for the analysis [26]. The eigenvalue criterion (eigenvalue of >1.0), which is commonly adopted for factor extraction, was used to select the number of factors. Finally, a shift in axes to principal component analysis was applied. The validity of conceptual construction was examined by correlating the questionnaire with related questionnaires, and emphasis was placed on subscales and dimensions that showed a statistically significant correlation at both $p < 0.05$ and $p < 0.01$.

3. Results

3.1. Demographic Characteristics of Participants

The mean age of the participants was 65 years, with sd = 14.8 years. Of the participants, 63% were female and 37% were male. A total of 44.5% of the participants had completed secondary education and 29% had completed university education, while 7% had completed compulsory education and 19.5% were technical education graduates. From the 50 patients who participated in the pilot phase, 30 were females (60%) and 20 were males (40%). In total, out of 200 participants, 37% (n = 74) were males and 63% (n = 126) were females. In both phases of the validation process, the pilot phase and the main phase, in addition to the SOPA-Brief, the Pain Beliefs Attitudes and Perceptions Inventory (PBAPI) and the Chronic Pain Coping Inventory were administered.

Asymmetry and SD item evaluation analysis of the questionnaire showed that skewness values for questionnaire items were to the left/negative side, albeit ranging close to values from −0.5 to +0.5, indicating a normal distribution. Extreme skewness was marked for seven items [2,3,5,7,12,13,25]. These were items involved in several SOPA subscales and were not removed in this stage of the analysis following Tait and Chibnall's initial structural use of the questionnaire, as well as other researchers' approach [27,28].

3.2. SOPA Brief Internal Reliability Index (30 Items)

The internal reliability of the SOPA Brief (30 items) was found to be Cronbach's a = 0.67 for all questions. For the individual scales, the index ranged from 0.506 (for the SOPAMedication scale) to 0.883 (for the SOPAEmotion scale). [Note that the scale has reversed items.] In the second phase, when the remaining patients in this study (n = 150) were included, the internal reliability of the SOPA Brief was calculated for all items of the scale and was Cronbach's a = 0.773 for the individual items (after reverse coding). For the subscales of the questionnaire, it ranged from 0.56 (for the SOPAMedication scale) to 0.78 (for the SOPASolicitude scale) (Table A1).

3.3. Reliability Index of Repeated Measures

In the third phase, the first 30 patients were given the SOPA-Brief and PBAPI questionnaires again after a long period of time to determine the test–retest reliability index. The original study design planned for a long interval of 3 months, suited for less stable constructs such as beliefs and attitudes [29]. The actual time interval was a lot longer than that. The back-to-back lockdowns following strict national health protocols in Greece due to COVID-19 pandemic resulted in time deviations from the original study design, and the test–retest sampling was performed a year later. The analysis was performed using Spearman's rho correlation coefficient, with the values being interpreted as very strong ($r > \pm0.8$), moderately strong ($r \pm 0.6$–0.8), fair ($r \pm 0.3$–0.6) and poor ($r < \pm0.3$). The SOPATreatment subscale had a $r = 0.813$, $p < 0.01$, the SOPAControl $r = 0.996$, $p < 0.01$, the SOPAHarm $r = 0.963$, $p < 0.01$, the SOPADisability subscale $r = 0.484$, $p < 0.01$, the SOPAMedication $r = 534$, $p < 0.01$, the SOPASolicitude $r = 465$, $p < 0.01$ and the SOPAEmotion $r = 433$, $p < 0.01$. Three of the subscales showed very strong reliability, whereas the other four subscales presented fair test–retest reliability.

3.4. Correlations with the Pain Beliefs and Attitudes Inventory and the Chronic Pain Coping Inventory

The SOPA Brief demonstrated positive correlations with some subscales of the Pain Beliefs and Attitudes Inventory-PBAPI and some subscales of the Chronic Pain Coping Inventory-CPCI, at both levels of statistical significance $p < 0.05$ and $p < 0.01$. In particular, the Solicitude subscale was found to be weakly positively correlated with the Mystery subscale and moderately positively correlated with the Self-Blame subscale of the PBAPI (Pearson's $r = 0.256$ $p < 0.01$ and $r = 0.351$ $p < 0.01$, respectively). The Emotion subscale had a weak positive correlation with the Time and Mystery subscales of the PBAPI ($r = 0.165$ $p < 0.05$ and $r = 0.247$ $p < 0.01$). This subscale also had a weak positive correlation with the Social Support subscale of the CPCI ($r = 0.146$ $p < 0.05$). Furthermore, the SOPA Brief Control subscale had a weak negative correlation with the Time subscale ($r = -0.252$ $p < 0.01$) and Mystery subscale ($r = 0.153$ $p < 0.05$). The Medication subscale presented a weak positive correlation with the Self-Blame subscale of the PBAPI ($r = 0.151$ $p < 0.05$) (see Tables A2 and A3).

3.5. Exploratory Factor Analysis (EFA)

The entire sample of data was checked for suitability to conduct exploratory factor analysis. To proceed with the analysis, it is necessary to meet the criterion of KMO > 0.5. For this dataset, the following was the case: the Kaiser–Meyer–Olkin Index (KMO) was calculated to be 0.632 (>0.5), which was considered sufficient for performing factor analysis on this dataset. Similarly, Bartlett's test of sphericity was statistically significant ($p < 0.01$), indicating that the choice of factor analysis was correct.

The exploratory factor analysis (EFA) was performed to reduce the number of items, as this questionnaire has already been adapted and validated in other languages and in some cases, it was necessary to adapt (and assimilate) a subscale for optimal adaptation to the target population. The application of the factor selection criterion (eigenvalue > 1) resulted in seven factors, exactly as in the original version of the questionnaire [16]. Table A4 shows the factors with eigenvalues above 1 (eigenvalue > 1), as well as the percentage of covariance they explain. Note that the resulting factors (subscales) explain 71.54% of the covariance of the individual items. Finally, Table A5 shows the resulting loadings per factor.

4. Discussion

The results of this study showed that the adaptation and validation of the SOPA-Brief presents with similar psychometric characteristics as the original version of Tait and Chibnall [16], consistent with its subscales and reliability and validity measures, respectively. The internal reliability of individual items and the seven subscales were satisfactory, with two less-than-satisfactory subscales, like the original version of the questionnaire. Furthermore, the SOPA-Brief had strong, positive correlations with several subscales with similar conceptual constructs from other scales, such as the PBAPI and CPI. Most importantly, the EFA came up with a similar structure for this set of data, validating that the subscales work well with the Greek target population as well. The two weak subscales, SOPAMedication and SOPADisability, had already been highlighted in the original work of Tait and Chibnall [16], and the possible explanation for their non-satisfactory internal reliability might be their number of items or their conceptual overlap with other subscales. This needs to be further investigated in a future multicenter study in Pain Unit patients, probably resulting in a modified version of the SOPA-Brief. In a corresponding study on the adaptation and weighting of the SOPA-B in the Portuguese language, the two scales were removed as they were not supported by the factor structure of the analysis performed [30]. In the present case, the removal of the two subscales did not improve the model. The internal consistency of the model was already satisfactory.

There are several advantages associated with the availability of a short scale measuring pain-related attitudes specifically in clinical context. Clearly, the primary one relates to the ease of administration but also to the usefulness of the information extracted from the interpretation of the scores on the subscales indicating patients' attitudes towards pain. Other advantages may arise from making it easier to provide a short scale assessing patients' attitudes, which can be tested in a wide range of treatment settings (e.g., work empowerment programs), to identify patients whose attitudes might interfere with a good response to the treatment in question.

The present study supports the conclusion that the Survey of Pain Attitudes (SOPA-Brief) is a reliable and valid tool in Greek and can be used in the Greek population. However, the limitations of this study should be mentioned. One limitation is that data were collected at a very difficult time for conducting studies, with some time intervals longer than the ones in the original design, due to the COVID-19 pandemic and all the restrictions it created. Until cross-validation research is conducted on the scale in Greek, it is too early to assume that it is as reliable and valid as it appears to be in its original form in English. Similarly, it could be potentially premature to assume that the SOPA Brief possesses the clinical value of the equivalent scale in English, the Survey of Pain Attitudes (SOPA, 57 items) [28]. Another drawback of the present study concerns the fixed order in which the questionnaires were given. The order was designed to start with the basic demographic data of the participants and finish with the scales and questionnaires to be used in the validation process. However, the participants (n = 30) who took part in the repeated test were not given one of the selected questionnaires for the sake of brevity. These effects may account for the improvements in the internal reliability values of the scale and merit further investigation in future cross-validation research of the psychometric properties of the scale. Finally, another limitation is that the SOPA Brief had weak positive, one weak negative and one moderate positive correlation to the PBAPI and CPI subscales, and this is another limitation indicating the possible inherent differences in the basic constructs of the questionnaires.

Despite the aforementioned limitations, the Survey of Pain Attitudes—30 items (SOPA-Brief) appears to be a feasible assessment tool for everyday clinical practice, either as a stand-alone test or as part of a battery of tools measuring and assessing the psychological dimensions of pain. A positive feature of the scale is its brevity and ease of use, and with further study, it may emerge as a useful tool for future research on patient attitudes and beliefs, flexible enough to be used by a variety of disciplines involved in chronic pain management.

5. Conclusions

In regards to the psychometric characteristics of the SOPA-Brief in the Greek language, the findings of this study show evidence of acceptable internal consistency for this tool to be used in Greek pain patients. As mentioned above, it is expected for tools that have not been widely used in clinical settings to result in a Cronbach's a ranging from 0.5 to 0.6 and still be considered acceptable for use. In our case, that only occurred for two out the seven subscales, same as for the original version of the SOPA-Brief. In addition, the tool appears to be comparable in terms of validity to those already existing and used in the Greek clinical context. In summary, the use of the SOPA-Brief in the Greek language can contribute substantially to chronic pain research and clinical practice as well. Its use can provide another validated tool for chronic pain assessment in Pain Units, therefore making it more possible to address patients' needs for pain diagnosis, treatment and management.

Author Contributions: Conceptualization and data collection: I.D.; data analysis, validation, writing—preparation of the original draft of the manuscript: N.M.; writing—review and editing: D.S., manuscript review: E.M.; supervision: A.A. All authors have read and agreed to the published version of the manuscript.

Funding: This research received no external funding.

Institutional Review Board Statement: This study was conducted as part of the PhD Thesis of Ioannis Dalakakis and was approved by the Ethics Committee of the School of Medicine, Aristotle University of Thessaloniki, Greece. Clinical Protocol Number 03/28/2 May 2018.

Informed Consent Statement: Informed consent was obtained from all subjects involved in this study.

Data Availability Statement: Data are available from the corresponding author on reasonable request.

Conflicts of Interest: The authors declare no conflicts of interest.

Abbreviations

The following abbreviations are used in this manuscript:

SOPA	Survey of Pain Attitudes
CPCI	Chronic Pain Coping Inventory
PBAPI	Pain Beliefs, Perceptions and Attitudes Inventory

Appendix A

Table A1. Internal relevance indicators of SOPA Brief subscales in Greek.

Survey of Pain Attitudes—Brief Version (30 Items)		
	Cronbach's a	
	Validation Phase	Test–Retest
Scale	n = 200	n = 30
Solicitude	0.78(5)	0.97(5)
Emotion	0.71(4)	0.99(4)
Control	0.69(5)	0.86(5)
Treatment	0.63(5)	0.87(5)
Medication	0.56(3)	0.64(3)
Harm	0.65(5)	0.98(5)
Disability	0.63(3)	0.79(3)

Table A2. Correlations of SOPA Brief subscales in Greek with CPCI subscales.

	Correlations SOPA-Brief with CPCI SOPA-Brief Subscales		
CPCI Subscale	Emotion	Treatment	Disability
CPCIAssistance		0.154 *	
CPCISocialSupport	0.146 *		0.154 *
CPCICopingSelfStatements			0.163 *

* $p < 0.05$; ** $p < 0.01$.

Table A3. Correlations of SOPA Brief subscales in Greek with PBAPI subscales.

	Correlations SOPA-Brief with PBAPI SOPA-Brief Subscales					
PBAPI Subscale	Control	Harm	Solicitude	Emotion	Medication	Disability
PBAPITime	−0.252	0.197 **				0.286 **
PBAPIMystery	0.153 *		0.253 *	0.165 *		
PBAPISelf-Blame			0.351 *	0.247 **	0.151 *	0.142 **

* $p < 0.05$; ** $p < 0.01$.

Table A4. Exploratory factor analysis (extraction method: principal component analysis).

Total Variance Explained									
	Initial Eigenvalues			Extraction Sums of Squared Loadings			Rotation Sums of Squared Loadings		
Component	Total	% of Variance	Cumulative %	Total	% of Variance	Cumulative %	Total	% of Variance	Cumulative %
1	5.649	18.830	18.830	5.649	18.830	18.830	5.136	17.119	17.119
2	5.271	17.569	36.399	5.271	17.569	36.399	4.008	13.360	30.478
3	3.251	10.838	47.237	3.251	10.838	47.237	3.641	12.138	42.616
4	2.723	9.075	56.313	2.723	9.075	56.313	3.215	10.717	53.333
5	2.275	7.582	63.894	2.275	7.582	63.894	1.938	6.459	59.791
6	1.255	4.182	68.076	1.255	4.182	68.076	1.888	6.294	66.086
7	1.040	3.467	71.543	1.040	3.467	71.543	1.637	5.457	71.543

Table A5. Exploratory factor analysis (principal component analysis—rotated component matrix).

Rotated Component Matrix [a]	Emotion	Control	Harm	Solicitude	Treatment	Disability	Medication
1. There are many times I can influence the amount of pain I feel	**0.373**	0.299	0.051	−0.544	−0.035	**0.332**	0.026
2. I will probably always have to take pain medication	0.121	−0.100	0.011	**0.778**	0.087	−0.026	0.129
3. When I hurt, I want my family to treat me better	0.113	0.014	−0.196	**0.831**	0.076	0.056	0.195
4. I don't expect a medical cure for my pain	−0.106	−0.022	**0.375**	0.211	**0.318**	−0.363	**0.501**
5. I have had the most relief from the pain with the use of medications	−0.075	**0.376**	**0.317**	**0.383**	−0.196	0.215	**0.469**
6. Anxiety increases the pain I feel	**0.493**	−0.202	**0.517**	0.277	0.145	0.194	0.044
7. When I am hurting, people should treat me with care and concern	0.250	−0.221	0.023	**0.763**	−0.254	0.107	−0.011
8. I have given up my search for the complete elimination of my pain through the work of the medical profession	0.168	0.253	−0.388	−0.217	**0.585**	0.017	0.021
9. It is the responsibility of my loved ones to help me when I feel pain	**0.809**	0.157	−0.190	0.259	0.007	−0.262	−0.032
10. Stress in my life increases my pain	**0.796**	−0.131	**0.310**	−0.152	−0.231	−0.007	−0.038
11. Exercise and movement are good for my pain problem	−0.064	0.127	**0.814**	−0.105	−0.072	0.227	−0.173
12. Just by concentrating or relaxing, I can 'take the edge' off my pain	0.156	**0.515**	0.278	−0.287	**0.306**	0.185	0.099
13. Medicine is one of the best treatments for chronic pain	−0.105	0.195	**0.358**	−0.014	0.132	**0.598**	−0.077
14. My family needs to learn how to take better care of me when I am in pain	**0.837**	0.132	−0.183	0.278	0.093	−0.096	0.001
15. Depression increases the pain I feel	**0.872**	0.035	0.125	0.047	0.135	0.219	−0.191
16. If I exercise. it can make my pain problem much worse	−0.117	−0.195	−0.322	0.125	0.202	−0.161	**0.653**
17. I believe that I can control how much pain I feel by changing my thoughts	0.268	**0.492**	−0.043	−0.200	0.212	0.157	−0.448
18. Often I need more tender loving care than I am now getting when I am in pain	**0.775**	−0.018	−0.168	**0.328**	0.096	0.095	−0.119
19. Something is wrong with my body that prevents movement and exercise	**0.695**	−0.049	−0.208	−0.080	0.123	−0.035	**0.319**
20. I have learned to control my pain	0.004	**0.838**	0.005	−0.057	−0.024	−0.071	−0.014
21. I trust that the medical profession can cure my pain	0.041	0.166	0.125	0.061	−0.255	0.769	−0.088
22. I know for sure that I can learn to control my pain	0.021	0.826	0.023	0.083	0.028	0.150	−0.123
23. My pain does not stop me from leading a physically active life	0.117	0.610	0.431	−0.216	0.044	0.129	−0.031
24. My physical pain will never be cured	0.192	−0.467	0.030	0.188	0.278	0.322	0.433
25. There is a strong relationship between my emotions and my level of pain	0.713	−0.131	0.246	−0.245	−0.225	−0.003	−0.120
26. I can do almost everything just as well as before my pain problem	−0.072	0.670	0.224	−0.282	0.192	0.050	−0.121
27. If I don't exercise regularly. my pain problem will continue to get worse	−0.093	0.151	0.882	0.053	0.125	−0.016	−0.026
28. Exercise can reduce the amount of pain I experience	0.059	0.113	0.774	−0.207	−0.087	0.108	0.107
29. I am convinced that there is no medical procedure that will help my pain	−0.036	−0.029	0.152	0.097	0.861	−0.165	0.129

Table A5. *Cont.*

Rotated Component Matrix [a]	Emotion	Control	Harm	Solicitude	Treatment	Disability	Medication
30. My pain would stop anyone from leading an active life	0.282	−0.666	0.037	−0.058	0.225	−0.369	−0.105
Extraction Method: Principal Component Analysis. Rotation Method: Varimax with Kaiser Normalization.a							
a. Rotation converged in 7 iterations.							

References

1. Hill, J.C.; Fritz, J.M. Psychosocial Influences on Low Back Pain, Disability, and Response to Treatment. *Phys. Ther.* **2011**, *91*, 712–721. [CrossRef] [PubMed]
2. Mills, S.E.; Nicolson, K.P.; Smith, B.H. Chronic pain: A review of its epidemiology and associated factors in population-based studies. *Br. J. Anaesth.* **2019**, *123*, e273–e283. [CrossRef] [PubMed]
3. Blyth, F.M.; March, L.M.; Nicholas, M.K.; Cousins, M.J. Self-management of chronic pain: A population-based study. *Pain* **2005**, *113*, 285–292. [CrossRef] [PubMed]
4. Butchart, A.; Kerr, E.A.; Heisler, M.M.; Piette, J.D.; Krein, S.L. Experience and Management of Chronic Pain Among Patients with Other Complex Chronic Conditions. *Clin. J. Pain* **2009**, *25*, 293–298. [CrossRef]
5. Gatchel, R.J.; Neblett, R.; Kishino, N.; Ray, C.T. Fear-Avoidance Beliefs and Chronic Pain. *J. Orthop. Sports Phys. Ther.* **2016**, *46*, 38–43. [CrossRef]
6. Vlaeyen, J.W.; Linton, S.J. Fear-avoidance model of chronic musculoskeletal pain: 12 years on. *Pain* **2012**, *153*, 1144–1147. [CrossRef]
7. Tan, G.P.; Teo, I.; Anderson, K.O.; Jensen, M.P. Adaptive Versus Maladaptive Coping and Beliefs and Their Relation to Chronic Pain Adjustment. *Clin. J. Pain* **2011**, *27*, 769–774. [CrossRef]
8. Sturgeon, J.A.; Zautra, A.J. Resilience: A new paradigm for adaptation to chronic pain. *Curr. Pain Headache Rep.* **2010**, *14*, 105–112. [CrossRef] [PubMed] [PubMed Central]
9. Strong, J.; Ashton, R.; Chant, D. The measurement of attitudes towards and beliefs about pain. *Pain* **1992**, *48*, 227–236. [CrossRef]
10. Moseley, G.L. Evidence for a direct relationship between cognitive and physical change during an education intervention in people with chronic low back pain. *Eur. J. Pain* **2004**, *8*, 39–45. [CrossRef]
11. Sturgeon, J.A. Psychological therapies for the management of chronic pain. *Psychol. Res. Behav. Manag.* **2014**, *7*, 115–124. [CrossRef] [PubMed] [PubMed Central]
12. Jensen, M.P.; Turner, J.A.; Romano, J.M. Pain belief assessment: A comparison of the short and long versions of the surgery of pain attitudes. *J. Pain* **2000**, *1*, 138–150. [CrossRef]
13. Jensen, M.P.; Turner, J.A.; Romano, J.M. Changes after multidisciplinary pain treatment in patient pain beliefs and coping are associated with concurrent changes in patient functioning. *Pain* **2007**, *131*, 38–47. [CrossRef] [PubMed]
14. Jensen, M.P.; Turner, J.A.; Romano, J.M.; Lawler, B.K. Relationship of pain-specific beliefs to chronic pain adjustment. *Pain* **1994**, *57*, 301–309. [CrossRef]
15. Jensen, M.P.; Karoly, P.; Huger, R. The development and preliminary validation of an instrument to assess patients' attitudes toward pain. *J. Psychosom. Res.* **1987**, *31*, 393–400. [CrossRef]
16. Tait, R.C.; Chibnall, J.T. Development of a brief version of the Survey of Pain Attitudes. *Pain* **1997**, *70*, 229–235. [CrossRef]
17. Christakou, A.; Sakellari, V. Validity and reliability of the Greek version of the Pain Beliefs and Perceptions Inventory for patients with chronic pain. *Int. J. Ther. Rehabil.* **2021**, *28*, 1–16. [CrossRef]
18. Dimitriadis, Z.; Kapreli, E.; Strimpakos, N.; Oldham, J. Psychometric properties of the Greek version of the Pain Catastro-phizing Scalein patients with chronic neck pain. *Arch. Hell. Med.* **2022**, *39*, 760–766.
19. Georgoudis, G.; Papathanasiou, G.; Spiropoulos, P.; Katsoulakis, K. Cognitive assessment of musculoskeletal pain with a newly validated Greek version of the Fear-Avoidance Beliefs Questionnaire (FABQ). *Eur. J. Pain* **2007**, *11*, 341–351. [CrossRef]
20. Hall, D.A.; Domingo, S.Z.; Hamdache, L.Z.; Manchaiah, V.; Thammaiah, S.; Evans, C.; Wong, L.L.V. A Good Practice Guide for Translating and Adapting Hearing-Related Questionnaires for Different Languages and Cultures. *Int. J. Audiol.* **2017**, *57*, 161–175. [CrossRef]
21. Tsang, S.; Royse, C.F.; Terkawi, A.S. Guidelines for developing, translating, and validating a questionnaire in perioperative and pain medicine. *Saudi J. Anaesth.* **2017**, *11*, S80–S89. [CrossRef] [PubMed]
22. Elfil, M.; Negida, A. Sampling methods in Clinical Research; an Educational Review. *Emergency* **2017**, *5*, e52. [PubMed]

23. Suen, L.J.; Huang, H.M.; Lee, H.H. A comparison of convenience sampling and purposive sampling. *Hu Li Za Zhi* **2014**, *61*, 105–111. (In Chinese) [CrossRef]
24. Taber, K.S. The Use of Cronbach's Alpha When Developing and Reporting Research Instruments in Science Education. *Res. Sci. Educ.* **2018**, *48*, 1273–1296. [CrossRef]
25. Chan, Y.H. Biostatistics 104: Correlational analysis. *Singap. Med. J.* **2003**, *44*, 614–619. [PubMed]
26. Watkins, M.W. Exploratory Factor Analysis: A Guide to Best Practice. *J. Black Psychol.* **2018**, *44*, 219–246. [CrossRef]
27. Pimenta, C.; Kurita GSilva, E.; Cruz, D. Validity and reliability of the Survey of Pain Attitudes (SOPA-28 items) in the Portuguese Language. *Revista da Escola de Enfermagem da USP* **2009**, *43*, 1070–1078.
28. Christakou, A.; Kapreli, E. Reliability and validity of the survey pain attitudes in Greek population. *Physiotherapy* **2015**, *101*, e721–e722. [CrossRef]
29. Quadri, N.; Wild, D.; Skerritt, B.; Muelhausen, W.; O'Donohoe, P. A literature review of the variance in interval length between administrations for assessment of test- retest reliability and equivalence of pro measures. *Value Health* **2013**, *16*, A40–A41.
30. Williams, D.A.; Thorn, B.E. An empirical assessment of pain beliefs. *Pain* **1989**, *36*, 351–358. [CrossRef]

MDPI AG
Grosspeteranlage 5
4052 Basel
Switzerland
Tel.: +41 61 683 77 34

Journal of Clinical Medicine Editorial Office
E-mail: jcm@mdpi.com
www.mdpi.com/journal/jcm

www.ingramcontent.com/pod-product-compliance
Lightning Source LLC
Chambersburg PA
CBHW040748250926
51850CB00007BB/1440
* 9 7 8 3 7 2 5 8 6 4 8 2 9 *